FUNDAMENTALS OF
Pain Medicine

How to Diagnose and Treat Your Patients

J.D. Hoppenfeld, MD
Interventional Pain Management
Southeast Pain Care
Charlotte, North Carolina

Wolters Kluwer
Health

Philadelphia • Baltimore • New York • London
Buenos Aires • Hong Kong • Sydney • Tokyo

Executive Editor: Rebecca Gaertner
Senior Product Development Editor: Kristina Oberle
Production Project Manager: David Saltzberg
Senior Manufacturing Manager: Beth Welsh
Marketing Manager: Stephanie Manzo
Design Coordinator: Teresa Mallon
Production Service: Aptara, Inc.

Library of Congress Cataloging-in-Publication Data

Hoppenfeld, J.D. (Jon-David), author.
  Fundamentals of pain medicine : how to diagnose and treat your
patients / J.D. Hoppenfeld.
       p. ; cm.
  Includes bibliographical references and index.
  ISBN 978-1-4511-4449-9 (hardback : alk. paper)
  I. Title.
  [DNLM: 1. Pain Management. 2. Pain—diagnosis. WL 704.6]
  RB127
  616'.0472—dc23
                                        2014000590

Care has been taken to confirm the accuracy of the information presented and to describe generally accepted practices. However, the authors, editors, and publisher are not responsible for errors or omissions or for any consequences from application of the information in this book and make no warranty, expressed or implied, with respect to the currency, completeness, or accuracy of the contents of the publication. Application of the information in a particular situation remains the professional responsibility of the practitioner.

The authors, editors, and publisher have exerted every effort to ensure that drug selection and dosage set forth in this text are in accordance with current recommendations and practice at the time of publication. However, in view of ongoing research, changes in government regulations, and the constant flow of information relating to drug therapy and drug reactions, the reader is urged to check the package insert for each drug for any change in indications and dosage and for added warnings and precautions. This is particularly important when the recommended agent is a new or infrequently employed drug.

Some drugs and medical devices presented in the publication have Food and Drug Administration (FDA) clearance for limited use in restricted research settings. It is the responsibility of the health care provider to ascertain the FDA status of each drug or device planned for use in their clinical practice.

To purchase additional copies of this book, call our customer service department at (800) 638-3030 or fax orders to (301) 223-2320. International customers should call (301) 223-2300.

Visit Lippincott Williams & Wilkins on the Internet: at LWW.com. Lippincott Williams & Wilkins customer service representatives are available from 8:30 am to 6 pm, EST.

Dedication

To my father who taught me the importance of the phrase that proceeded all of his books. "To all the men who preserved this body of knowledge, added to it and passed it on for another generation." To my mother for her continued love and support.

To my wife, Brie, you bring happiness to every aspect of my life. To my son Palmer who I am proud of every day

To Eileen Wolfberg who has been making generations of Hoppenfeld's look good.

To the Chicago Medical School

To the NYU Department of Neurology who provides superb training and a wonderful environment to grow.

To Dr. Kate Henry who exemplifies how influential a teacher can be in each of her students' lives.

To Dr. Russ Portonoy, for giving me a chance to prove myself.

To Dr. Jay Bakshi, for his technical training and life lessons, as well as, the fabulous team at Manhattan Spine and Pain.

To my colleagues at Southeast Pain Care. The level to which you take care of our patients on a daily basis exemplifies the best of medicine.

To my direct partner Dr. Tom Heil, I could not ask for a better teammate.

To my colleagues who have reviewed the chapters of this book: Dr. Bert Vargas, Dr. Elizabeth Morgan, Dr. General Hood, Dr. Dave Hergan, Dr. Brian Thoma, Dr. Felix Muniz, Dr. Tom Heil, Dr. Kathyrn Chance, Dr. Aaron Sharma, Dave Binkney, Katrina Traverso Justin Miller and Anne DePriest.

To my illustration team: Lead by Mike De La Flor a pioneer in medical illustration. Allison Keel, Melisa Silva, Ashley Helms, Renée Cauble, Denise Bowman, and "Big Mike" Erico.

—J.D. Hoppenfeld, M.D.

For Larry and Sylvia Gatzke.
—Mike de la Flor

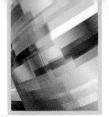

Preface

This book is designed to be used by all healthcare professionals to improve the quality of life of their patients. Pain is ubiquitous and presents itself in the practices of every doctor. Whether your practice is primary care, general surgery, or a specialty, you have patients with pain. No matter how different our practices may be, we all have patients who need better pain management. This book will present the basics of pain management, currently not a mainstay of medical school curricula or most residency training programs. The principles provided here will give you the tools to understand, work up, and alleviate your patient's pain. Multiple case examples are provided to make the book relevant and applicable. This book by no means is comprehensive; however, its purpose is to cover the most common causes of pain, those you will encounter frequently in your practice, and the most common treatment options. You will understand when and how to use pain medications as well as when a patient can benefit from a procedure.

Some patients present with a primary complaint of pain while others complain of pain secondary to a more generalized disease process or procedure. As a healthcare professional, you are trained to diagnose the pathology and then treat it. However, another layer of patient care needs more focus in the medical community. Our actions to alleviate pain will not hinder our ability to treat the underlying disease. Yet modern medicine often considers these goals mutually exclusive, with pain management a distant second. As medical professionals, when we have an incomplete understanding of how to treat a condition, we undertreat it, erring on the side of "do no harm." This book will give you the confidence to confront your patient's discomfort and succeed in conquering the pain.

The anatomical reasons for some causes of pain are well established, while other causes are not. In some cases we can identify the exact pathologic causes of the patient's pain, for example, lumbar radiculopathy, a fractured fibula, pancreatic cancer, and so on. In other cases, pain symptoms can be analyzed and lead us to the pain generator that cannot be detected by MRI or lab tests, for example, muscle spasm, abdominal adhesions, and peripheral neuropathy of unknown etiology.

It is frustrating that we cannot measure pain as objectively as we can, for example, systolic blood pressure in hypertension or white matter lesions in multiple sclerosis. This is a fact that we simply have to accept, at this point, in order to take better care of our patients. In medicine we are constantly dealing with modalities we do not completely understand. We do not know the exact mechanism of action of a number of our most common medications, but we know that they work and that we can help our patients with them. When a patient presents with hypertension we begin our workup, knowing there is a high likelihood that we are not going to find a cause and effect for the diagnosis. When we cannot find the cause, we label the patient as having essential hypertension. Our foundation of medicine stresses that while we do not completely understand the cause of hypertension, it is imperative to treat it. Another common example is multiple sclerosis—we do not know what causes it yet we must treat it, and do so with medications whose mechanisms are currently not completely comprehended. We should function the same way in the case of pain.

While we cannot always make the anatomical diagnosis until science advances, we understand the symptoms and what treatment modalities work well for those symptoms. Your patient's symptoms can establish a general pain diagnosis, such as muscular spasm. As long as the symptoms are well understood, you can properly treat the pain. Treatment modalities for pain may include physical therapy, lifestyle modification, yoga, nonsteroidal anti-inflammatory medication, an injection, or possibly surgery.

If we understood pain completely, we could explain why some patients with an abnormal examination or abnormal images that normally represent a painful condition are pain free. A good example of this is that some patients with cervical spondylolisthesis (slippage of the vertebral bodies) who have both abnormal imaging and signs of myelopathy on examination (hyperreflexive, increased muscle tone) often can be pain free. People have different responses to the same pathology. It is not uncommon for two people to have different subjective responses to the same stimuli. The temperature from a faucet may be fixed, but you may think the water feels cool while another thinks the water feels hot. This is how we are built.

At times we apply a cause and effect to something seen on imaging when one may not exist. Modern imaging has given us an unprecedented ability to understand the cause of pain, but it has also reinforced our known limitation in understanding pain. While pathology may be discernible on imaging, it may not be the cause of the patient's pain. A good example of this is as follows: If 100 people randomly selected off the street, age 40 years, are sent for an MRI regardless of whether they have back pain, 35% will have a herniated disc. Many asymptomatic people have a herniated disc. If a patient presents with nonspecific low back pain, a CT scan and/or MRI may be ordered to find the cause. There is a 35% chance that the patient will have a herniated disc regardless of whether pain is present. A 1994 *New England Journal of Medicine* study showed that over half the people observed with no back pain had at least one bulging disc.[1] This book will help you interpret test results and show you how to apply them to your patients with pain.

We should use a patient's history, physical examination, and our proper interpretation of imaging to guide us to a generator of the pain. We then can target therapy toward that generator. We have specific treatment modalities that work based on the pain generator. The treatment of pain that may have stumped us in the past now becomes much more manageable. We will know what to do and how to do it, and be better physicians for it.

There are three hurdles that the practitioner faces upon encountering a patient with pain. The first is uncertainty as to why the patient has pain. The second not knowing how to treat it properly. The third is knowing why the patient has pain and being aware of appropriate treatment, but not treating for fear of taking action. Pain does not always get better on its own, and is considered chronic after 3 months. The longer treatment is delayed, the harder pain is to alleviate. Only 50% of people return to work when they are out for 6 months. Only 25% return to work when they are out for 1 year. After reading this book, you will be better motivated to diagnose and properly treat your patient's pain in a reasonable timely fashion.

There are instances in which the proper choice and use of a medication or procedure is critical. For example, it has been well demonstrated that the use of tricyclic antidepressants (TCA) such as Elavil-is an effective treatment for postherpetic neuralgia. Stellate ganglion block for complex regional pain syndrome of the upper extremity is a proven treatment for painful symptoms. When pain is not controlled early, it can become chronic. The brain internalizes the pain in an area of the cortex that represents the area experiencing it. Once the brain's cortex undergoes synaptic modulation,

further treatment of the pain can become very difficult. This can be seen in phantom limb pain.

There are five common scenarios you will encounter when treating patients with pain.

First scenario: *The source of pain does not warrant a diagnostic work-up the pain is temporary and will subside on it's own.* Your goal is to manage the painful symptoms until the underlying pain pathology corrects itself on its own. An example of this is after the first snowfall of the year, a patient presents with new low back pain. The pain is without radiation and occurred after shoveling his driveway. After a full history and physical examination, the diagnosis is nonspecific myofascial low back pain. Even with this nonspecific diagnosis, we can treat the patient's symptoms of low back pain with a nonsteroidal anti-inflammatory drug (NSAID) and some rest. You may not have a specific diagnosis, but you still have the ability to properly treat your patient. This book will provide guidelines on appropriate use of NSAIDs and other pain medications, so that your patients can obtain the best results. It will give you the starting doses of medications and tell you how to titrate them.

Second scenario: *The source of pain warrants a diagnostic work-up, the work-up shows the pathology and necessitates intervention because the pain will not resolve on its own.* Severe osteoarthritis of the hip is a good example of this. After seeing the patient you astutely order an MRI, which shows severe arthritis of the right hip. You try conservative treatment: Physical therapy and an NSAID. The pain does not improve with these conservative measures and surely will not improve on its own. A surgical option to control the underlying cause of the pain exists. The patient wants the surgery and the surgeon is willing to do it. A hip replacement is done correctly and the patient's pain improves.

Third scenario: *The source of pain warrants a diagnostic work-up, the work-up does not show the source of pathology and the pain necessitates intervention because the pain will not resolve on it's own.* An example of this is the patient presenting with symptoms that indicate a painful peripheral neuropathy. A work-up should always be done looking for correctable causes of such a neuropathy, including alcohol, diabetes, HIV, and medications. Even though a work-up is justified, however, be aware that most likely the cause of the peripheral neuropathy will not be determined. Peripheral neuropathy can be easily identified on history, and you can implement a treatment plan tailored to it. Guidelines for the appropriate use of neuropathic pain medications are fully covered in this book.

Fourth scenario: *Everything is done right – work-up, diagnosis, treatment – yet the pain does not get better.* A good example of this is spine fusion surgery for low back pain. The surgery is done correctly, but the patient does not get completely better. The patient is now given the diagnosis of failed back surgery syndrome. Some patients have great results, but some continue to experience significant pain despite a technically well-performed surgery. This book presents the best pain management options currently available for this type of situation including spinal cord stimulation therapy.

Fifth scenario: *The palliative setting.* You see a patient who presents with hemoptysis; after a full work-up you determine that the patient has lung cancer. She is pain free for 6 months but develops pain as the cancer metastasizes to her thoracic spine. Despite treatment, the cancer continues to spread. While you eventually will not be able to treat the cause of the pain, in this case Stage IV lung cancer, you understand the painful symptoms it will generate—for example, bone pain from metastasis and nerve pain from chemotherapy. This book will help you target treatment for the pain generators to control the painful symptoms effectively.

Our goal of treating disease has not changed, but our intrinsic knowledge of controlling pain has. With the principles outlined in this book, you will have a strong grasp on how to treat pain. You will be able to overcome any fear of mishandling treatment of pain, knowing you can set a safe and effective pain management plan into motion including spinal cord stimulation therapy.

REFERENCE

1. Jensen MC, Brant-Zawadski MN, Obuchowski N, et al. Magnetic resonance imaging of the lumbar spine in people without back pain. *New Engl J Med.* 1994;331(2):69–73. *Study found that over half of people with no low back pain that were imaged had a least one bulging disc.*

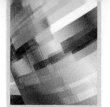

Contents

PART I

Symptoms and Conditions

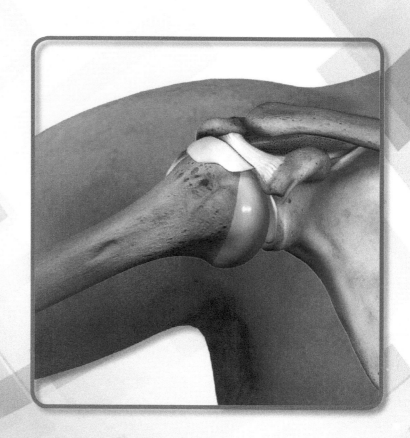

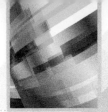

CHAPTER 1

Musculoskeletal Pain

PAIN IN THE SHOULDER
- Bursitis
- Arthritis
- Rotator Cuff Injury
- Adhesive Capsulitis

PAIN IN THE ELBOW
- Tendinitis
- Olecranon Bursitis
- Traumatic Arthritis

PAIN IN THE NECK
  (CERVICAL SPINE)

PAIN IN THE LOWER BACK
  (LUMBAR SPINE)
- Muscles and Ligaments
- Vertebral Bodies
- Facet Joints
- Vertebral Discs

PAIN IN THE HIP
- Arthritis
- Ischemic (Avascular) Necrosis
- Fractures

PAIN IN THE BUTTOCK
- The Sacroiliac Joint
- Greater Trochanteric Bursitis
- Ischiogluteal Bursitis

PAIN IN THE KNEE
- Arthritis
- Meniscal Tear
- Patellar Tendonitis
- Osteochondritis

PAIN IN THE SHOULDER

The shoulder is a common location of pain. In this ball-and-socket joint, the ball is the top, rounded part of the humerus, and the socket is the outer edge of the scapula (the glenoid fossa, Fig. 1-1). The joint is held together by muscles, ligaments, and tendons. The ball is too big for the relatively flat socket. This design allows the shoulder to be the most movable joint in the body but at the same time most prone to dislocation. Pain can come from the shoulder joint itself or may be

Figure 1-1 Anatomy of the shoulder. ▶

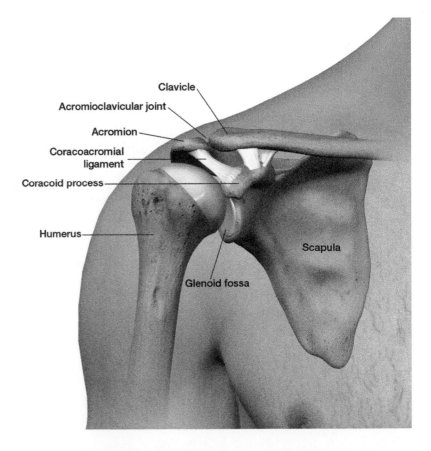

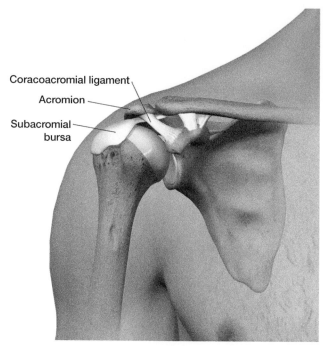

Figure 1-2 The subacromial bursa.

acromioclavicular (AC), (3) rotator cuff injury, and (4) adhesive capsulitis (frozen shoulder).

Bursitis

A bursa is a, fluid-filled sac that functions as a gliding surface to reduce friction between tissues of the body. The major bursa of the shoulder is the subacromial bursa. The shoulder's subacromial bursa (Fig. 1-2) separates the supraspinatus tendon (one of the four tendons of the rotator cuff) from the coracoacromial ligament. When the arm is resting at the side, the bursa lies laterally below the acromion. When the arm is abducted, it moves medially beneath the acromion (Fig. 1-3). When subjected to increase friction and overuse the subacromial bursa can become inflamed. Pain is usually of slow onset. Discomfort occurs in the shoulder or upper arm at the site of the bursa. On examination, the pain is worse when the patient abducts the arm, specifically from 70 to 100 degrees.

Treatment involves rest and a nonsteroidal antiinflammatory drug (NSAID). A cortisone injection at the bursa effectively reduces inflammation and pain.

Arthritis

Glenohumeral: The primary cause of osteoarthritis is normal wear and tear. It can also occur when a significant trauma disrupts the cartilage covering the proximal humerus. In osteoarthritis, the joint surface degenerates and the subchondral bone remodels,

referred—from diseases affecting the gallbladder, heart, or cervical spine.

This section will focus on common sources of chronic pain originating from the shoulder itself. They include (1) bursitis, (2) arthritis—both glenohumeral and

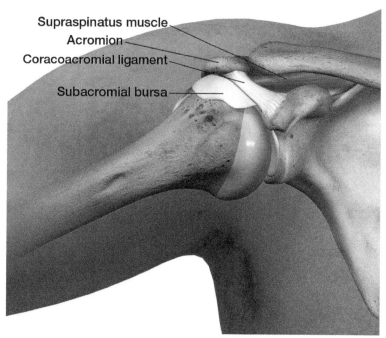

Figure 1-3 Subacromial bursa movement. The bursa lies in a lateral position when the arm is at rest; as the arm is abducted the bursa moves medially. Subacromial bursitis pain is worse as the arm is abducted.

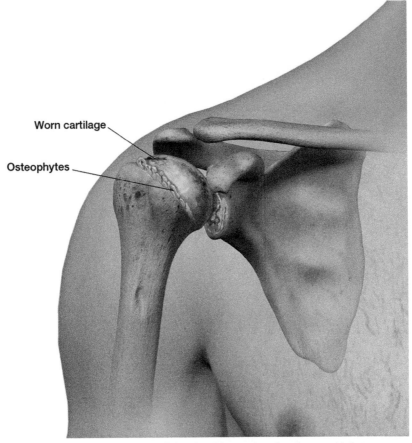

Figure 1-4 Arthritis of the shoulder at the glenohumeral joint.

leading to pain and decreased range of motion (Fig. 1-4). Patients describe the pain as slowly progressive, diffuse, and deep in the joint; movement makes it worse. Physical examination may reveal crepitus and, in advanced cases, decreased range of motion. Radiography may show only subtle changes to the bone in a patient with clinical manifestations of pain from arthritis. Until there is more advanced destruction, x-ray results may be underwhelming. Magnetic resonance imaging (MRI) can provide greater evidence of articular cartilage wear.

Painful symptoms are treated with NSAIDs and/or a cortisone injection and physical therapy. If conservative means do not control the shoulder pain, shoulder replacement may be a proper treatment option.

Acromioclavicular: Arthritis in the shoulder can also develop between the acromion and the clavicle (Fig. 1-5). The AC joint is superior to the glenohumeral junction. On examination, to elicit AC joint pain, have the patient bring the affected arm across the chest, which compresses the AC joint.

Treatment of AC arthritis is the same as for glenohumeral arthritis except that the cortisone injection is placed into the AC joint.

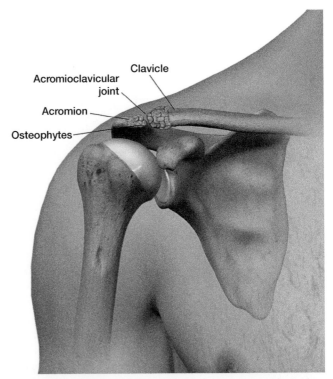

Figure 1-5 Arthritis of the shoulder at the acromioclavicular joint.

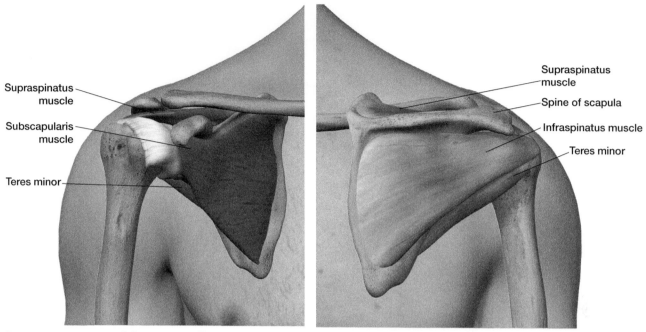

Figure 1-6 Anatomy of the rotator cuff. The supraspinatus, infraspinatus, teres minor, and subscapularis. The supraspinatus is most prone to pathology.

Rotator Cuff Injury

The rotator cuff is a group of four tendons that attach the scapula to the humerus: The supraspinatus, infraspinatus, teres minor, and subscapularis. They form a "cuff" over the posterior aspect of the proximal humerus (Fig. 1-6). The supraspinatus tendon is most frequently involved in tears. Rotator cuff injuries span a spectrum of pathologies, from mild tendinitis to massive tears. Younger patients usually report a history of trauma, whereas older patients present with a gradual onset of shoulder pain. They often describe pain as being located over the posterior aspect of the shoulder; overhead activities make it worse. The drop arm test helps detect rotator cuff pathology: The patient fully abducts the arm in the extended position (Fig. 1-7). The patient is asked to slowly lower the arm to the side. If the patient is not able to lower the arm slowly and smoothly to the side, it may be because of rotator cuff dysfunction. MRI is the imaging technique of choice.

NSAIDs and muscle relaxants remain the first-line symptomatic treatment. Physical therapy is also important. It may be necessary to consider a corticosteroid injection to decrease pain and inflammation as well as allow further advancement in physical therapy treatment. The patient should limit activity that involves high-tensile loads for 2 weeks after injection, because the tendon is potentially at risk for further tearing; common daily activities are not limited. Whether to proceed with surgical repair of the rotator cuff depends on the age, activity level, and functional needs of the patient.

Adhesive Capsulitis

In adhesive capsulitis, abnormal bands of fibrous tissue grow within the joint capsule. There is also a lack

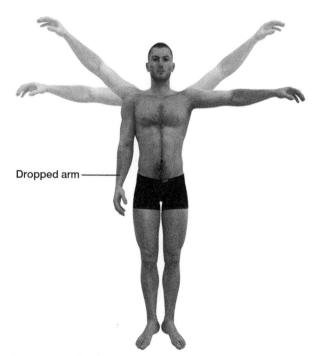

Figure 1-7 The drop arm test. The patient slowly lowers the arm from an abducted extended position. Problems performing this task can indicate rotator cuff pathology. This test is most accurate if pathology is moderate to severe.

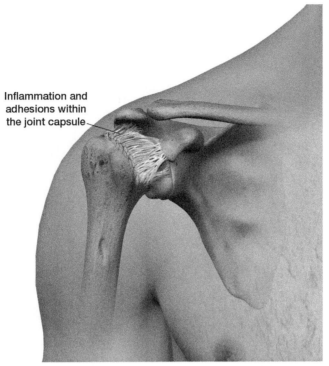

Inflammation and adhesions within the joint capsule

Figure 1-8 Adhesive capsulitis. Abnormal bands of fibrous tissue grow within the joint capsule.

of synovial fluid, which lubricates the joint (Fig. 1-8). This condition affects about 2% of the general population and occurs most frequently in women between the ages of 40 and 70. It affects 10% to 15% of people with diabetes. This disorder is characterized by a restricted range of motion and pain. It is known to develop after a shoulder is injured or immobilized for an extended period of time. Arthrography shows diminished joint volume. Routine radiographs are generally normal.

Muscle relaxants in combination with an opioid can be helpful. Physical therapy is useful. Cortisone injections with a local anesthetic usually allow the patient to participate more fully in physical therapy. However, because the joint space is so narrow, insertion of medication into the joint can be difficult. Therefore, a suprascapular nerve block may be advisable. The suprascapular nerve provides both motor and sensory innervation to the shoulder. Blocking this nerve alleviates pain so that physical therapy is less of a problem. If participation in physical therapy is limited, even with a pre-physical therapy shoulder injection or suprascapular nerve block, gentle manipulation under anesthesia to increase range of motion may be necessary.

PAIN IN THE ELBOW

Tendinitis

Lateral Epicondylitis (tennis elbow): Tennis elbow is an idiopathic condition of middle-aged people in which the outer part of the elbow becomes painful and tender (Fig. 1-9). It is commonly associated with playing

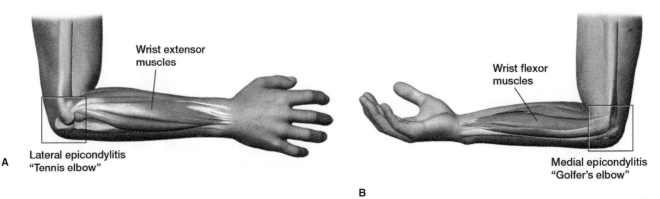

Wrist extensor muscles

Wrist flexor muscles

A Lateral epicondylitis "Tennis elbow"

Medial epicondylitis "Golfer's elbow"

B

Figure 1-9 A: Tennis elbow (lateral epicondylitis). **B:** Golfer's elbow (medial epicondylitis).

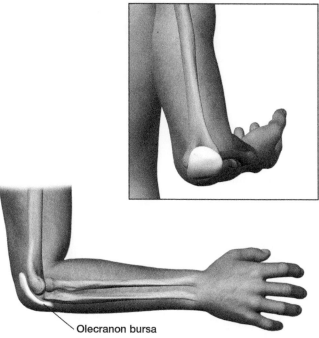

Figure 1-10 The olecranon bursa.

tennis, although the condition can occur in nontennis players. The lateral epicondyle is the site of origin of the wrist extensor muscles. Gripping and resistance to wrist extension movement are painful.

NSAIDs combined with a brace to reduce strain at the elbow epicondyle is the treatment of choice. A counterforce tennis elbow strap can reduce tension of the muscles as they attach to the lateral epicondyle, especially the carpi radialis brevis. A cortisone injection can be beneficial.

Medial Epicondylitis (golfer's elbow): This syndrome is analogous to lateral epicondylitis and involves the wrist flexors on the medial side of the elbow (Fig. 1-9). Pain is exacerbated by offering resistance to wrist flexion.

Treatment is the same as for tennis elbow.

Olecranon Bursitis

The olecranon bursa is a fluid filled sac that lies on the back of the elbow to allow smooth movement of the joint (Fig. 1-10). When the bursa becomes inflamed, it fills with extra fluid and causes pain at the back of the elbow, often accompanied by noticeable swelling at the bony part of the elbow.

An NSAID and a compression bandage are usually all that is necessary. If this is insufficient, the next step is a simple in-office procedure: Drainage of fluid and an injection of cortisone at the bursa followed by a compression bandage.

Traumatic Arthritis

Osteoarthritis is more common in weight-bearing joints, such as the hips or knees. Traumatic arthritis is common in non–weight-bearing joints such as the elbow. The cause is a previous injury—a dislocation or fracture. Patients commonly complain of a locking or grinding sensation.

NSAIDs are usually the treatment of choice, with cortisone injections when needed.

PAIN IN THE NECK (CERVICAL SPINE)

The common sources of pain in the cervical spine are the same as those in the lumbar spine. The treatment algorithms are typically the same as well.

PAIN IN THE LOWER BACK (LUMBAR SPINE)

Isolated low back pain is a complaint all practitioners face. In the majority of patients, the pain usually resolves on its own. A patient may need supportive treatment such as over-the-counter Tylenol or ibuprofen for a couple of days until the pain subsides. However, there are people who suffer from low back pain that does not resolve with time and over-the-counter medication. For these patients, it can be difficult to pinpoint the exact cause of chronic low back pain.

Although there is a limit to practitioners' understanding of certain types of pain, this does not mean that patients do not experience them. It is usually possible to tease out a generator or multiple generators of a patient's low back pain. There are specific treatment modalities tailored to specific pain generators. As long as practitioners understand pain generators well, they can properly treat back pain.

Four of the main generators of isolated low back pain are (1) muscle and ligaments, (2) vertebral bodies, (3) facet joints, and (4) vertebral discs. A patient may have one of these four as the source of low back pain or a combination of more than one. Low back pain that radiates into the leg is usually caused by compression or inflammation of a lumbar nerve root. This is covered in Chapter 2, Neuropathic Pain.

Muscles and Ligaments

Myofascial pain is probably the most common reason for isolated low back pain. Axial load is the tension administered along the spine when force is applied. The highest percentage of axial weight is carried in the lower back. With increased tension patients may develop muscle spasm (a painful and involuntary muscular contraction) or strain (an acute tearing injury to muscle). These pathological changes can become chronic. Muscle changes include the formation of taut muscle bands, painful taut muscle bands are known as trigger points (Fig. 1-11). Trigger points are thought to exist because of an abnormal neuromuscular junction, which is where the nerve and the muscle connect. This junction is a hyperexcitable region, where each strand of muscle tissue gets information on when to contract. If this charged region becomes overexcited, the muscle remains contracted. Actin and myosin strands remain pulled over each other in a pathological full contraction.

A good analogy for visualizing this is the effect of static cling on pants. Too much electric charge causes pants to become bunched up in certain regions whereas sitting flush in others. With careful palpation trigger points may be palpated, an increase in muscle tone is detected.

Ligaments support the spinal canal, forming a continuous, dense connective-tissue "stocking" around the spine. When the spine is aligned and mechanical forces optimized, supporting ligaments are not overly stressed. When the vertebral bodies lose their exact alignment (spondylolisthesis—slipping of one vertebra on another) or muscles go into spasm, stress is transmitted to the ligaments. Patients may complain of an achy, dull pain. They may have trigger points on examination.

A muscle relaxant is a good treatment option. Trigger point injections can be very effective at treating muscular pain from taut muscle bands as they disrupt the trigger points, allowing the muscles to regain their normal contraction sequence. Returning to the static cling analogy, the needle diffuses the charge, allowing the muscle to sit flush again. Physical therapy is a valuable tool for treating myofascial pain.

Vertebral Bodies

A person who "breaks" his or her back has fractured a vertebral bone. Vertebral compression fractures (VCFs) occur in both traumatic setting and nontraumatic settings. The most common cause of VCFs in the elderly is

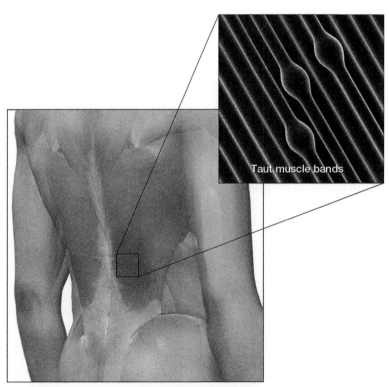

Figure 1-11 Taut muscle bands in the lumbar paraspinal region.

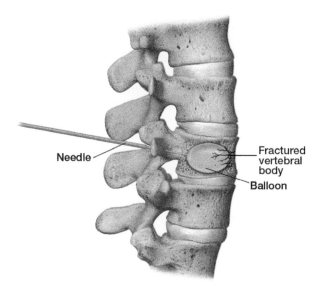

Figure 1-12 Kyphoplasty being used to treat a vertebral compression fracture. After a trochanter is inserted into the center of the fractured vertebral body, a balloon is inflated. The balloon makes a cavity by pushing out trabecular bone. Into this cavity bone cement is injected.

osteoporosis. In the United States, more than 500,000 age-related osteoporotic compression fractures occur every year.[1] The second most common cause of VCFs is metastatic cancer to the bone, with breast cancer being a notorious primary source, and the third most common cause is trauma. If back pain is preceded by trauma, it is due diligence to rule out a vertebral compression fracture.

VCFs are a significant problem. The lifetime risk for a VCF is 16% in women and 5% in men.[2] Patients with one VCF are at risk for sustaining future VCFs. If a patient loses mobility secondary to pain from a VCF, this can lead to a downward spiral: Loss of mobility, further osteoporosis, and fracture of another vertebra. Improving bone quality by treating the underlying osteoporosis is crucial in preventing this vicious cycle.

Treatment includes the use of an NSAID and, if needed, an opioid. Interventionally an injection of bone cement, a procedure known as vertebroplasty, stabilizes the fracture and helps with pain. If a balloon makes a cavity for the cement before injection, the procedure is known as kyphoplasty (Fig. 1-12). If the spine is not stable, surgery is necessary. Using rods and screws, a fusion is performed to secure the fractured vertebrae to the adjacent vertebra.

Facet Joints

The facet joints are synovial lined joints that help lock the posterior aspect of two vertebrae together (Fig. 1-13). The wear and tear from everyday movement can cause these joints to become arthritic and painful over time. Typically, patients with facet joint pain are of age 65 years or older. Two particular subsets of younger patients present with facet joint pain[1]: Young athletes participating in sports that involve repetitive spinal motion, especially lumbar flexion/extension, and to a lesser degree, rotation, and[2] those that have had mechanical trauma. Patients often report that the pain is in the midline of the spine but may be more on the right or left side. The pain is

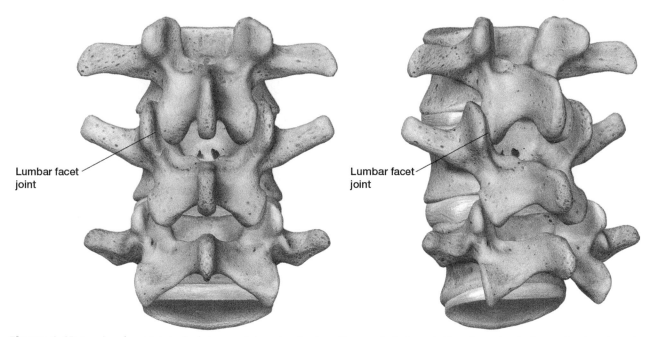

Figure 1-13 Lumbar facet joints, lock two vertebrae bodies together posteriorly and allow the spine to flex, extend and rotate.

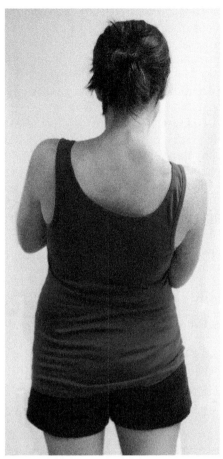

Figure 1-14 Facet joint pain caused by extension and rotation simultaneously toward the painful side of the body on examination.

deep and achy in nature. When the patient extends and rotates at the same time toward the painful side, the pain may worsen (Fig. 1-14). Some physicians use this maneuver as a mechanism to stress the facet joints to test for facet pathology. From a mechanical point of view, extension and extension rotation stress facet joints but also probably stress discs and ligaments more.[3] Computed tomography (CT) or MRI can reveal which facet joints have arthropathy. In general, the last three joints (L3/L4, L4/L5, and L5/S1) tend to be affected, because the maximum amount of lumbar motion and axial force is located there (Fig. 1-15). It is necessary to keep in mind that imaging alone showing facet arthropathy is a poor predictor of response to diagnostic blocks.[4] The combination of facet pain on history and examination, combined with imaging that corresponds to the pain, is a much more reliable predictor.

Treatment includes weight loss, along with strengthening and stretching the supporting muscles. This is key in reducing axial load so that the facet joints are exposed to less stress. Medical management for painful arthritic facet joints includes an NSAID and, if needed, an NSAID–opioid combination. In addition, it is possible to block the nerves that innervate the facet joint with a local anesthetic to see whether the joint is the source of pain. Cortisone injected directly into the joint also alleviates pain. If this decreases the pain, a more permanent block may be necessary, known as radiofrequency ablation.

Figure 1-15 Arthritis of the L3/L4, L4/L5, ▶ and L5/S1 facet joints on the right.

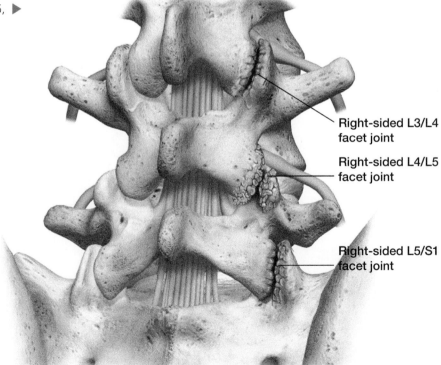

Right-sided L3/L4 facet joint

Right-sided L4/L5 facet joint

Right-sided L5/S1 facet joint

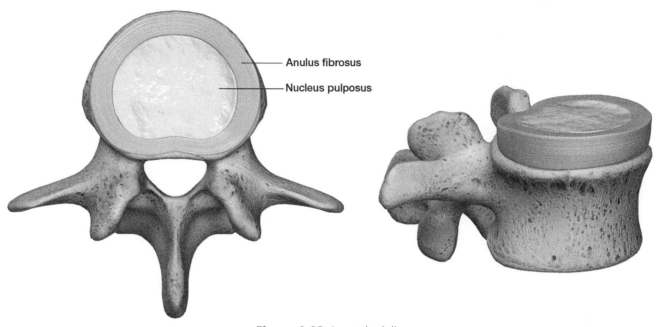

Figure 1-16 A vertebral disc

Vertebral Discs

A vertebral disc is constructed like a jelly donut. The outer layer (anulus fibrosus) is innervated with sensory fibers, whereas the inside layer (nucleus pulposus) is not (Fig. 1-16). Over time, the anulus fibrosus develops cracks (Fig. 1-17). It is thought these cracks (radial tears) are a source of low back pain. Patients often complain of a nondescript axial low back pain that is made worse with prolonged sitting or standing. MRI results show loss of properly hydrated discs; structures containing water appear white on T2-weighted MRIs, whereas a degenerated disc that has lost hydration

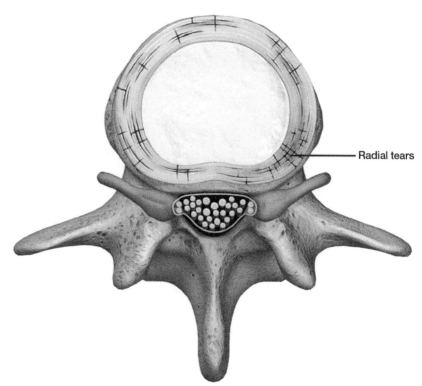

Figure 1-17 Cracks (radial tears) in the anulus fibrosus.

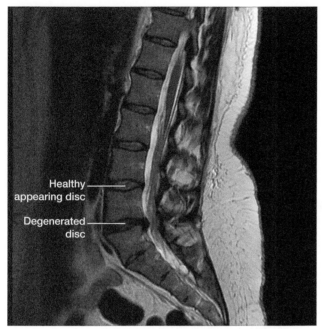

Figure 1-18 On a T2-weighted MRI things that contain water look white and bright. Discs that are healthy and have good amount of water content are bright whereas discs that are dehydrated and degenerated appear black.

appears black and may be referred to as a "black" disc (Fig. 1-18). Patients may have one or more black discs. An abnormal signal focus at the disc margin on MRI may indicate a disruption of concentric fibers comprising the anulus fibrosus. Not all degenerative

black discs seen on MRI are painful—on occasion they are simply a radiologic finding.

Weight loss is key to reducing axial load and the stress applied to the discs. Medical management includes an NSAID and, when needed, an opioid. Lumbar epidural steroids have been used to successfully treat the pain from lumbar degenerative disc disease. It may be necessary to remove the disc if conservative options fail, which may necessitate the use of a discogram to determine which black disc on the MRI is the actual source of pain. The practitioner inserts a needle into the disc and slowly injects contrast solution, adding volume to put pressure on the disc. The patient then reports if this pressure reproduces the pain. A discogram helps differentiate which discs are degenerated and painful as opposed to those that are only degenerated.

PAIN IN THE HIP

Three of the most common causes of hip pain that originate from the hip are (1) arthritis, (2) ischemic (avascular) necrosis, and (3) femoral neck stress fracture. Lumbar spine and sacroiliac (SI) joint pathology can also radiate into the hip, mimicking true hip pathology.

Arthritis

Patients with arthritis may report locking, clicking, and catching of the hip (Fig. 1-19). Groin pain is a typical complaint, whereas lateral buttock pain is more indicative of greater trochanteric bursitis. The Stinchfield test is used to test for arthritis. The patient is asked to

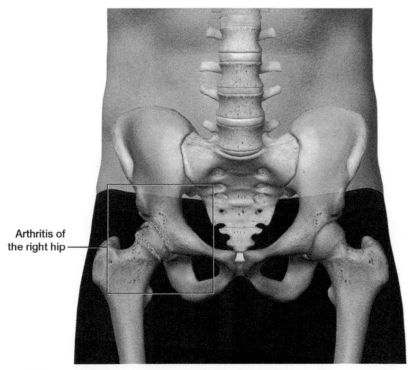

Figure 1-19 Arthritis of the right hip. Patients often report groin pain.

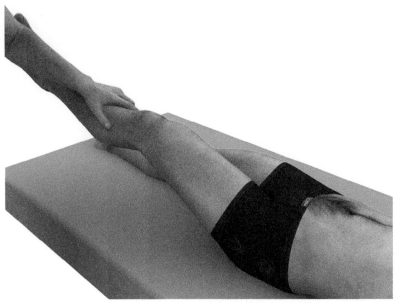

Figure 1-20 The Stinchfield test. When the patient lifts their leg to 30 degrees, hip pathology will be felt in the groin whereas lumbar or sacroiliac pathology will be felt in the back.

elevate a straight leg off the table against the resistance of the doctor's hand (Fig. 1-20). The test is positive if it brings about the patient's typical groin, or thigh pain. A key feature on physical examination is decreased rotation, particularly internal rotation, which causes pain. Radiographs show asymmetric joint space narrowing and sclerosis of the weight-bearing portion of the joint (Fig. 1-21).

Arthritic hip pain typically responds well to a steroid injection; performance of these injections is best under x-ray guidance. Medically, an NSAID may be effective with the addition of an opioid if the pain is not alleviated. When conservative options fail, it is necessary to consider a hip replacement.

Ischemic (Avascular) Necrosis

The femoral head is the most frequent site of osteonecrosis. The death of bone tissue in the head of the femur is caused by an inadequate blood supply. Common causes include sickle cell disease, systemic lupus erythematosus (especially when treated with chronic steroids), femoral head fractures, and radiation exposure. Complaints of pain are the same as for osteoarthritis of the hip. Early in the course of the pathology, radiographs are normal; gradually nonspecific osteopenia develops. If clinical suspicion is high, the most useful diagnostic test is an MRI, which is a sensitive indicator for early stages of ischemic necrosis.

Management includes reducing the causative agent as much as possible; in overweight patients this means weight loss especially. In advanced cases, in which

collapse of the femoral head has begun, total hip arthroplasty is the treatment of choice.

Fractures

Hip fractures should be strongly suspected in patients with hip pain after trauma. They are more likely to

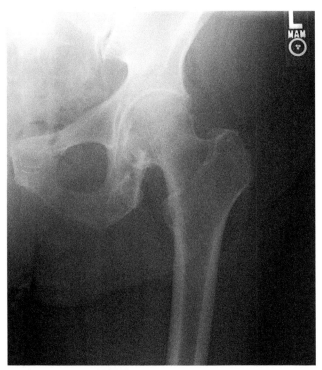

Figure 1-21 X-ray of the left hip showing arthritis, asymmetric joint space narrowing and sclerosis.

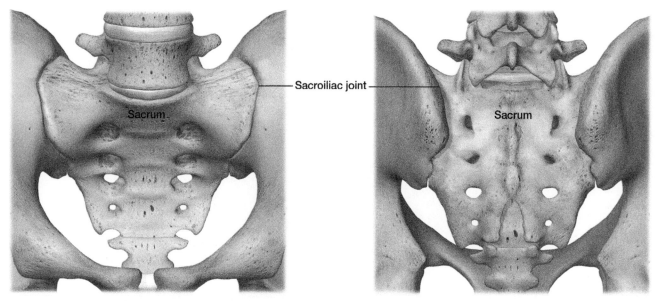

Figure 1-22 Anatomy of the sacroiliac joint, where the spine and the pelvis connect.

occur in people with osteoporosis as well as in young women with amenorrhea.[4] In 1996, of the 340,000 hospitalizations for hip fractures, 80% were women.[5] Anteroposterior views of the pelvis and hip, as well as a cross-table lateral view, are usually sufficient to show femoral neck stress fractures. If the x-rays are not conclusive, a bone scan can sufficiently rule out fractures.

Femoral neck fractures usually require surgical stabilization.

PAIN IN THE BUTTOCK

The Sacroiliac Joint

The SI joint is the weight-bearing joint between the sacrum at the base of the spine and its connection to the ileum of the pelvis (Fig. 1-22). It is where the spine and the pelvis connect. Pain from the SI joint is often manifested at the gluteal dimple, which corresponds to the S2 foramen (Fig. 1-23). The pain is usually sharp and may radiate into the thigh or groin. Patients may report that the pain is worsened while climbing stairs. SI joint degeneration develops more often in patients who have had lumbosacral fusion regardless of the number of fusion segments. Physical examination is notoriously unreliable for teasing out SI joint pain, which may affect one SI joint or both. A diagnostic injection under fluoroscopic guidance is often needed to confirm or refute the diagnosis. If the injection of local anesthetic into the joint does not alter the patient's pain, it is necessary to consider another source of pain.

First-line medication treatment is an NSAID. Interventionally, patients often will respond to an SI joint injection of a steroid and anesthetic combination.

Greater Trochanteric Bursitis

A bursa is a fluid-filled sac that functions as a gliding surface to reduce friction between tissues of the

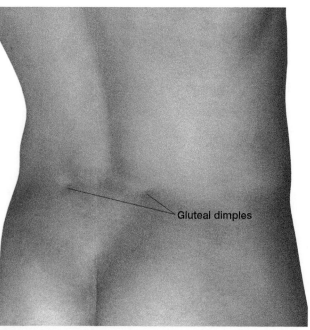

Figure 1-23 Pain from the SI joint is often manifested at the gluteal dimple.

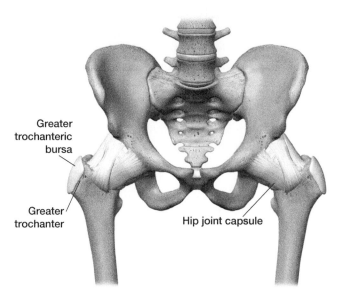

Figure 1-24 The greater trochanteric bursa is located over the lateral posterior aspect of the greater trochanter of the femur.

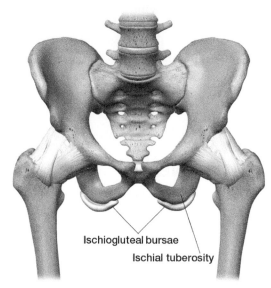

Figure 1-26 The ischiogluteal bursae are located at the ischiogluteal tuberosity where the hamstring muscles originate from the pelvis. This condition is commonly know as weavers bottom.

body. The greater trochanteric bursa is located on the lower outer area of the buttock (Fig. 1-24). The muscles and tendons that come in contact may inflame this bursa. It is possible to reproduce pain by directly palpating the bare posterior portion of the trochanter (Fig. 1-25).

Greater trochanteric bursitis typically responds very well to a cortisone injection.

Ischiogluteal Bursitis

Ischiogluteal bursitis is also referred to as weaver's bottom because traditionally weavers would sit in a position that aggravates the ischiogluteal bursa. The ischiogluteal bursa lies between the hamstring tendon and the pelvic bone (ischial tuberosity, Fig. 1-26). Patients typically experience pain in the lower buttock,

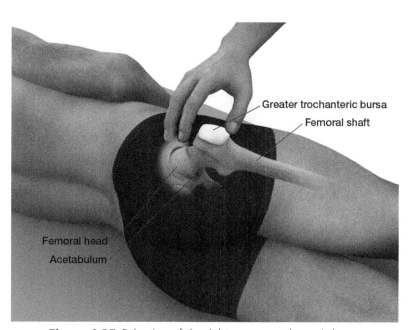

Figure 1-25 Palpation of the right greater trochanteric bursa.

which is exacerbated with direct pressure over the ischium. To properly palpate the area, it is necessary to flex the leg, pulling the gluteus maximus upward to expose the ischial bursa.

Treatment begins with stopping any activity that increases pain until the symptoms dissipate. If this does not work, the next option is an ischiogluteal bursa cortisone injection.

PAIN IN THE KNEE

Chronic knee pain is commonly caused by arthritis, chronic meniscal tear, tendonitis or osteochondritis. Pain can also be referred from the hips or lumbar spine to the knee.

Arthritis

Arthritis of the Knee Joint: Over time, the cartilage of the joint wears thin. The meniscus, or joint cushion, thins and wears away (Fig. 1-27). Arthritis is common in this weight-bearing joint, especially in patients who are overweight or who have had significant knee injuries. There is also a large genetic component to arthritis of the knee. Patients complain of pain with activities, decreased range of motion, stiffness, and tenderness along the joint line. The knee has three compartments: The medial, the lateral, and the patellofemoral. Weight-bearing x-rays show joint space narrowing in one or all three compartments of the knee. MRI is more sensitive than x-rays and CT for assessing the extent and severity of osteoarthritic changes.

Medically, NSAIDs are the preferred treatment. Weight loss is key in obese patients. Interventionally, a cortisone injection into the joint itself can provide significant pain relief. Viscosupplementation—that is, injecting a lubricant—has also been shown to be effective in treating osteoarthritic knee pain.[6] If conservative options fail, a knee replacement may be necessary.

Patellofemoral Arthritis: Patients with this condition report pain that is located above the kneecap as it connects to the femur. The practitioner may elicit pain using the patellofemoral grind test, which evaluates the quality of the articulating surfaces of the patella and the

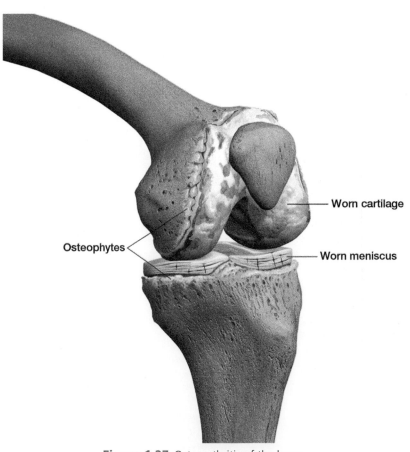

Figure 1-27 Osteoarthritis of the knee.

Worn cartilage

Worn meniscus

Osteophytes

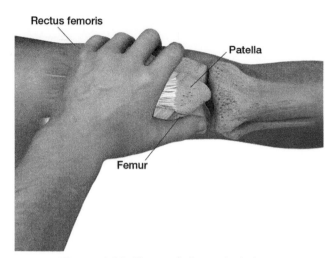

Figure 1-28 The patellofemoral grind test.

trochlear groove of the femur (Fig. 1-28). It is necessary first to apply pressure to the superior aspect of the patella, pushing inferiorly with the leg in the neutral position. Then the patient tightens the quadriceps muscles by extending the leg; this enables the practitioner to feel how the patella glides and if it causes pain.

Conservative treatment includes avoiding activities that require extensive knee flexion, such as deep knee bends. Quadriceps strengthening is the focus in physical therapy. NSAIDs can be used medically. As described previously, both a cortisone injection and viscosupplementation can be helpful interventionally.

Meniscal Tear

A meniscus is the thick, crescent-shaped cartilage in the knee, a pad between the femur and the tibia. There is a meniscus on both the lateral and medial aspect of the knee joint, which provides a gliding surface for joint movement. These menisci also function to distribute body weight evenly across the knee joint. Meniscus tears occur frequently following trauma and sport injuries. The meniscus can tear peripherally or more centrally. Peripheral tears can heal on their own. However, larger, more central tears do not often heal and can often lead to chronic pain. The periphery of the meniscus is nourished by small blood vessels, the center of the meniscus has no direct blood supply therefore heals poorly. Patients report pain along the medial or lateral aspect of the knee joint line depending on which meniscus is torn; the medial meniscus is most commonly torn. Because the smooth gliding surface no longer exists, patients also report a clicking with movement. On examination, an audible click may be heard. A definitive diagnosis is achieved with an MRI.

Conservative treatment is the same as for osteoarthritis of the knee. This includes treatment with anti-inflammatory medication, physical therapy, and cortisone injections. To prevent further deterioration and relieve

pain symptoms, arthroscopic debridement of the torn edge of the meniscus may be necessary.

Patellar Tendonitis

Patellar tendonitis, also called jumper's knee, is pain in the band of tissue (patellar tendon) that connects the patella (kneecap) to the tibia (Fig. 1-29). This pain is typically worse with jumping, as the name implies, as well as rising or walking after sitting. Patellar tendonitis is often seen in basketball players. The key is preventing overuse of the patellar tendon.

Wearing a band across the patellar tendon (an infrapatellar strap) can be helpful. It alters the weight-bearing surface of the patella presented to the intertrochlear groove.

Osteochondritis

Osteochondritis is a disorder in which fragments of bone or cartilage come loose around the knee joint. The underlying bone from which the fragment separates is normal, as opposed to osteonecrosis, in which the underlying bone is avascular. Osteochondritis occurs most frequently in the knee, followed distantly by the elbow. The medial aspect of the knee is affected in 75% of cases. MRI is helpful in supporting the clinical diagnosis. Symptoms are usually vague and poorly localized. It may be possible to feel fragments along the joint line. Knee arthroscopy is both diagnostic and therapeutic.

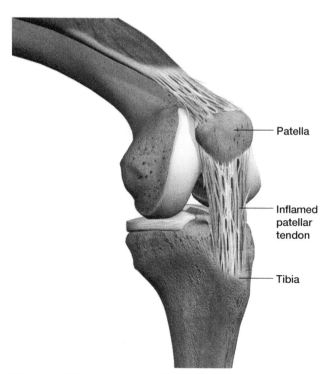

Figure 1-29 Patellar tendonitis, also known as jumper's knee.

CASE STUDIES

A 53-year-old, overweight woman presents complaining of a 2-year history of right knee pain. She states that the knee pain has increased over the past 6 months and denies any specific trauma to the knee. She describes the pain as constant, and walking or prolonged standing makes it worse. The pain is deep, dull, and achy. She has no back pain. On examination, she has no weakness and the right knee does not appear to be grossly unstable. X-rays, which she has brought to the office, show joint space narrowing.

You diagnose the patient with osteoarthritis of the right knee and prescribe an NSAID and physical therapy. At a 1-month follow-up examination, the woman states that the NSAID helps but that she went to physical therapy only once because it made her right knee worse. You both agree that proceeding with a knee injection would both help the pain and allow her to participate in physical therapy. The knee is draped and prepped in sterile fashion; via a lateral approach, you inject 40 mg of Kenalog in 4 mL of 0.25% bupivacaine. You stress diet to reduce weight bearing on the knee and the importance of resuming physical therapy.

A 61-year-old man presents with lower back pain, which he has had for at least the past year. However, it has increased in intensity over the past 3 months. No specific trauma is associated with the start of the pain. The pain occurs daily, despite the use of ibuprofen. It is axial in nature, with no radiation into the leg. The man describes the pain as deep, dull, and achy, and it is worse on the right side of the spine. The pain radiates out toward the flank. He has no bowel or bladder problems. The patient believes that he has sciatica.

You astutely recognize that his axial low back pain is most likely caused by facet arthropathy, a degenerative disc, or a combination of both. On examination, he has full strength in his extremities, and there is no pain on palpation of the SI joints. The patient does have pain over the lower facet joints, particularly on the right. The patient's constant back pain despite the use of an NSAID prompts you to get an MRI of the lumbar spine. The MRI shows facet arthropathy and degenerative disc disease with no foraminal compression (nerve root impingement as it exits the spinal canal).

You decide to send the patient for diagnostic/therapeutic lumbar facet joint injections and physical therapy. The patient has a lumbar facet joint injection under fluoroscopic guidance at L3/L4, L4/L5, and L5/S1 on the right. This results in near resolution of his pain.

A 22-year-old male college senior complains of elbow pain. He plays on his college golf team. The patient states that the pain is on the lateral aspect of his elbow. He has had the pain for the past 2 months, and the elbow is becoming more tender. He notes no specific trauma, and there is normal motion of the elbow on examination. With palpation of the lateral epicondyle, the pain is exquisite. You diagnose tennis elbow, lateral epicondylitis. The patient responds, "How can I have tennis elbow? I'm a golfer!" You explain that tennis elbow is so prevalent that it is actually more common in golfers than golfer's elbow (medial epicondylitis).

You prescribe Celebrex 100 mg twice a day and a brace to reduce strain on the elbow. Within 2 weeks the painful symptoms abate.

REFERENCES

1. Scane AC, Sutcliffe AM, Francis RM. The sequelae of vertebral compression fractures in men. *Osteoporos Int.* 1994;4:89–92.
2. McGraw JK, Cardella J, Barr JD, et al. Society of Interventional Radiology quality improvement guidelines for percutaneous vertebroplasty. *J Vasc Interv Radiol.* 2003;14(7):827–831.
3. Revel M, Poiraudeau S, Auleley GR, et al. Capacity of the clinical picture to characterize low back pain relieved by facet joint anesthesia. Proposed criteria to identify patients with painful facet joints. *Spine.* 1998;23(18):1972–1977.
4. Teitz CC, Hu SS, Arendt EA. The female athlete: Evaluation and treatment of sports-related problems. *J Am Acad Orthop Surg.* 1997;5(2):87–96.
5. Stevens JA, Olson S. Reducing falls and resulting hip fractures among older women. *Home Care Provid.* 2000;5(4):134–141.
6. Strauss EJ, Hart JA, Miller MD, et al. Hyaluronic acid viscosupplementation and osteoarthritis: Current uses and future directions. *AM J Sports Med.* 2009;37(8):1636–1644.

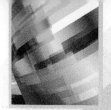

CHAPTER 2

Neuropathic Pain

Nerves send sensory impulses to the brain for interpretation. These impulses travel in a regular pattern when the nervous system is working properly. When injured, this regular controlled transmission of impulses fails and nerves fires aberrantly. Injured nerves, no longer triggered solely by appropriate stimuli, develop pathologic activity manifesting as abnormal excitability to normal chemical, thermal, and mechanical stimuli. The brain interprets this aberrant nerve firing as pain. With neuropathic pain, the patient usually reports an electric, shooting, burning pain rather than an achy, dull pain.

This chapter presents the most universal high-yield causes of neuropathic pain in different parts of the body. To learn the particulars of how to properly prescribe medications or perform procedures mentioned in this chapter, it is necessary to refer to the chapter dedicated to the specific subject.

PAIN IN THE FACE: TRIGEMINAL NEURALGIA

In the world of pain, one of the most severe forms is trigeminal neuralgia (tic douloureux, meaning painful spasm). This pain can be so severe that it has been known to cause suicide. The trigeminal nerve, or the fifth cranial nerve, which is responsible for sensory impulses originating from the face above the jaw line, has three branches: Ophthalmic (V1), maxillary (V2), and mandibular (V3) (Fig. 2-1). The pain of trigeminal neuralgia is most common in the V2 and V3 branches of the trigeminal nerve. It is a sharp, electric pain that radiates deep into the cheek, lips, and tongue, typically on one side of the face. During an attack, any sensory stimuli, even a stream of fast-moving air, may exacerbate the pain. Theories about the cause of trigeminal neuralgia remain controversial. One prevailing theory is that a small blood vessel wrapped around the branches of the trigeminal nerve causes periodic compression, leading to aberrant nerve firing.

History and Examination

The diagnosis is primarily based on history. Patients describe the pain as brief, stabbing, and shock-like. Exacerbations often come in clusters, with complete remission that may last months to years. Pain is

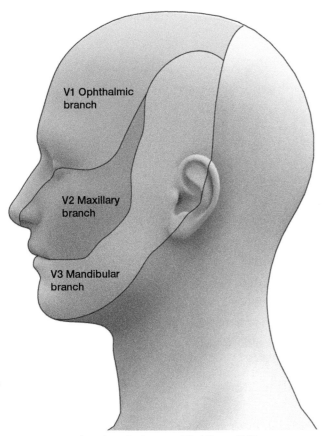

Figure 2-1 The trigeminal nerve: V1, V2, and V3 sensory distribution.

PAIN IN THE THUMB, INDEX, MIDDLE, AND HALF OF THE RING FINGER: CARPAL TUNNEL SYNDROME

Carpal tunnel syndrome (CTS) is one of the most common causes of pain in the hand. It results from compression of the median nerve under the transverse carpal ligament (Fig. 2-2). CTS leads to an irritable electric sensation in the distribution of the median nerve (Fig. 2-3). Symptoms may be unilateral or bilateral. Upon waking, people may feel as if the affected hand is asleep. In severe cases, atrophy of the thenar eminence (muscle at the base of the thumb) may eventually occur. Two medical conditions associated with CTS are pregnancy and hypothyroidism. In these conditions fluid retention in tissues may exacerbate this compressive neuropathy.

History and Examination

Patients describe an electric, painful sensation in the palm, thumb, index, middle, and half of the ring finger. If a patient has pain in the neck that radiates down through the arm into the hand, the diagnosis of cervical radiculopathy should be entertained. If there is numbness of the whole hand bilaterally, it is necessary

unilateral; examination should confirm that pain is in the distribution of the trigeminal nerve. When patients present with symptoms that go past the midline of the face or the jaw line, it is important to check for another cause of the pain. When a young person presents with trigeminal neuralgia, this may be the first sign of multiple sclerosis; a magnetic resonance imaging (MRI) of the brain with contrast is used to investigate this possibility. Other than pain, physical examination findings are normal. The practitioner should ask about a vesicular outbreak in the area to rule out postherpetic neuralgia (PHN).

Treatment

Tegretol (carbamazepine) and Lyrica (pregabalin) are useful in the treatment of trigeminal neuralgia. Baclofen, a muscle relaxant, can be very beneficial. Opioids have been employed in combination with the above medications. Trigeminal nerve blocks can provide relief during painful exacerbations. In microvascular decompression, also known as the Jannetta procedure, a surgeon explores the nerve for an encroaching blood vessel. If found, it is necessary to separate ("decompress") the vessel and nerve with a surgical pad.

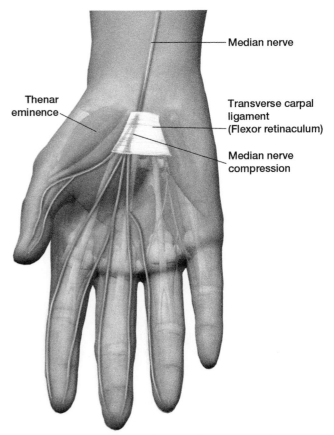

Figure 2-2 Compression of the median nerve, under the transverse carpal ligament (flexor retinaculum). Carpal Tunnel Syndrome (CTS).

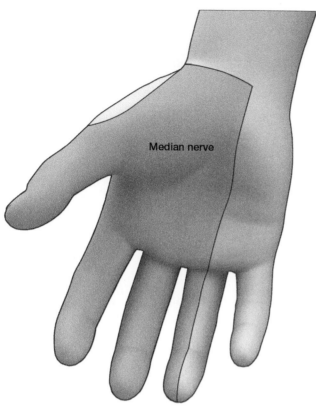

Figure 2-3 Territory of the median nerve. Carpal Tunnel syndrome.

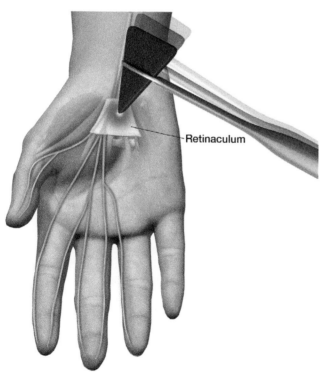

Figure 2-4 Tinel sign. Percussion at the transverse carpal ligament (flexor retinaculum) produces paresthesia along the path of the median nerve.

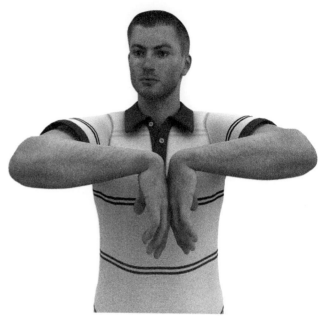

Figure 2-5 Phalen maneuver. This position should be held for at least 1 minute to check if median nerve irritation is felt.

to consider peripheral neuropathy. The existence of paresthesia (an abnormal sensation in the skin, such as numbness, tingling, pricking, or burning) in the pinky and ring finger is more indicative of ulnar neuropathy. On examination, tapping on the median nerve (Tinel sign, Fig. 2-4) or compressing the nerve using Phalen maneuver (Fig. 2-5) can elicit the symptoms of CTS. A nerve conduction study shows increased latency of the median nerve.

Treatment

Because CTS is a mechanical problem, wrist splints may relieve the compression. Wrist splints are available at most pharmacies. Normally, when people sleep, the wrist is in a flexed position, narrowing the carpal tunnel for hours. To alleviate symptoms patients wear a wrist splint at night, placing the wrist in a neutral position. Typically, antiseizure and antidepressant medications used to treat neuropathic pain can also help. An injection into the area of compression, a steroid mixed with a local anesthetic, can provide pain relief as well. Some 25% of patients will have long-term relief of their symptoms following a CTS nerve block.[1] Surgery consists of cutting the transverse carpal ligament to relieve the compressive neuropathy.

PAIN IN THE THORACIC REGION: POSTHERPETIC NEURALGIA

A common, often missed, cause of burning pain across the abdomen or chest is PHN. This type of neuralgia (pain along the course of the nerve) begins after an outbreak of herpes zoster (shingles). The cause of herpes zoster is a dormant varicella virus harbored in the

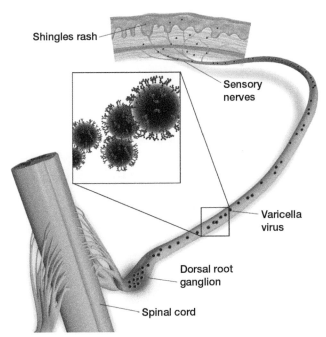

Shingles rash

Sensory nerves

Varicella virus

Dorsal root ganglion

Spinal cord

Figure 2-6 The varicella virus lays dormant in the dorsal root ganglion. When activated it spreads along the corresponding nerve eventually reaching the skin. A vesicular rash is seen at the skin level.

dorsal root ganglion that is reactivated (Fig. 2-6). The virus spreads along the nerve, presenting as pain, itching, and tingling along the dermatome in which it spreads. Vesicle formation follows (Fig. 2-7). After the acute phase, the vesicles from the herpes rash begin to crust over. For most people, this is the end of the painful symptoms, but roughly 20% go on to develop PHN. Less than 10% of people younger than age 60 develop PHN, whereas about 40% of people older than 60 do. African Americans are 75% less likely than whites to develop this condition. Typically, the pain follows a thoracic

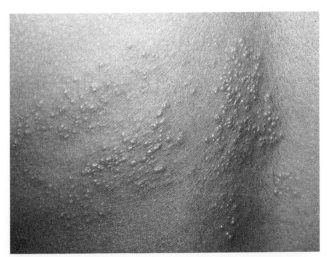

Figure 2-7 Shingles rash. (From: Craft N, Fox LP, Goldsmith LA, et al. Visual Dx: Essential Adult Dermatology. Philadelphia, PA: Lippincott Williams & Wilkins; 2010.)

dermatome, but it can follow any dermatome. If the pain lasts more than a month, it is defined as PHN. Sensation may be altered over this area, with the patient experiencing either hypersensitivity or decreased sensation.

History and Examination

Patients describe a burning pain, electric in nature with exquisite sensitivity of the skin that follows a dermatome. Often patients have a significant deterioration in quality of life. On examination, the patient may have scars from previous vesicles. However, it is important to remember that on rare occasions, PHN can occur without any previous vascular rash. In this instance, the nerve is affected by reaction of the virus, but it never clinically manifests at the skin level.

Treatment

Aggressive treatment during the acute outbreak can sometimes prevent progression to PHN. Acyclovir is effective in reducing the length of time of the acute outbreak of lesions and in decreasing pain and promoting healing.[2,3] Antiseizure and antidepressant medications used for neuropathic pain are first-line treatment. A 5% Lidoderm (lidocaine) patch over the area is a reasonable treatment option with a low–side-effect profile. Epidural steroid injections may be effective. (The author often performs a series of three epidural steroid injections, 1 to 2 weeks apart.) In Forrest's study, the use of epidural steroid injections at weekly intervals for people who have had PHN for more than 6 months provided 89% of the patients complete relief from their pain at 1 year. This study did not have a control group.[4] For patients who do not respond to medications and injections, a spinal cord stimulator trial is a reasonable next step.

PAIN IN THE BACK OR NECK AND DOWN THE LEG OR ARM: RADICULAR PAIN

One of the most common pain complaints is radicular pain (irritation of a nerve root). When the spinal cord is affected, this is referred to as a myelopathy. If only the nerve root is involved, it is radiculopathy without signs of myelopathy. (When radiculopathy occurs in the lumbar spine, some refer to this as sciatica.) The pain radiates along the path of the nerve root being irritated. In the lower extremities, people may describe it as pain that starts in the lower back/buttocks and radiates down one or both legs. In the upper extremities, people may describe it as cervical pain that radiates down one or both arms. The most common cause of radicular pain is a herniated disc that affects a nerve root.

To better understand this, it helps to take a closer look at the anatomy involved with radicular pain from

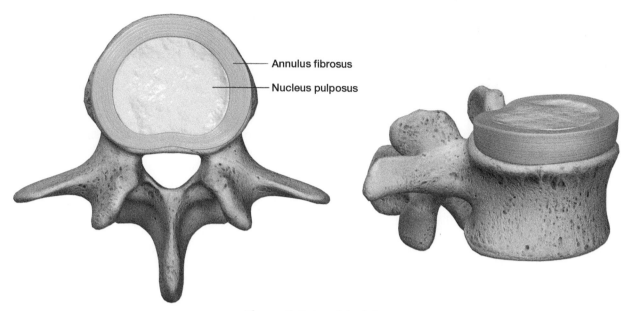

Annulus fibrosus

Nucleus pulposus

Figure 2-8 A vertebral disc.

a herniated disc. A vertebral disc is shaped like a jelly donut; the jelly-like inner part is the nucleus pulposus and the thick outer part is the anular fibrosus (Fig. 2-8). The nucleus pulposus, the jelly-like inner part of a vertebral disc, contains inflammatory factors such as substance P and nitrous oxide. When the nucleus pulposus starts to leak out through the outer layer of the disc (annular fibrosus), it results in an inflammatory reaction around the nerve root (Fig. 2-9).[5] When a disc herniates out of its normal position and/or releases its inner inflammatory content, it can affect the nerve root at that location. If the disc or the inflammatory content is herniating to just one side of the spinal column, it can affect only the ipsilateral nerve root, leaving the contralateral nerve root alone. This is why some people have pain radiating down both legs and some down one leg only (Fig. 2-10). It is generally theorized that either physically compressing the nerve root and/or bathing it in this inflammatory matrix is the cause of radicular pain. Inflammation and physical protrusion of the disc can go on to cause pressure on the epidural venous plexus, causing venous obstruction.[6] When the venous side backs up, it can lead to decreased perfusion of the nerve root from the arterial side. Prolonged irritation and poor blood circulation appear to make these nerve roots hypersensitive,[7] further contributing to prolonged radicular pain.

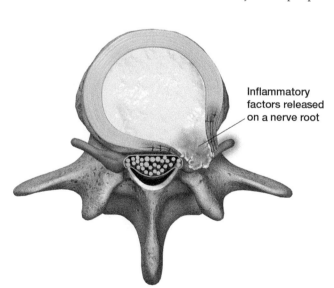

Inflammatory factors released on a nerve root

Figure 2-9 Herniated disc with inflammatory factors being released on the nerve root.

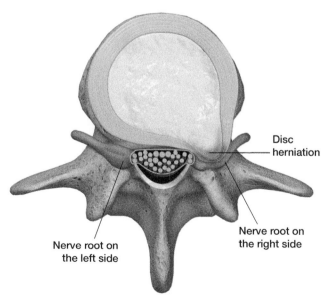

Disc herniation

Nerve root on the right side

Nerve root on the left side

Figure 2-10 Right-sided disc herniation, affecting only the ipsilateral nerve root. In this case the patient would have only right leg symptoms with the left leg being unaffected.

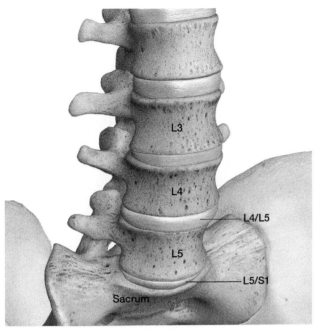

Figure 2-11 The L4/L5 and L5–S1 disc level. Ninety percent of, lumbar disc herniations occur at these two levels.

Ninety percent of lumbar disc herniations occur between the fourth and fifth lumbar vertebral bodies (L4–L5) and between the fifth lumbar vertebral body and the sacrum (L5–S1) (Fig. 2-11). This is a matter of physics. The greatest range of motion in the spine is at the L4–L5 and L5–S1 levels, which makes these discs most vulnerable to herniation. The irritation of a specific nerve root or roots by these discs sends a signal to the brain, which interprets this as pain along the entire nerve. For example, irritation of the L5 nerve root tricks the brain, which senses that the entire nerve, not just the nerve root, is affected.

History and Examination

On history, patients often report their radicular pain as being burning, electric, sharp, and lancinating. The symptoms can be constant or come and go. It is possible to make the pain worse by leaning forward, because this position may put more pressure on the nerve root by further herniating the disc against the nerve root. On examination, the course that the pain travels helps identify which nerve root is affected (Fig. 2-12). The

Figure 2-12 Dermatome map. A dermatome is an area of skin that is mainly supplied by a single nerve. ▶

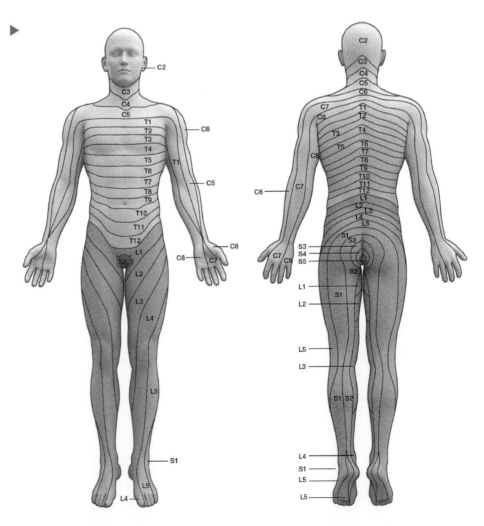

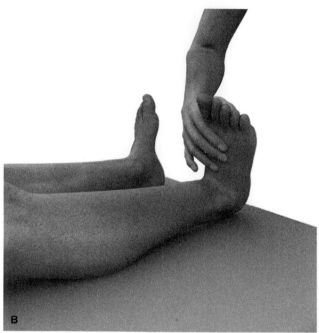

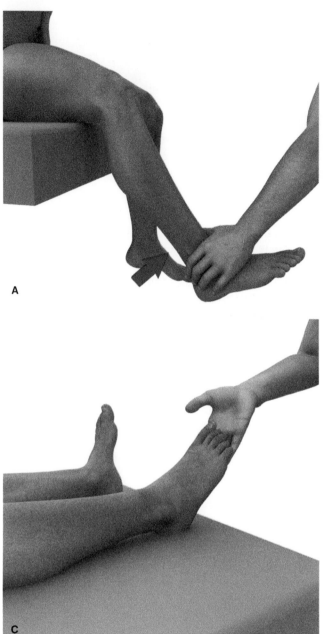

Figure 2-13 Motor testing for lower-extremity radicular level. **A:** Quad strength corresponding to the L4 nerve root. **B:** Dorsiflexion corresponding to L5 nerve root. **C:** Plantar flexion corresponding to the S1 nerve root.

longitudinal extent of the pain appears to be proportional to the amount of pressure exerted on the nerve root,[7] thus the further down toward the toes the pain spreads along the nerve root, the more affected it is. Motor testing also helps identify which nerve root may be the source of the problem. If there is weakness in quadriceps strength, it indicates that the L4 nerve root may be affected. Weakness on dorsiflexion indicates that the L5 nerve root may be affected,

whereas plantar flexion weakness is indicative of an S1 radiculopathy (Fig. 2-13). A good way to help remember these is as follows. "Quad" means four—L4. Bending five toes toward the patient (dorsiflexion) tests L5. Pressing down on the gas (plantar flexion) of a new S1 Porsche tests S1. A positive straight-leg test is a nonspecific sign for lumbar disc herniation. The patient experiences pain in the back when the leg is extended. Normally, patients can elevate the leg 60 to

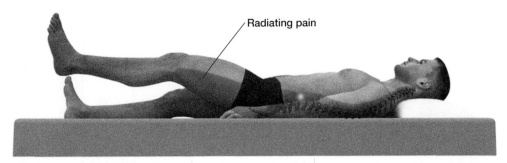

Figure 2-14 Straight-leg test. Elevation of the leg can reproduce concordant radicular symptoms.

90 degrees on this test, which is positive if an elevation of 40 degrees or less produces pain (Fig. 2-14).

This phenomenon can also occur in the cervical spine. Cervical discs can herniate, causing cervical radiculopathy with paresthesia (a skin sensation of tingling or prickling) radiating down the arm. On history, when paresthesia is felt into the thumb, it is the C6 nerve root; when it goes into the middle finger, it is the C7 nerve root; and when paresthesia is felt into the pinky, it is the C8 nerve root (Fig. 2-15). Pain, however, often may follow a different distribution or pattern than paresthesia in the cervical spine.[8] A patient thus may have paresthesia all the way to the pinky in a C8 radiculopathy but generalized pain in the shoulder and triceps. Motor testing on physical examination also helps identify which nerve root may be affected. If there is weakness in the biceps, this indicates C5 and C6, whereas triceps weakness is C7. If a patient also has upper motor neuron signs on examination (increased reflexes, increased tone, fasciculations, clonus), it indicates that not only the nerve root is affected but the spinal cord may be involved.

This section focuses on the most common causes of radiculopathy and in 98% of cases, the cause is a disc herniation.[9] Work-up should include an MRI of the affected spinal segments. If the patient has had surgery, it is necessary to order an MRI with contrast to help differentiate between new pathology and scar tissue. Although a herniated disc is by far the most common

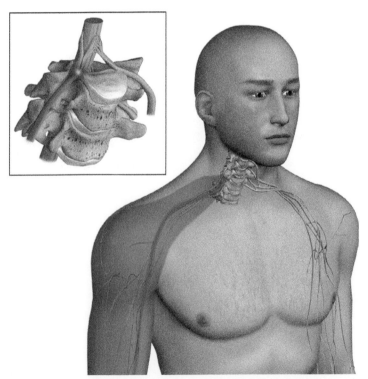

Figure 2-15 Cervical radiculopathy. In this case a cervical disc is herniated toward the right producing pain down the right arm.

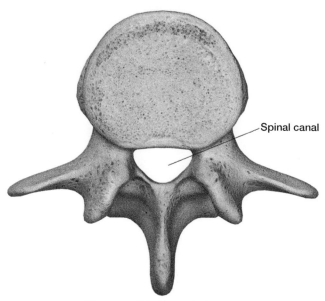

Figure 2-16 The spinal canal.

cause of radiculopathy, there are differential diagnoses. With a history of cancer or constitutional symptoms, a tumor is a possibility. With fever, night sweats, or chills, infection is a possibility. With a history of radiation, radiation plexitis is a consideration.

Treatment

The painful symptoms of radiculopathy tend to resolve over time. Radiculopathy caused by a herniated disc may be treated with a series of epidural steroid injections,

which decrease inflammation at the site of injury. Epidural steroids can improve the patient's quality of life while a natural resolution of symptoms occur. First-line medication treatments include antiseizure and/or antidepressant medications used for neuropathic pain. Second-line medications include an opioid added to the neuropathic pain medication. Physical therapy can help alleviate pressure on the spine by strengthening core muscles and increasing flexibility. More aggressive treatment includes surgical removal of the disc.

PAIN IN THE BACK OR NECK AND POSSIBLY DOWN THE LEGS OR ARMS: SPINAL CANAL STENOSIS

Spinal canal stenosis is a reduction in the anterior–posterior and lateral diameters of the spinal canal (Fig. 2-16). This condition occurs both in the lumbar and cervical spine, rarely in the thoracic spine. When the spinal cord and/or nerve roots that travel through the canal are compressed, the body interprets this as pain. Spinal canal stenosis is part of the normal aging process but can be accelerated in some individuals. Patients with a congenitally narrowed spine are at higher risk for symptomatic stenosis. Advanced degenerative changes of the spine can lead to symptomatic spinal canal stenosis. The vertebrae are lined up to create the oval that is the spinal canal—when a vertebral body slips out of alignment, perfect symmetry is lost and the spinal canal becomes narrowed at that area (Fig. 2-17). This phenomenon is known as

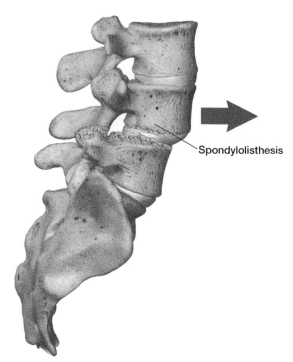

Figure 2-17 Spondylolisthesis: A forward dislocation of one vertebra over the one beneath it producing pressure on spinal nerves.

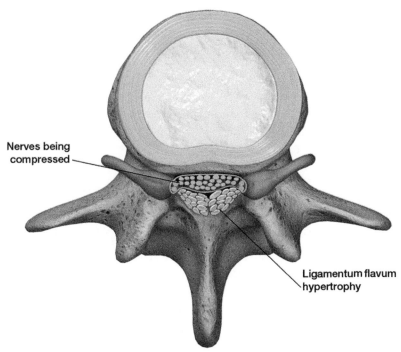

Figure 2-18 Ligamentum flavum hypertrophy leading to spinal canal stenosis. Fibrosis is the main cause of ligamentum flavum hypertrophy, and fibrosis is caused by the accumulation of mechanical stress with time. Ligamentum flavum hypertrophy tends to be disproportionately increased at the L4/L5 and L3/L4 levels.

spondylolisthesis (spon-dee-low-lis-THEE-sis), *spondylo* meaning spine, and *listhesis* meaning slippage. Spondylolisthesis may vary from mild to severe. Another source of spinal canal stenosis is thickening of the ligament that runs in the posterior aspect of the spinal canal, the liga-mentum flavum; if its degree of hypertrophy increases beyond a critical amount, the spinal canal starts to narrow (Fig. 2-18). The facet joints that link the vertebral bodies posteriorly can hypertrophy, which leads to both central canal and foraminal stenosis (Fig. 2-19).

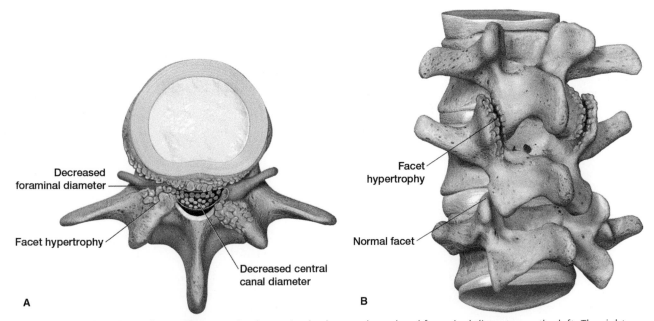

Figure 2-19 A (axial view): Facet hypertrophy decreasing both central canal and foraminal diameter on the left. The right foraminal diameter is minimally affected. **B (oblique view):** Facet hypertrophy.

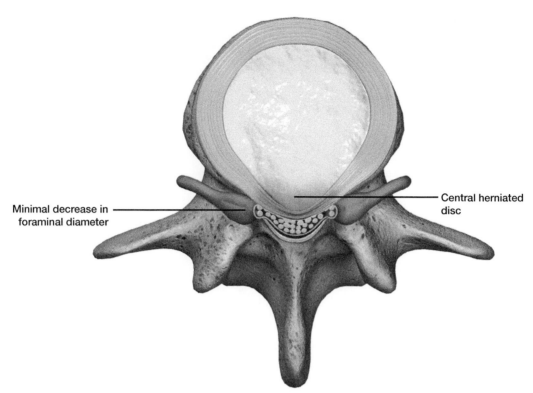

Minimal decrease in foraminal diameter

Central herniated disc

Figure 2-20 Centrally herniated disc decreasing central spinal canal diameter with minimal effect of foraminal diameter.

A vertebral disc can herniate centrally rather than laterally and contribute to central canal stenosis (Fig. 2-20).

The most common sites of spinal canal stenosis in the lower lumbar region are L4–L5 and L5–S1. There is no cord to be impinged at these levels, as the spinal cord usually ends at L1, thus the nerve roots only are impinged. Lumbar spine stenosis may result in radicular pain, neurogenic claudication, or both by compressing the exiting nerve roots. Neurogenic claudication is pain and paresthesia in the back, buttocks, and legs that is relieved by rest. Spinal canal stenosis in the cervical as compared to the lumbar spine may result in radicular pain but also, if severe enough, cause myelopathy from cord compression. Myelopathy is any functional disturbance and/or pathologic change in the spinal cord.

History and Examination

The history presented is often very similar to that of radicular pain as described in that section, sometimes with slight differences. Symptoms are usually bilateral rather than unilateral. Patients can have a greater degree of back pain compared to leg or arm pain. Pain is usually worse with walking and relieved with rest in lumbar stenosis. If the spinal canal becomes critically stenotic, it can lead to changes in the spinal cord and the presence of myelopathy on examination.

Signs of myelopathy include increased reflexes, increased muscle tone, fasciculation, and clonus. MRI can evaluate both the diameter of the spinal canal and the integrity of the underlying spinal structures.

Treatment

Spinal canal stenosis causing myelopathy is a surgical indication; thus, it is necessary to refer patients directly to a spine surgeon. For lesser degrees of spinal canal stenosis, the same modalities used to treat lumbar and cervical radiculopathy are useful. The natural history of spinal stenosis is not well understood. A slow progression seems to occur in affected individuals. Even with significant stenosis, many individuals have only mild symptoms and very little clinical progression of symptoms.

PAIN ON THE TOP AND LATERAL ASPECT OF THE THIGH: LATERAL FEMORAL CUTANEOUS NEUROPATHY (MERALGIA PARESTHETICA)

The lateral femoral cutaneous nerve is purely sensory, derived from the L2 and L3 nerve root. It passes just medial and inferior to the anterior superior iliac spine, where it is accessed for a nerve block. The nerve then passes beneath the inguinal ligament. It enters the

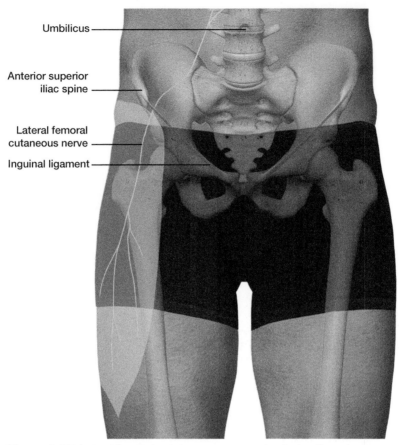

Umbilicus

Anterior superior
iliac spine

Lateral femoral
cutaneous nerve

Inguinal ligament

Figure 2-21 Lateral femoral cutaneous nerve; anatomical path and sensory area innervation. Lateral femoral cutaneous neuropathy is also known as meralgia paresthetica.

thigh and supplies sensation to the anterolateral aspect of the thigh, starting just below the hip (Fig. 2-21).

When the nerve becomes compressed or irritated, it causes pain in the anterior lateral thigh. This is commonly referred to as meralgia paresthetica. The word is derived from the Greek word *meros,* meaning thigh, and also meaning pain. Paresthesia is an altered sensation, which people often describe as burning, tingling, or pinpricks. Entrapment of the lateral femoral cutaneous nerve can occur anywhere along its path but is common near the anterior superior iliac spine or the inguinal ligament. The most common cause is pregnancy; other causes are abdominal tumors, uterine fibroids, ascites, and trauma (seat belt injury). Obesity is also a common cause; ironically, rapid weight loss may remove protective fat layers and lead to compression.

History and Examination

Patients complain of anterior and lateral thigh burning and/or tingling. Unlike lumbar radiculopathy, buttock and back pain are absent, and the pain does not exist below the knee. The pain can increase with standing and walking. The symptoms are primarily unilateral but can occur bilaterally. On examination,

hip extension can exacerbate the symptoms, and hip flexion can relieve them. In cases for which the clinical diagnosis is in doubt, electrodiagnostic testing can be helpful.

Treatment

Treatment for meralgia paresthetica is primarily conservative. In pregnancy the symptoms usually resolve after the birth of the child. If the symptoms do not resolve on their own, a nerve block using corticosteroids and a local anesthetic may be necessary. The nerve block can both help relieve the symptoms and help alleviate the compression. Physical therapy can also be of benefit.

PAIN IN THE FEET OR HANDS: PERIPHERAL NEUROPATHY

Peripheral neuropathy (also known as distal axonopathy) often presents as a burning, electric feeling in the feet. The presentation is symmetrical, with possible sensory loss and paresthesia. The pain is typically of slow onset and progressive. Walking may exacerbate the pain. The feet are the most common origin of peripheral neuropathy; the longest nerve fibers from the heart are most vulnerable. Peripheral neuropathy as it spreads upward may go on to affect the ankles and beyond. Peripheral neuropathy can also affect the hands. It is possible to differentiate peripheral neuropathy from a nerve root problem (radiculopathy), because both cause paresthesia in the feet or the hands, but peripheral neuropathy is not accompanied by back or neck pain that radiates to the extremity. Rather, the pain is distal only, symmetrical, and ascends rather than descends.

History and Examination

Patients complain of a symmetrical pain in their feet, which they often describe as burning or a feeling of pins and needles. On examination, patients may have no clinical findings. However, as the disease progresses, they develop sensory deficits to light touch. Decreased Achilles reflex, the ability to sense vibration (128-Hz tuning fork perceived for <10 seconds), and position sense at the toe can all decrease. It is also important to examine the feet for abnormal skin breakdown in patients with deep sensory deficits. Ulceration followed by infection, and finally amputation, is a known sequela.

The most common causes of peripheral neuropathy are uncontrolled diabetes, alcohol abuse, human immunodeficiency virus, peripheral vascular disease, and idiopathic conditions. Medications, such as isoniazid and chemotherapy may also induce peripheral neuropathy. A less likely cause is a vitamin deficiency, such as B_{12}. A work-up is necessary to rule out these underlying causes.

Treatment

Correction of the underlying cause, if possible, is important. It is essential to tell patients that the medication prescribed for painful symptoms does not alter the clinical progression of the disease. In cases of diabetic peripheral neuropathy, proper glycemic control, not pain medication, is the treatment. Antiseizure and antidepressant medications used to treat neuropathic pain are useful in the management of the painful burning symptoms of peripheral neuropathy. A topical anesthetic is another option for treating the pain. Interventionally, a spinal cord stimulator is Food and Drug Administration approved for the treatment of the pain from peripheral neuropathy. On top of pain control, small studies have shown that patients with good outcomes from spinal cord stimulation have an increase in their microcirculatory blood flow as measured by Doppler laser flow in the symptomatic legs, because the device creates a partial sympathetic block leading to vascular dilatation. It may be necessary to consider a spinal cord stimulator trial if neuropathic pain medications are not controlling the symptoms.

PAIN IN THE STUMP AND PHANTOM LIMB PAIN

Pain in a stump following amputation is common. Roughly 50% of amputees have stump pain, which may occur upon postsurgical healing. Patients often describe this as a burning, sharp pain made worse by compression. Neuroma formation at the site is a frequent cause. Stump pain, unlike phantom limb pain, occurs in a still-intact body part.

After amputation, patients may experience both phantom sensation and phantom limb pain. Phantom sensation is any nonpainful sensation of an absent limb. Phantom limb pain is the sensation of pain in an absent limb. Postoperative studies have shown that 85% to 90% of patients experience phantom limb pain in the first month postamputation.[10] At 1-year follow-up, 60% of patients continue to have pain. However, only 5% to 10% of those 60% have severe pain at 1 year.[11] Phantom limb pain is often undiagnosed and therefore is undertreated. Even when diagnosed, practitioners often underestimate the severity of pain and do not offer treatment. In one study, 61% of amputees with phantom pain discussed the problem with their physicians, who offered treatment to only 17%.[12]

Severe preamputation pain may be a risk factor for phantom limb pain. In some but not all surveys, chronic pain in the body part to be amputated was a risk factor for phantom limb pain. It is hypothesized that high preoperative pain levels may sensitize the central nervous system. However, phantom limb pain has occurred in amputations secondary to acute trauma when the patient had no history of preamputation pain. Conversely, some patients with a history of severe chronic pain in an extremity before amputation never develop phantom limb pain.

Phantom limb pain occurs in equal frequency in men and women. The level or side of amputation does not play a role. The pain usually presents within the first week after amputation.[11] However, there is anecdotal evidence of presentation being delayed for months and even years. Patients often describe phantom limb pain as a burning or crushing sensation in the missing limb; alternatively, they may feel as if the (missing) limb is being stabbed with needles.[10] Patients with missing lower extremities often describe the pain as if their toes were tightly flexed, and those with missing upper extremities as if their fingers were tightly clenched.[13] Patients report that the pain is more frequently episodic rather than constant.

Phantom pain is primarily located in the distal part of the limb. It has been theorized that the large cortical representation of the hand and foot may contribute to the sensitivity of the distal part of the missing extremity as being more susceptible to phantom limb pain.

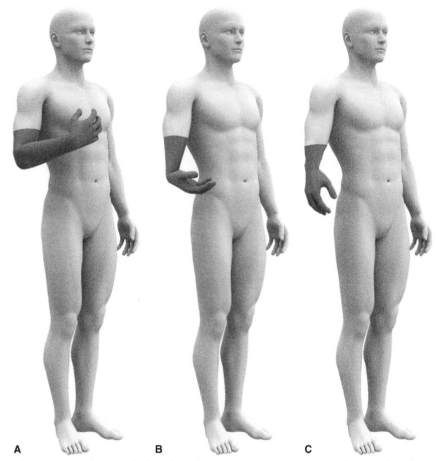

Figure 2-22 Phantom limb pain, telescoping. In telescoping the phantom hand gradually approaches the residual limb and eventually becomes located inside the stump.

The gradual improvement of phantom limb pain occurs proximal to distal, with pain in the toes and fingers being the last to dissipate. This is known as telescoping. The patient feels as if the toes are located at the stump as the more proximal pain dissipates. As the proximal pain improves further, the toes or fingers of the phantom limb may even be experienced at or in the stump (Fig. 2-22).

History and Examination

Typically, imaging, laboratory work, and electrodiagnostic studies are not indicated in the work-up of phantom limb pain. Diagnosis remains clinical: The stump should be examined fully; obviously, one cannot examine the missing limb. Often, findings at the stump are nonsignificant. There may be trigger points, however. Skin abrasions, blisters, or breakdown may be present. They are often caused by a poor-fitting prosthesis. It is necessary to be especially vigilant for signs of local infection. Local trauma may exist at the stump of the amputated limb.

It is important to note that stump pain and phantom limb pain are commonly seen together. Sherman and Glenda[12] reported that stump pain was present in 61% of amputees with phantom pain but in only 39% of those without phantom limb pain.

Treatment

Stump Pain: Stump pain is most commonly caused by a poor-fitting prosthesis. Therefore, proper fitting can eliminate the majority of stump pain complaints. If a patient has a trigger point caused by a neuroma formation, a neuroma injection may be necessary. Surgical treatment is typically useful only when it is apparent that the stump has not healed properly. Proximal extension is not indicated for amputation pain.

Phantom Limb Pain: Mirror box manipulation is a novel approach to treating phantom limb pain and has shown significant promise. A loss of sensory input from the limb to the somatosensory cortex alters motor output. It is hypothesized that the motor system needs sensory input to make the limb move—without it, the motor system perceives the missing limb to be paralyzed and contracted. This constant contracted feeling

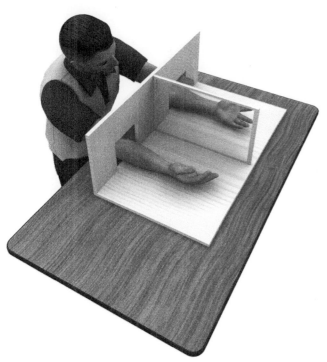

Figure 2-23 Mirror box manipulation for the treatment of phantom limb pain.

may be the precursor of pain. The premise of mirror box manipulation is that the missing afferent sensory input is provided so that the missing limb can be moved and pain relieved. A mirror is held to the side of the intact limb. When the patient moves the intact limb, the patient perceives the phantom limb to be moving in the mirror, providing the missing sensory input (Fig. 2-23). Small studies have shown this to be a successful treatment of phantom limb pain, but it is unclear whether mirror therapy is better than motor imagery alone.

Multiple medications may be useful for the treatment of phantom limb pain. To date, studies have shown that no medication is superior. It is thought that phantom limb pain is of neuropathic origin (that is, pain originating from the peripheral or central nervous system). Commonly, antidepressants and anticonvulsants used to treat neuropathic pain may be effective in phantom limb pain. In addition, in cases of severe pain, narcotic therapy may be useful.

As shown in anecdotal evidence, transcutaneous electrical nerve stimulation (TENS) placed at the stump of the missing limb can be helpful for phantom limb pain. It is inherently safe, which adds to its value as a treatment modality. A significant limitation to the use of TENS is the need for electrode placement and use of a prosthesis. Spinal cord stimulation may also be a successful remedy for the treatment of phantom limb pain. Sympathetic nerve blocks may provide pain relief. If helpful, sympathetic nerve blocks are usually transitory

for phantom limb pain; however, some patients experience long-term benefit. Invasive procedures such as cordotomy, dorsal root entry lesions, and sympathectomy have not produced encouraging results.

Studies have shown that 20% to 60% of amputees may be clinically depressed, between three and five times greater than that of the general population.[14] The loss of a limb has social, economic, and psychological implications. Depression and anxiety further exacerbate phantom limb pain, as they do other painful conditions. A multimodal approach to the patient's pain, including psychological care should be strongly considered.

POSTSURGICAL NEUROPATHIC PAIN SYNDROMES

Post-thoracotomy Pain Syndrome

A thoracotomy involves making an incision into the chest to gain access to the lungs, heart, esophagus, aorta, or thoracic spine. Retractors, sutures, wires, or incisions can damage the intercostal nerves during this procedure (Fig. 2-24). Post-thoracotomy pain syndrome (PTPS) usually develops 1 to 2 months postoperatively.[15] It is necessary to monitor pain closely in the immediate postoperative period because it predicts the development of PTPS. Some 56% of patients with moderate to severe acute postoperative pain develop PTPS, whereas 36% of patients with minor postoperative pain experience it.[16,17]

History and Examination: Patients report that pain is electric and burning in the area of the incision.

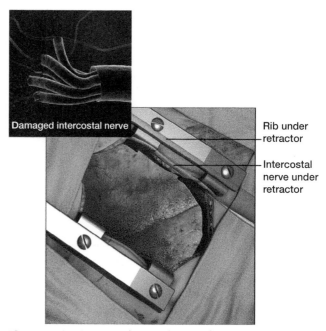

Figure 2-24 Intercostal nerve damage from a thoracotomy.

Although post-thoracotomy pain is often severe at 1 month, it usually subsides by 1 year.[18] In approximately 3% to 5% of individuals, the pain remains severe 1 year postop.[19] On examination touching the skin may elicit pain.

Treatment: Advanced surgical techniques, including using video assistance during thoracotomy, have not decreased the incidence of PTPS.[17] The most effective treatment/prevention remains the use of intraoperative and postoperative epidural catheter analgesia with local anesthetics.[20] Antidepressant and antiseizure medications used for neuropathic pain can also be effective. If the patient continues to have pain, intercostal nerve blocks can be effective.

Postsurgical Pelvic Nerve Pain

In a small number of patients, an electric, burning groin pain develops after transverse lower abdominal procedures, hernia repairs, or hysterectomies. It is theorized that one of the pelvic nerves in the sutures, mesh, or scar tissue becomes entrapped. As a result of the development of laparoscopic approaches for these procedures, the incidence of pelvic nerve entrapment has significantly decreased. Neuralgia may occur immediately or up to several years after the procedure. Three pelvic nerves can be affected: The iliohypogastric nerve, the ilioinguinal nerve, and the genitofemoral nerve. Because they are located so close to each other, one nerve or a combination of nerves can be affected.

Clinically, there is also overlap in the sensory supply of these nerves.

The iliohypogastric nerve: The iliohypogastric nerve arises primarily from the L1 nerve root and in some cases a twig of the T12 nerve root. This nerve transverses the psoas muscle and then travels anteriorly, penetrating the transverse abdominal muscle near the iliac crest. It comes to lie superiorly and medially to the anterior superior iliac spine just superior to the ilioinguinal nerve, where it can be accessed for a nerve block. It supplies the lower abdominal wall muscles and a region just superior to the pubis (Fig. 2-25).

The ilioinguinal nerve: The ilioinguinal nerve arises from the T12 and L1 nerve roots. This nerve transverses the psoas muscle, wraps around toward the iliac crest, and lies superiorly and medial to the anterior superior iliac spine, where it can be accessed for a nerve block. It supplies sensory branches to the pubic symphysis, as well as the superior and medial aspect of the femoral triangle. In males, it innervates the shaft of the penis and anterior scrotum. In females, it innervates the mons pubis and labia majora (Fig. 2-25).

The genitofemoral nerve: The genitofemoral nerve arises from the L1 and L2 nerve root. It transverses the psoas muscle and then splits into the genital and femoral branches near the inguinal ligament. The femoral branch provides skin sensation in the upper part of the femoral triangle. In males, the genital branch innervates the cremasteric muscle and the scrotal skin. In females,

Figure 2-25 Iliohypogastric and ilioinguinal nerve path and sensory innervation. ▶

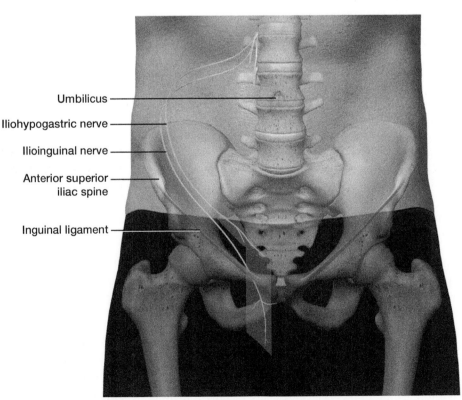

Umbilicus

Iliohypogastric nerve

Ilioinguinal nerve

Anterior superior iliac spine

Inguinal ligament

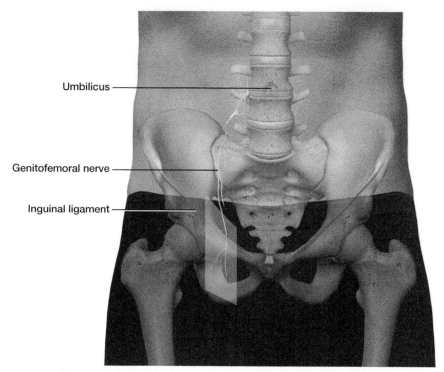

Umbilicus

Genitofemoral nerve

Inguinal ligament

Figure 2-26 Genitofemoral nerve path and sensory innervation.

this branch innervates the mons pubis and labia majora (along with the ilioinguinal nerve; Fig. 2-26).

History and Examination: Patients complain of a unilateral sharp, shooting pelvic pain. Pain may be made worse with light touch in the area of scarring or entrapment. Hyperesthesia (excessive sensitivity) or hypoesthesia (decreased sensitivity) may occur in the cutaneous area supplied by the nerve. Imaging is usually negative. No reliable electrodiagnostic test exists for the diagnosis of injury to these nerves.

Treatment: In some patients, pain may be from inflammatory or nerve entrapment origin. Removing the mesh or scar tissue to facilitate nerve decompression may be entertained. However, little data about how to diagnose these conditions are available, and information about the success of mesh removal or scar decompression is also scarce. Symptomatic medical treatment involves antiseizure drugs and antidepressants used to treat neuropathic pain. A block of any of these nerves can be both diagnostic and therapeutic.

CASE STUDIES

Case 1

A 61-year-old man with diabetes presents with pain in his gluteal region that radiates down both legs. He reports having a burning sensation that radiates down his legs to both feet. History reveals that the symptoms have been present for the past year and have been progressive. He has been taking the neuropathic pain medication Cymbalta (duloxetine) 30 mg daily for 6 months. The medication helps, but he still has pain. He has been working with his primary care physician to control his blood sugar but admits that he needs to change his diet. He wants to know if he should increase his Cymbalta dose.

On examination, the patient has normal sensation to light touch in both feet. He has full strength in his lower extremities. His Achilles reflex is normal bilaterally. He has no skin breakdown. Straight-leg test is positive bilaterally.

You explain to the patient that he most likely has pain from a herniated disc in his back affecting the nerves that run down his legs. It helps to explain this using the following analogy: The back is the control center for the legs in the same way that the light switch in the examination room is the control center for the light in the room. Flicking the switch turns on the lights. The effects are not visible at the actual switch but rather at the light. The same way that pain from a herniated disc may be not felt at the disc itself but rather in the buttock and legs. When a disc pushes on a nerve, it "turns on" the pain down into the legs, as it were.

An MRI of the lumbar spine reveals an L5–S1 herniated disc that pushes on both L5 nerve roots (the left and right). Treatment options include physical therapy, increasing the Cymbalta dose, epidural steroid injections, and surgical removal. After discussing these choices with the patient, the practitioner decides to increase the patient's Cymbalta dose to 60 mg—the standard therapeutic dose—and send him for an epidural steroid injection under fluoroscopic guidance, hoping to decrease his pain.

The patient obtains good relief of his radicular pain after two epidural steroid injections and is participating in physical therapy. He continues to work with his primary care physician to control his blood sugar (in this case, a "red herring").

Case 2

A 49-year-old man presents with pain in his right hand. He reports that the pain used to come and go but is now constant. It is sharp and electric in nature. He has no pain in his left hand, neck, or either arm. He notices no specific trigger. Ibuprofen is somewhat helpful. He thinks that he was told that the pain was referred from a herniated disc in his neck, but he is not sure.

On examination, the patient has full strength, and his sensation to light touch is intact and his reflexes are normal. When questioned in depth, he characterizes the pain as strongest in his thumb, index, middle, and part of the ring finger. At this point, carpal tunnel syndrome CTS is your working diagnosis.

You send the patient for a nerve conduction study and prescribe a splint for the right wrist. It is to be worn at night to keep the wrist in the neutral position, which should relieve pressure on the median nerve. The nerve conduction study comes back positive for CTS and negative for radiculopathy. When you call the patient with the results of the nerve conduction study, he reports that the wrist splint is already starting to help. The patient is scheduled for a follow-up visit in 1 month, at which time if the symptoms have not resolved you are considering a carpal tunnel injection.

REFERENCES

1. Gelberman, RH, Aronson D, Weisman MH. Carpal-tunnel syndrome: Results of a prospective trial of steroid injecting and splinting. *J Bone Joint Surg Am.* 1980;62:1181–1184.
2. Peterslund NA, Seyer-Hansen K, Ipsen J, et al. Acyclovir in herpes zoster. *Lancet.* 1981;2(8251):827–830.
3. McKendrick MW, McGill JI, White JE, et al. Oral acyclovir in acute herpes zoster. *BMJ Neurology.* 1989;39(suppl 1):327.
4. Forrest JB. The response to epidural steroid injections in chronic dorsal root pain. *Can Anaesth Soc J.* 1980;27(1):40–46.
5. Saal JS. The role of inflammation in lumbar pain. *Phys Med Rehab: State Art Rev.* 1990;4:191–199.
6. Hoyland JA, Freemont AJ, Jayson MI. Intervertebral foramen venous obstruction. A cause of periradicular fibrosis? *Spine.* 1989;14(6):558–568.
7. Smyth MJ, Wright V. Sciatica and the intervertebral disc; an experimental study. *J Bone Joint Surg Am.* 1958;40-A:1401–1418.
8. Slipman CW, Plastaras CT, Palmitier RA, et al. Symptom provocation of fluoroscopically guided cervical nerve root stimulation. Are dynatomal maps identical to dermatomal maps? *Spine.* 1998;23(20):2235–2242.
9. Bogduk N, Govinda J. *Medical management of acute lumbar radicular pain: An evidence based approach.* Newcastle, Australia: Newcastle Bone and Joint Institute; 1999.
10. Parkes CM. Factors determining the persistence of phantom pain in the amputee. *J Psychosom Res.* 1973;17(2):97–108.
11. Nikolajsen L, Ilkjaer S, Kroner K, et al. The influence of preamputation pain on postamputation stump and phantom pain. *Pain.* 1997;72:393–405.
12. Sherman RA, Glenda GM. Concurrent variation of burning phantom limb and stump pain with near surface blood flow in the stump. *Orthopedics.* 1987;(10):1395–1402.
13. Wilkins KL, McGrath PJ, Finley GA, et al. Phantom limb sensations and phantom limb pain in child and adolescent amputees. *Pain.* 1998;78(1):7–12.
14. Ephraim PL, Wegener ST, MacKenzie EJ, et al. Phantom pain, residual limb pain, and back pain in amputees: Results of a national survey. *Arch Phys Med Rehabil.* 2005;86(10):1910–1919.
15. Kanner R. Postsurgical pain syndromes. In: Foley KM, ed. *Management of cancer pain. Syllabus of the postgraduate course of Memorial Sloan-Kettering Cancer Center.* New York, NY; 1985:65–72.
16. Perkins FM, Kehlet H. Chronic pain as an outcome of surgery. *Anesthesiology.* 2000;93(4):1123–1133.
17. Obata H, Saito S, Fujita N, et al. Epidural block with mepivacaine before surgery reduces long term post-thoracotomy pain. *Can J Anesth.* 1999;46(12):1127–1132.
18. Gotoda Y, Kambara N, Sakai T, et al. The morbidity, time course and predictive factors for persistent post-thoracotomy pain. *Eur J Pain.* 2001;5:89–96.
19. Perttunen K, Tasmuth T, Kalso E. Chronic pain after thoracic surgery: A follow up study. *Acta Anaesthesiol Scand.* 1999;43:563–567.
20. Senturk M, Ozcan PE, Talu GK, et al. The effects of three different analgesia techniques on long-term postthoracotomy pain. *Anesth Analg.* 2002;94(1):11–15.

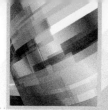

CHAPTER 3

Cancer Pain

COMMON CAUSES OF CANCER PAIN
▶ Metastatic Bone Pain
▶ Visceral Pain
▶ Neuropathic Pain
▶ Headache
▶ Spinal Cord Compression due to Tumor
▶ Pain Caused by Surgery for Cancer

PRE-EXISTING PAINFUL CONDITIONS

TREATMENT
▶ Clinical WHO Analgesic Guidelines
▶ Spinal Cord Compression due to Tumor
▶ Cancer Blocks
▶ Radiation

Pain management is of particular importance in cancer patients. Extensive research has shown that pain is the symptom that cancer patients fear most. Up to 50% of patients undergoing cancer treatment and up to 90% of patients with advanced cancer have debilitating pain.[1] Effectively managing your patients' pain will dramatically improve their quality of life while enduring cancer treatment. Though the top priority is to cure or put the cancer in remission, proper pain management should be provided concurrently from the beginning of treatment. This chapter will help you do that, your goal being to develop a regimen that prevents baseline pain and is flexible enough to treat breakthrough pain. Breakthrough pain is defined as episodic exacerbations of pain above the established baseline.[2] Both the medical and procedural management of cancer pain will be reviewed here.

The first step in setting up a proper pain plan is to determine all potential individual sources of pain. I say "sources" in the plural as a cancer patient commonly may have more than one type of pain. Both the cancer itself and its treatment can cause pain. The patient's type of cancer, location of the pain, how the pain feels (electric, dull, sharp), and treatments administered (chemotherapy, radiation therapy, surgery) will help you identify the pain generators. Once you have established the pain generators, determine the severity of each instance. In terms of pain, the focus should be on how functional the patient is. Does the patient have trouble walking or dressing because of pain? Does the pain medication affect mental status? The following list provides the most common pain generators in cancer patients; it is not all consuming but touches on the most prevalent.

Metastatic Bone Pain

The most common cause of pain in cancer patients is bone metastases—70% of patients with bone metastasis have bone pain. The pain is caused by stretching of the periosteum (the membrane that lines the outer surface of all bones; Fig. 3-1) and nerve irritation in the endosteum (the tissue lining the medullary cavity of the bone; see Fig. 3-1). If you have ever been kicked in the shin, you have an understanding of what bone pain feels like.

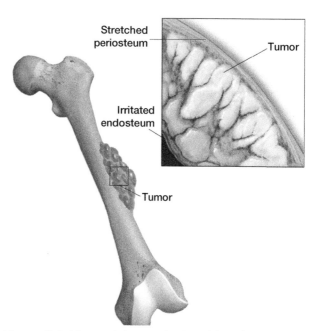

Figure 3-1 Metastatic bone pain: Stretching of the periosteum, irritation of the endosteum.

When evaluating any patient with cancer pain it is necessary to consider bone metastasis. The patient may have pain from metastatic bone destruction from a lung primary or possibly a pathologic fracture. Cancers that tend to metastasize to the bone are: Breast, lung, thyroid, kidney, and prostate. The ribs, pelvis, and spine are normally the first bones involved. Pathologic fractures are common in breast cancer due to the lytic nature of the lesions. They are less common in lung cancer due to short life span and rare in prostate cancer, which tends to involve osteoblastic lesions.

Imaging can help you confirm your diagnosis of metastatic bone pain. A bone scan is very sensitive in detecting osseous metastases and is recommended as the imaging study of choice. Laboratory studies should be performed as well to identify anemia, thrombocytopenia, and hypercalcemia that can be seen with metastatic bone disease.

Visceral Pain

Visceral pain (internal organ pain) occurs when pain fibers around organs are activated. Tumors cause pain by invasion, obstruction, distension, or compression of an organ (Fig. 3-2). Organs that are hollow are more likely to be painful than solid organs. Hollow organs include the uterus, ureter, fallopian tubes, colon, rectum, stomach, bladder, bile duct, and gallbladder. Visceral pain is not well localized—patients often complain of a deep, gnawing, or dull pain of unspecified location. This is because there are a small number of visceral afferent nerves covering a large area. Visceral pain can be referred to the back, groin, or shoulder. Pancreatic and uterine cancers are especially known for their painful attack of abdominal/pelvic organs.

Neuropathic Pain

Neuropathic pain in cancer patients is often not caused by the cancer itself; instead, it may be a side effect of treatment.

Chemotherapy: Chemotherapy can cause a painful sensory neuropathy (Fig. 3-3). Patients often describe this neuropathy as a burning electric pain in the distal extremities. The symptoms usually begin during chemotherapy but may have a delayed onset. Three of the most common offending agents are vincristine (used for hematologic cancer), cisplatin, and paclitaxel (used for breast and ovarian cancer).[1,3]

Radiation: Targeted radiation used to treat cancer can also cause neuropathic pain (Fig. 3-4). Radiation injury to the brachial or lumbosacral plexus can occur with direct exposure. The mechanism of

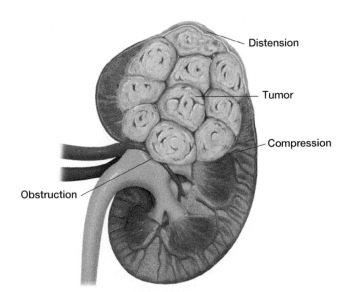

Figure 3-2 Visceral pain, internal organ pain. Pain is caused by invasion, obstruction, distension, or compression of an organ.

radiation-induced neuropathy may be related to a combination of localized ischemia and subsequent fibrosis due to microvascular insufficiency. Radiation injury to the plexus may present 1 to 30 years following radiation treatment. For the brachial plexus, pain is commonly described as aching in the shoulder or hand. Other symptoms include paresthesia in the lateral fingers or entire hand. For the lumbosacral region, presenting symptoms include weakness of the legs associated with sensory symptoms, paresthesia, and numbness. Weakness starts distally in the L5 to S1 segments and slowly progresses. Magnetic Resonance Imaging (MRI) and/or Electromyography (EMG) can help establish the diagnosis. MRI features suggestive of radiation-induced plexopathy include diffuse, uniform, symmetric swelling, and T2 hyperintensity of the plexus as compared to nonuniform, asymmetric, focal enlargement, and the presence of a mass with postcontrast enhancement, which is indicative of tumor recurrence. The EMG feature suggestive of radiation-induced plexopathy is myokymia. Myokymia is a brief spontaneous tetanic contraction of motor units or groups of muscle fibers.

Headache

Metastatic brain tumors are more common than primary brain tumor with lung cancer being the main source. Meningiomas are the most common primary brain tumor and are typically benign. While gliomas (tumor arising from glial cells) represent 80% of all malignant primary brain tumors. Parenchymal brain tissue has no pain receptors; pain is generated when vessels and/or the meninges are stretched by a mass

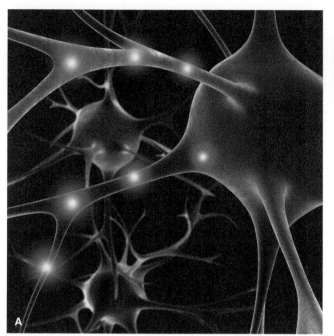
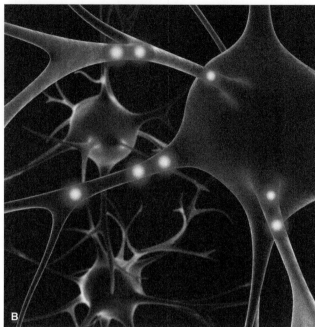

Figure 3-3 Chemotherapy-induced peripheral nerve dysfunction. **A.** Nerves send impulses in a regular controlled pattern. **B.** When nerves are injured they fire aberrantly which is interpreted by the brain as burning, electric neuropathic pain.

(Fig. 3-5). The meninges and blood vessels are innervated by both cervical and cranial (primarily trigeminal) nerves. Headache due to tumor is typically worse in the morning, and may be accompanied by vomiting, confusion, double vision, numbness, or weakness. The headache can worsen with increase of intracranial pressure as a result of sneezing or a bowel movement. Cancer patients with a long history of headache pre dating the cancer who present with different headache symptoms are of a great concern. On ophthalmoscopic examination, if the intracranial pressure is raised enough, bilateral papilledema and optic disc swelling can be seen.

Spinal Cord Compression due to Tumor

Spinal cord compression occurs in roughly 2% to 5% of cancer patients. A tumor produces edema, inflammation,

Figure 3-4 Radiation-induced neuropathic pain. Brachial plexopathy and lumbosacral plexopathy.

Brachial plexus

Lumbosacral plexus

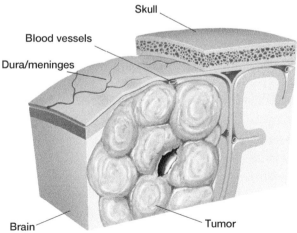

Skull
Blood vessels
Dura/meninges
Brain
Tumor

Figure 3-5 Cranial tumor pain. Vessels and meninges being stretched by a mass.

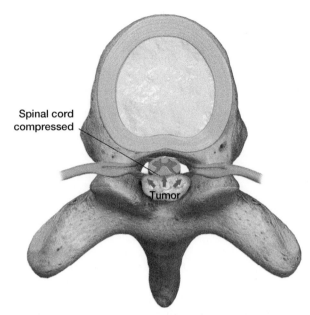

Figure 3-6 Spinal cord compression.

and mechanical compression, with direct neural injury to the cord, as well as vascular damage and impairment of oxygenation (Fig. 3-6). Patients present with acute back pain and neurologic deficits in the lower extremities, which may include sensory changes and/or weakness. They also may present with bowel or bladder incontinence. This is a neurologic emergency, as patient outcomes can often be determined by the care provided in the first hours of onset. Treatment guidelines are covered in the latter part of this chapter.

Pain Caused by Surgery for Cancer

Pain after Thoracotomy: A thoracotomy is a chest incision to gain access to the lungs, heart, esophagus, aorta, or thoracic spine. A thoracotomy may be needed for tumor debulking. Damage to the intercostal nerves may occur as a result of retractors, sutures, wires, or cutting (Fig. 3-7). It is not uncommon for the nerve to be totally severed or included in a suture when closing the chest. The incidence of severe pain is 3% to 5% one year post of, and pain that interferes with activities of daily living is reported by about 50% of patients.[4] Pain is described as electric and lancinating. Pain can be elicited on examination by touching the skin. It usually develops 1 to 2 months after the procedure.[5]

Pain after Mastectomy: A mastectomy is surgical removal of all or part of the breast. One in eight women will develop breast cancer; approximately 60% are treated surgically for axillary node staging and primary breast tumor resection. It is estimated

Figure 3-7 Post-thoracotomy pain syndrome cause by intercostal nerve damage. A neuropathic pain alone the course of one or more intercostal nerves.

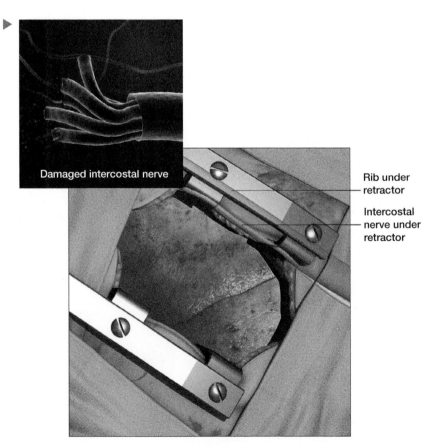

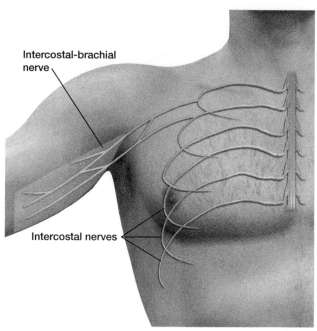

Figure 3-8 Intercostal-brachial nerve innervating the posterior arm, axial and anterior chest wall.

that over 50% of women suffer chronic pain following the treatment for breast cancer surgery.[6] The procedure may cause damage to the intercostobrachial nerve that innervates the posterior part of the arm, axial, and anterior chest wall (Fig. 3-8).[5] Patients may present holding their arm tight to their chest, as movement can exacerbate the pain.

PRE-EXISTING PAINFUL CONDITIONS

Ten percent of people with cancer pain have a preexisting painful condition such as degenerative arthritis and diabetic peripheral neuropathy. Always ask about this in your history: "Do you have any painful conditions that existed before cancer?" Not every type of pain a cancer patient has is cancer related.

TREATMENT

The first step in treating cancer pain is to ask patients what their goals and expectations are in terms of pain control. Some patients would like you to be more aggressive, some less so. When developing your treatment plan, target each of the pain generators. Your treatment plan may include a mixture of nonopioids, opioids, injections, radiation, and surgery.

The World Health Organization (WHO) has introduced a three-step analgesic ladder in treating cancer pain (http://www.who.int/cancer/palliative/painladder/en/). This is the gold standard and backbone of treating cancer pain. Step 1 includes nonopioid medication for mild pain. Step 2 includes a short-acting, moderate-strength opioid with or without a nonopioid medication. Step 3 includes a stronger opioid with or without a nonopioid medication. It is important to remember that opioids are the mainstay of cancer pain treatment. The ladder is vague in terms of medications and doses.

Clinical WHO Analgesic Guidelines

This is a how-to book for practical and functional use, because you need to know what to do and how, quickly and easily. Table 3-1 is a variant of the WHO analgesic ladder, developed for this book for enhanced functionality. It includes doses to be used as a guide, more direction on adjuvant medical therapy, and when to consider a procedure. If your patient presents in moderate to severe pain, it is appropriate to start at Step 2 or 3. The choice of treatment should be based on the severity of the pain, not the stage of the disease.[7] Cancer pain is dynamic and while patients experience periods of stability, those with advancing disease will need adjustments in their regimen. Tolerance to medications is rarely seen in cancer patients. The need for increasing doses of opioids is usually explained by progression of disease rather than tolerance.[7] It is important to remember that many more treatment options exist outside of this table, which covers the basics per the mission of this book. More detail about each of the medications or procedures can be found in the latter part of this book.

If your patient has metastatic bone pain, two useful adjuvant therapies are nonsteroidal anti-inflammatory drugs (NSAIDs) and bisphosphonates. NSAIDs not only provide a synergistic effect when combined with opioids but have the added benefit of blocking prostaglandin E_2, a growth factor for metastatic bone disease. Bisphosphonates are a class of drugs that inhibit osteoclast action and the resorption of bone. They are commonly used for the treatment of osteoporosis but can be very helpful in treating bone pain. Bone resorption can lead to increased pain through sensitization and activation of pain-messaging fibers in and around the periosteum. A bisphosphonate has been shown to be beneficial in the treatment of bone pain from metastatic disease, especially from multiple myeloma.[7] Pamidronate (Aredia), a bisphosphonate, can be given as an infusion. The standard protocol is 90 mg via IV infusion delivered over at least 2 hours, repeated every 3 to 4 weeks as needed. Before infusions a baseline creatinine, calcium, electrolyte, magnesium, and phosphate level should be drawn.

If your patient has cancer related pain from a bowel obstruction, consider using octreotide (Sandostatin). It reduces gastric secretions and motility, and can be very helpful in reducing not only pain but nausea, vomiting, and diarrhea. A typical starting dose is 150 μg SC or IV q8.

TABLE 3-1 Three-step Analgesic Ladder for Cancer Pain

Step 1: Nonopioid medication

1. Acetaminophen (Tylenol) 650 mg every 6 h as needed
2. A nonsteroidal anti-inflammatory drug (NSAID), which may include Celebrex 100 twice a day as needed or ibuprofen 400 mg every 6 h as needed
3. If nerve pain is present: A neuropathic pain medication for a burning, electric pain (see Chapter 13, Antidepressant Medications Used for Neuropathic Pain; or Chapter 14, Antiseizure Medications Used for Neuropathic Pain)

Step 2: Short-acting opioid medication, procedures & radiation

Add a short-acting opioid with or without a nonopioid medication. For certain types of cancer, consider an injection; consider radiation therapy.

Short-acting opioid medications

- Vicodin (hydrocodone/acetaminophen) 5 mg/325 mg
- Percocet (oxycodone/acetaminophen) 5 mg/325 mg
- Dilaudid (hydromorphone) 2 mg
- Nucynta (tapentadol) 50 mg

Take one tablet every 6 h as needed

If your patient is still in pain, increase the dose. For Vicodin and Percocet, you can increase the opioid dose (from 5 mg to 10 mg) without increasing the acetaminophen component.

- Vicodin 10 mg/325 mg
- Percocet 10 mg/325 mg
- Dilaudid 4 mg
- Nucynta 100 mg

Consider an injection for cancer pain

- Superior hypogastric block for prostate, rectal, bladder, or cervical cancer
- Celiac plexus block for pancreatic cancer
- Kyphoplasty/vertebroplasty for vertebral compression fractures
- Intercostal nerve block for metastatic pain to the chest wall

Consider radiation therapy

- Targeted radiation can help reduce pain from a focal region of tumor cells

Step 3: Long-acting opioid medication

Use stronger opioid pain medication with or without a nonopioid medication.

If the patient is using short-acting pain medication around the clock and is still in pain, add a long-acting pain medication, titrating it until the patient no longer needs to use the short-acting medication around the clock (see Chapter 15, Opioids).

1. **Long-acting opioid medication choices**
   Long-acting morphine (MS Contin) 15 mg po twice a day or every 8 h
   - Next step: MS Contin 30 mg po twice a day or every 8 h
   - Next step: MS Contin 60 mg po twice a day or every 8 h
   Long-acting oxycodone (OxyContin) 10 mg po twice a day or every 8 h
   - Next step: OxyContin 20 mg po twice a day or every 8 h
   - Next step: OxyContin 40 mg twice a day or every 8 h
   Fentanyl patch 25 µg every 72 h (useful in patients with swallowing difficulties)
   - Next step: Fentanyl patch 50 µg every 72 h
   - Next step: Fentanyl patch 100 µg every 72 h
   Consider an intrathecal pain pump

Spinal Cord Compression due to Tumor

Treatment for spinal cord compression includes high-dose corticosteroids and radiation as well as possible surgical decompression. The typical initial corticosteroid, dexamethasone, dose is 96- or 100-mg intravenous bolus followed by 24 mg orally four times daily for 3 days, then taper over 10 days. Radiation treatment for spinal cord compression is covered in Chapter 18, Radiation Therapy. The key is early recognition and addressing it as an emergency. Table 3-2 outlines treatment efficacy in relation to point of intervention.

TABLE 3-2 Chance of Remaining Ambulatory with Treatment for Spinal Cord Compression

Point of Intervention	Chance of Remaining Ambulatory
If treatment starts while patient is still able to walk	75%
If treatment starts with partial or incomplete weakness	30–50%
If patient is already paralyzed	10–20%

Cancer Blocks

Three procedures that have gained wide acceptance for the treatment of cancer pain include a celiac plexus block, intercostal nerve block, and a superior hypogastric plexus block. The goal is to stop the transmission of painful impulses from reaching the brain. The celiac plexus block is used for pancreatic cancer, the intercostal nerve block for chest wall metastasis, while the hypogastric plexus block is used for pelvic cancer pain.[8,9] To learn how a celiac plexus block or superior hypogastric block is done see Chapter 24, the Plexus and Sympathetic Block chapter. To learn how an intercostal nerve block is done see Chapter 27, Common Nerve Blocks.

Radiation

Radiation therapy works by damaging the DNA of cancerous cells. It can be used to help reduce pain from cancer by shrinking the tumor. The most sensitive cancers are most lymphomas and germ cell tumors. Melanoma and renal cell cancer are generally considered radioresistant. To learn more about radiation therapy see Chapter 18, Radiation Therapy.

CASE STUDY

Case

You are treating a patient with advanced lung cancer. Your patient has undergone two rounds of chemotherapy and radiation as well as a video-assisted thoracoscopic surgery (VATS) to help remove the primary source. At this point, your patient has deep pleural pain from the primary source of the cancer. The pleural pain is rated a 6 out of 10 on a visual analog pain scale and dull in nature. The patient has intercostal burning–electric pain at the site of the thoracotomy. This pain is rated 5 out of 10. He has thoracic back pain from a T9 vertebral compression fracture caused by metastatic disease to the spine. This pain he rates as a 7 out of 10 and describes it as duly deep, achy, and constant. He has some numbness mixed with a burning pain in his feet from the chemotherapy, which he rates as 3 out of 10. He also has long-standing osteoarthritis of the right knee. The patient is currently on Percocet 5/325 one tablet every 6 hours, which he is taking around the clock.

Begin with using an NSAID for metastatic bone pain and osteoarthritis, for example, Celebrex 100 po bid. This should help with his periosteum pain.

He has burning neuropathic pain in his feet from the chemotherapy and at the chest wall from the thoracotomy.

For this, start the patient on an antiseizure or antidepressant medication used for neuropathic pain. In this case study, we are going to start the patient on Cymbalta 30 mg once a day and titrate it to 60 mg once a day in 1 week.

The patient is taking a short-acting opioid around the clock and is still in pain. You now need to increase his opioid as well—from Percocet 5/325, every 6 hours, to Percocet 10/325 every 6 hours as needed. You should also prescribe a laxative to prevent opioid-induced constipation. You explain the kyphoplasty procedure to the patient; he decides to have the procedure as it may help alleviate the back pain he is having from the T9 vertebral compression fracture.

A month later, the patient returns stating that the medication adjustments as well as the kyphoplasty have been very helpful for his pain. You see him 1 month later and he is still stable. You see him 2 months later and his pleuritic pain has increased as well as his tumor burden. You start OxyContin 10 mg every 8 hours and leave him on Celebrex, Cymbalta, and Percocet at their current doses. Hospice is contacted; eventually the patient dies in hospice.

REFERENCES

1. Quasthoff S, Hartung HP. Chemotherapy-induced peripheral neuropathy. *J Neurol.* 2002;249:9–17.
2. Agency for Health Care Policy and Research (USPHS). *Clinical Practice Guideline number 9 on Management of Cancer Pain.* Washington, DC: U.S. Department of Health and Human Services, 1994; AHCPR Pub. No. 94-0592
3. Windbreak AJ. Chemotherapeutic neuropathy. *Curr Opin Neurol.* 1999;12(5):565–571.
4. Perttunen K, Tasmuth T, Kalso E. Chronic pain after thoracic surgery: a follow-up study. *Acta Anaesthesiol Scand.* 1999;43(5):563–567.
5. Kanner R. Post-surgical pain syndromes. *Management of cancer pain: syllabus of the postgraduate course, Memorial Sloan-Kettering Cancer Center.* 1985 Nov 14–16. New York, NY: Memorial Sloan-Kettering Cancer Center; 1985:65–72.
6. Lau B, Blyth F, Cousins M. Persistent pain after breast cancer surgery. *Pain Med.* 2007;8(7):611.
7. Fallon M, Hanks G, Cherny N. Principles of control of cancer pain. *BMJ.* 2006;332:1022–1024.
8. Brown DL, Bulley CK, Quiel EL. Neurolytic celiac plexus block for pancreatic cancer pain. *Anesth Analg.* 1987;66:869–873.
9. de Leon-Casasola OA, Kent E, Lema MJ. Neurolytic superior hypogastric plexus block for chronic pain associated with cancer. *Pain.* 1993;54(2):145–151.

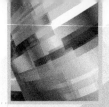

CHAPTER 4

Abdominal Pain

COMMON CAUSES OF CHRONIC ABDOMINAL PAIN
▶ Visceral
▶ Somatic
▶ Chronic Pain Post Abdominal Surgery
▶ Referred Pain

TREATMENT
▶ Lifestyle Modification
▶ Treatment by Category

Establishing a proper differential diagnosis, ordering a workup, making a diagnosis, then medically or surgically treating the underlying cause of a patient's abdominal pain is reserved for general medicine texts and is beyond the scope of this book. This chapter will focus on symptom-oriented chronic pain management. How to analyze symptoms, and how to treat those symptoms. The focus of this section is not to help you diagnose the many causes of abdominal pain but rather to help you understand the painful symptoms. History taking and thorough examination are critical in understanding the nature of those painful symptoms that can be tied to a diagnosis and those that can not.

The pain can best be addressed by careful characterization of the symptoms. A pain history includes the PQRST:

P	*Palliate or provoking factors.*
Q	*Qualities—burning, electric, sharp, dull.*
R	*Radiation—for example, pancreatic pain may radiate to the back.*
S	*Severity of pain. Usually done on a visual analog scale of 0 to 10.*
T	*Temporal events associated with the pain—is the pain constant or does it come and go?*

Teasing out the aggravating and relieving factors is critically important, especially in chronic abdominal pain. Patients with chronic abdominal pain may have an exacerbation of their symptoms with certain types of food or medication. Certain activities may trigger the patient's abdominal pain. Stressful life events often precede an exacerbation of symptoms. Stress, which is defined as an acute threat to homeostasis, shows both short- and long-term effects on the functions of the gastrointestinal tract. Stress leads to an alteration of the brain–gut interactions ("brain–gut axis"), ultimately contributing to the development of a broad array of gastrointestinal disorders. Major effects of stress on gut physiology include (1) alterations in gastrointestinal motility; (2) increase in visceral perception; (3) changes in gastrointestinal secretion; (4) increase in intestinal permeability; (5) negative effects on regenerative capacity of gastrointestinal mucosa and mucosal blood flow; and (6) negative effects on intestinal microbiota.[1] Aggravating factors should be targeted in the treatment plan.

When the symptoms of abdominal pain have been worked up and there is still no known diagnosis, the goal of examination is to determine if the pain is visceral or somatic. In Carnett test, the site of maximal abdominal pain is identified. The patient is asked to tense the abdominal musculature by attempting to sit up. Increased pain with tension of the abdominal musculature suggests abdominal wall etiology (Fig. 4-1). In one common scenario, patients develop abdominal wall neuromas after surgery. There is no diagnostic imaging test for abdominal wall neuromas.

The principles provided here will give you the tools to alleviate your patient's pain without hindering your ability to treat the disease generating it. Primary care doctors, GI specialists, urologists, and general surgeons are trained to evaluate the causes of abdominal pain and treat the underlying condition. The goal will be to correct the root of the underlying problem while managing the patient's pain. Statistically, there are a number of chronic cases you will encounter for which we currently do not have the ability to establish a cause-and-effect diagnosis. Despite the best diagnostic tools available, the cause of a patient's chronic abdominal pain often remains unclear. Chronic abdominal pain is

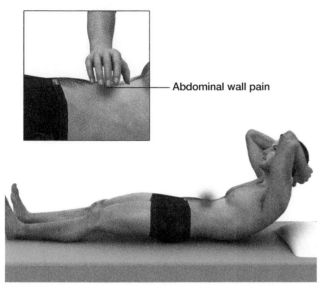

Abdominal wall pain

Figure 4-1 Carnett test. The abdomen is palpated while the patient holds the anterior abdominal muscles tense; the tense muscles prevent the examiner's fingers from coming in contact with the underlying viscera and any tenderness elicited over them will be somatic in location.

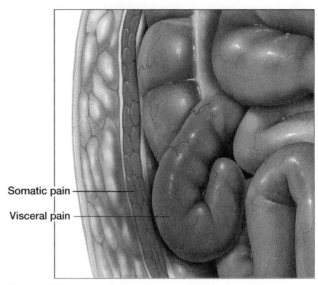

Somatic pain

Visceral pain

Figure 4-2 Abdominal wall pressed against an inflamed appendix. Somatic pain from the abdominal wall and visceral pain from the appendix.

less likely than acute abdominal pain to reveal underlying organic pathology. In those cases, we understand the nature of the symptoms and can employ treatment modalities that work well for those symptoms. Be forewarned, however, that some chronic abdominal pain—such as that of unknown etiology despite full medical workup—is difficult to treat. Abdominal pain caused by cancer is covered in Chapter 3, Cancer Pain.

There are four basic sources of abdominal pain. They are visceral, somatic, chronic pain post abdominal surgery and referred.

Visceral

Visceral abdominal pain is pain that comes from an organ. Organs that are hollow—like the intestine—are much more likely to generate pain than a solid organ, like the liver. Unlike pain in other parts of your body, cutting a visceral organ—like the intestines—during surgery is not painful. Visceral pain is elicited with distension, compression, or torsion of an organ. Visceral pain is not well localized and often described as dull and achy. This is because there are a small number of visceral afferent nerves covering a large area. In contrast to this, when a painful sensation is felt at the pad of a finger it is sharp and detailed; in the finger there are a large number of nerves to cover a small area. A larger visceral area, such as the liver, has many less afferent nerves to help the body localize the pain.

Somatic

Somatic structures are the underlining support structures of the abdominal cavity—for example, the fascia,

muscles, and peritoneum. Somatic pain is often well localized, and typically described as sharp and focal. A common aggravating factor is movement. An example of somatic abdominal pain is an abdominal wall neuroma, which is entrapment of a branch of the anterior cutaneous nerve as it courses through the abdominal wall muscle. A good example of the interplay of visceral and somatic pain is appendicitis. When the appendix is inflamed, the visceral pain is not well localized. The pain may be described as deep and dull. As the abdominal wall later comes in contact with the inflamed appendix, the pain becomes sharp and localized (Fig. 4-2).

Chronic Pain Post Abdominal Surgery

Many patients with chronic abdominal pain have had abdominal surgery. For some, this was the start of their pain; others have had surgery to ameliorate the pain without any change in their symptoms. Understanding the symptoms before and after surgery is crucial. The pain generator before and after surgery may be completely different. Several months post surgery, patients who continue to have abdominal pain despite normal postsurgical workup are diagnosed with functional abdominal pain. The pain generator may be from abdominal adhesions. An adhesion is a band of scar tissue that binds two parts of tissue together. Abdominal adhesions develop when the body's repair mechanisms respond to any tissue disturbance, such as surgery, trauma, infection, or radiation. After surgery, adhesions typically begin to form within the first few days. Adhesions are a common effect of surgery, occurring in up to 90% of people who undergo abdominal surgery. Most postoperative adhesions are not painful. It is theorized that adhesions can cause pain by pulling on nerves; nerves can get caught within the adhesion. Adhesions above the liver may cause pain with deep breathing. Intestinal adhesions may cause pain because of obstruction. The use of laparoscopy can often reveal adhesions, which can be lysed then and there. Diagnostic laparoscopies are performed when noninvasive tests do not yield a cause of the patient's abdominal pain. The value of laparoscopy for treating abdominal adhesions has been difficult to determine as patients who undergo a successful adhesiolysis may still have chronic pain and patients found to have no adhesions have been shown to report pain relief (most likely a placebo effect) after diagnostic laparoscopy.

Referred Pain

Referred pain occurs when a pain generator sends a signal back to the spinal cord for transmission up to the brain. The brain becomes confused and interprets pain as coming not from the actual pain generator but rather from another source that happens to enter the spinal cord at the same level. The classic example of this is the transmission of gallbladder pain signals interpreted by the brain as shoulder pain (Fig. 4-3). Referred pain to the abdomen may come from the thoracic spine. Spinal structures with a nerve supply originating from T7 to T12 refer pain to the abdomen.

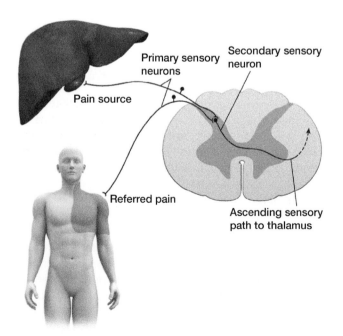

Figure 4-3 Referred pain. Gallbladder pain signals can be confused by the brain and interpreted as shoulder pain.

TREATMENT

Chronic abdominal pain is treated in the outpatient setting medically with lifestyle modification, nonopioids and/or opioids, and possibly an injection. If a patient has chronic abdominal pain and the underlying condition cannot be determined, you treat the symptoms directly. Even if the diagnosis has been determined and the pain remains despite best medical effort in treating the underlying condition, you treat the symptoms directly. The symptoms can best be organized into categories. The patient may fit perfectly into one treatment category or may need a multidisciplinary approach.

Lifestyle Modification

Different types of food and medication can cause abdominal pain. A food and medication diary can help reveal an illusive irritant. Abdominal pain of unknown etiology can often cause high stress levels and be caused by high stress levels. Many patients have poor coping styles and a significant amount of anxiety. Complete care involves addressing these issues.

Treatment by Category

Category 1: Spasm: A patient complains of a tight, squeezing pain. The patient may use the word *spasm*. The location of the pain is typically more generalized. For this type of pain, a muscle relaxant should be prescribed. See Chapter 12, Muscle Relaxants, to learn how to dose and titrate these medications.

Category 2: Neuropathic Pain: Your patient complains of an electric, burning pain, which is characteristic of neuropathic pain. One of the antidepressant or antiseizure medications used for neuropathic pain is appropriate in this instance. See the chapters on these medications for coverage of dosage and titration. These medications do not work instantly—time is required to titrate to a therapeutic level.

Category 3: Nonspecific Pain; Without Gastrointestinal Irritation: The patient's pain is described as being nonspecific, deep, and achy. It can be episodic. For these symptoms, an NSAID could be effective. It is important when using an NSAID to make sure that the patient does not have any bowel or kidney disease.

Category 4: Referred Pain: When a patient presents with both back pain and abdominal pain, it is due diligence to consider the diagnoses of referred pain. The onset of symptoms should coincide. Long-term back pain and new-onset abdominal pain are most likely not related, but when the timing between the two is close, a thoracic pain generator may be the source of both. Conversely, an abdominal pain generator, pancreatic pain, can refer to the back. If the abdominal workup is negative and symptoms continue, an MRI of the thoracic spine should be considered.

Category 5: Abdominal Wall Pain Generator:
The patient's pain is sharp, well localized, and seems to be somatic in origin. The patient reports often being able to push into the abdomen and locate exactly where it hurts. There is also a positive Carnett sign. This type of pain is commonly caused by entrapment of the anterior cutaneous branch of a thoracic nerve but also may be from a surgical scar neuroma or myofascial trigger points. For this type of pain, an injection directly into the area—using a local anesthetic coupled with a steroid—can be effective. For reasons that are not clearly understood, this type of injection provides long-term pain relief in a majority of patients. The theory is that the anesthetic breaks a chronic pain cycle and the steroids enhance the anesthetic effect by leading to neuronal membrane stabilization. Experimental models have shown that these injections reduce ectopic neural discharge from neuromas.[2]

Category 6: Severe Abdominal Pain That Does Not Respond to Conservative Measures:
Opioids can play a role in treating the symptoms of chronic abdominal pain. Opiates activate receptors that modulate our perception of painful stimuli. They act within the brain and spinal cord to alter pain transmission. Opioids are neither organ nor disease specific: For example, Dilaudid is not specifically for liver pain, whereas morphine is not specific for kidney pain. The side effect of all opioids is alteration of GI motility. Opioids decrease GI motility and secretory functions, which can potentially exacerbate existing issues in patients with GI motility problems. Another important aspect to be evaluated is that the absorption of opioids may be altered in patients who have had a partial or full colon resection. Because of alteration in gut length, a fentanyl patch that delivers opioids via a transdermal mechanism, bypassing the gut, is a preferable mechanism for treating chronic abdominal pain with an opioid. See Chapter 15, Opioids to learn how to properly use this type of medication. The utility of opioids should be constantly evaluated as their use can produce problems in patients with chronic abdominal pain. In an attempt to control this pain, the physician prescribes increasing doses of narcotic analgesics. Despite this, the pain can persist and can even worsen. Narcotic bowel syndrome is defined as chronic or frequently recurring abdominal pain that has persisted or worsened despite treatment with increasing doses of narcotics. Symptoms include a combination of abdominal pain, nausea, vomiting, bloating, and constipation. If opioid therapy does not decrease the patient's pain and improve both functionality and quality of life, alternative treatment options should be explored.

CASE STUDIES

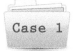
Case 1

Your partner asks you for a second opinion about one of her patients. The patient is a 37-year-old female with abdominal pain for the last year. Your partner has done a full history and examination, has run blood tests, gotten a number of medical images, and has done a colonoscopy and endoscopy—all negative. The pain is unrelated to bowel function. Your partner has prescribed an NSAID as well as a muscle relaxant, which the patient has been on for the last month and a half—both only slightly helpful.

When you meet the patient for the first time, you find that the abdominal pain is not diffuse but rather concentrated in the lower right quadrant. When you palpate the abdomen, you are not able to elicit any specific tender point. You then ask the patient if she can find the exact location of maximum tenderness with the pad of her index finger, which she is able to do. When she does a half

sit up and keeps the pad of her finger on the same spot, the pain becomes slightly more defined. You explain to the patient that you do not know the exact cause of her abdominal pain but it most likely is coming from a specific point in her abdominal wall. Patients have responded very well to an injection into the area. You let your partner's patient know that an injection in some cases has been shown to provide long-term pain relief but that there is no guarantee this will help. The patient wishes to go forward with the injection; an informed consent form is signed. After cleaning the skin, you advance a 2.5-in, 25G needle to the maximum site of pain. After negative aspiration, you inject 40 mg of Kenalog (a steroid) in 5 mL of 0.5% bupivacaine (a local anesthetic). The patient follows up 1 month later, reporting that her pain is about 70% less and that she would like to repeat the injection to see if the pain can be reduced further.

Case 2

A 30-year-old female presents with generalized abdominal pain. She has already seen an internist and two gastroenterologists for this. She has lived with the pain for the last 2 years with no specific inciting event. The pain is spasmodic in nature and episodic. The patient has had no changes in her menstrual cycle and the pain is not associated with it. She reports periodic episodes of diarrhea but for the most part her stool is normal. There is no history of any abdominal surgery. There is no family history of abdominal pathology. On examination, there is diffuse moderate tenderness with no specific trigger points or abdominal masses. Previous generalized blood work and a CT scan of the abdomen are normal. The patient had a colonoscopy and endoscopy with her second gastroenterologist, which were also normal. You review a food log the patient has been keeping and no specific trigger is seen. The patient admits to depression when asked directly if she has depression.

You have no diagnosis for the cause of the patient's pain, but based on the symptoms of cramping as tight pain you prescribe a muscle relaxant, tizanidine 4 mg po bid. During the interview it is clear that the patient is emotionally fragile, and based on your interaction it is apparent that psychological counseling is needed as part of a multimodal approach to patient care. Based on your experience, you understand that with some patients a referral to psychology can be made during an initial consult but for others a doctor–patient therapeutic relationship needs to be established before a patient will accept a psychological referral. You provide positive feedback that you are going to work with the patient. The patient is scheduled to see you again in 2 weeks, at which time you plan to broach the subjects of both treating her abdominal pain and referring her to a psychologist. The patient does not return for her follow up appointment and your office is late asked to release the patients medical records to another primary care doctor in town.

REFERENCES

1. Konturek PC, Brzozowski T, Konturek SJ. Stress and the gut: Pathophysiology, clinical consequences, diagnostic approach and treatment options. *J Physiol Pharmacol.* 2011;62(6):591–599.

2. Devor M, Govrin-Lippmann R, Raber P. Corticosteroids suppress ectopic neural discharge originating in experimental neuromas. *Pain.* 1985;22(2):127–137.

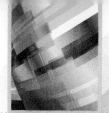

CHAPTER 5

Pelvic Pain

COMMON CAUSES OF CHRONIC PELVIC PAIN
- Common Known Diagnosis of Chronic Pelvic Pain
- Visceral Pelvic Pain
- Somatic Pelvic Pain
- Neuropathic Pelvic Pain

TREATMENT
- Medications
- Injections
- Surgery

This chapter presents the most common causes of chronic pelvic pain (CPP). CPP is a prevalent and challenging disorder to manage. CPP is a noncyclic pain of 6 or more months' duration that localizes to the anatomic pelvic, anterior abdominal wall at or below the umbilicus, the lumbosacral back, or the buttocks and is of sufficient severity to cause functional disability or lead to care. Roughly 38 of 1,000 visits in the primary care setting among women aged 15 to 73 is for CPP, comparable to the incidence of asthma visits.[1] CPP is the most common reason for referral to gynecology clinics, accounting for 20% of all appointments.[2] In one-third to one-half of these cases, the pathology cannot be identified.[3] To make treatment even more challenging, CPP may occur in 50% of patients with a history of physical or sexual abuse.[4]

This chapter covers diagnosis and treatment modalities for the most common causes of CPP. Treatment for known diagnoses is explored first. These common causes of CPP, for which the diagnosis is known, are described in Table 5-1. It is important to remember that patients with CPP may have more than one disease that may lead to pain.

In fact, endometriosis and interstitial cystitis (IC) are commonly referred as the evil twins. Cancer as a cause of pelvic pain is covered in Chapter 3, Cancer Pain. Some of the most challenging CPP cases are those for which the diagnosis cannot be determined.

How to determine the cause of CPP when the diagnosis is not readily known is beyond the scope of this book. Although we cannot currently make the diagnosis, we understand the painful symptoms and what treatment modalities work well for those symptoms. In these cases, the therapeutic plan will be treating the symptoms. Treating pelvic pain of unknown etiology can be frustrating to both the patient and the physician.

COMMON CAUSES OF CHRONIC PELVIC PAIN

Common Known Diagnosis of Chronic Pelvic Pain

If the diagnosis is known, you have the pain generator. Table 5-1 lists the most common, high-yield causes of CPP, and how they present.

If the diagnosis is unknown, it is important to determine whether the pain is visceral, somatic, neuropathic, or a combination.

Visceral Pelvic Pain

Visceral pain is pain that comes from an organ, such as the bladder or rectum, or in females the uterus, ovaries, and fallopian tubes. Pain is elicited with distension, compression, or torsion of an organ. Visceral pain is not well localized and often described as dull and achy. This is because there are a small number of visceral afferent nerves covering a large area (e.g., the bladder), thus many fewer nerves to help pinpoint the exact pain location.

Somatic Pelvic Pain

Somatic structures are the support structure of the pelvic cavity, which include fascia, muscles, and the pelvic floor. Somatic pain is often well localized and typically described as sharp and focal.

Neuropathic Pelvic Pain

Nerves send sensory impulses to the brain for interpretation. These impulses travel along a nerve axon in a regular pattern when the nervous system is working correctly. When a nerve is injured, this regular controlled transmission of impulses fails and the nerve

TABLE 5-1 Most Common High-yield Causes of CPP and their Pathology and Presentation

Diagnosis	Pathology and Presentation
Postoperative pelvic adhesions	Abnormal bands of scar tissue. Typically, adhesions show no symptoms. Adhesions may cause visceral pain by impairing organ mobility. Of open gynecologic procedures, ovarian surgery carries the highest risk of readmissions directly related to adhesions (7.5/100).[5] When symptomatic they can present as deep, dull, achy pain. Adhesions involving the vagina or uterus may cause pain during intercourse.
Endometriosis	Collection of endometrial cells that develop remote from the uterus. During hormonal stimulation, the endometrial tissue triggers an inflammatory response. This is a surgical diagnosis confirmed by pathology. The degree of visible endometriosis has no correlation with the degree of pain, because location is more predictive than total volume. Increased pain usually occurs a few days before menses and begins to resolve 1–2 d into the menses. Pain during or after sex is common with endometriosis and usually predictive of deep rectovaginal endometriosis. Sonographic findings may include cysts in the ovaries, referred to as endometriomas. Patients may present with problems becoming pregnant.
Pelvic congestion syndrome (pelvic varices)	Overfilling of the pelvic venous system. This can be a result of pregnancy or of unknown origin. This pain is not related to the menstrual cycle. Pain is constant and worse with standing; patients may get some relief when they lie down. Pain is worse as the day goes on. Patients often complain of postcoital ache and may have heavy vaginal discharge.
Leiomyoma (fibroid)	A commonly benign tumor that occurs within the uterus. The pathogenesis of pain associated with these lesions is unclear. They are more common in African-Americans than Whites. Increased menstrual bleeding, known as menorrhagia occurs. Pain can be spontaneous or induced by tactile pressure. Symptoms often become worse during pregnancy.
Interstitial cystitis (IC)	Inflammation of the bladder wall. The cause is unknown. It is more common in women than men. There are no radiographic, laboratory, or serologic findings; and no biopsy patterns that are pathognomonic for interstitial cystitis. Daytime and nighttime urinary frequency, urgency, and pelvic pain for at least 6 wks are characteristic. The cystitis may be worse around the menstrual cycle. There is an absence of proven urinary infection. There are intermittent periods of exacerbations and remissions. Approximately 90% of cases are female.
Chronic prostatitis	Found in males, this term is a misnomer as there is no evidence, it is associated with infection. Nonetheless it is usually treated with oral antibiotics. This condition involves intermittent dysuria and pelvic pain or discomfort, for more than 3 of the previous 6 mos without documented urinary tract infections. Patients may have ejaculatory pain and erectile dysfunction.
Irritable bowel syndrome	Irritable bowel syndrome (IBS) is a functional GI disorder characterized by abdominal pain and altered bowel habits in the absence of specific and unique organic pathology. Spasmodic pelvic and abdominal cramping that varies in location. Often associated with pain relief with defecation. May be associated with constipation, diarrhea, or mixed picture. Symptoms may increase with menses.
Extra-pelvic referred pain	E.g., thoracic–lumbar spine pathology. Symptoms vary.

fires aberrantly. Injured nerves develop pathologic activity, manifesting as abnormal excitability. They have an elevated sensitivity to normal chemical, thermal, and mechanical stimuli that would not typically trigger a

TABLE 5-2 Evaluation of Pain History

P	*Palliative* or *Provoking* factors.
Q	*Qualities*—burning, electric, sharp, dull.
R	*Radiation*.
S	*Severity*—usually done on a visual analog scale 0 to 10.
T	*Temporal* events associated with the pain: Is the pain constant or does it come and go?

nerve to fire. This aberrant nerve firing is interpreted by the brain as neuropathic pain. Nerves can be damaged in a number of ways: Mechanically, via infection, from metabolic conditions, toxins, radiation, and idiopathically. In neuropathic pain, the patient usually reports an electric, shooting, burning pain rather than an achy, dull pain.

The goal in taking a pain history is to understand the parameters of the pain as detailed above. The second part of taking a pain history includes evaluating the specific details surrounding the pain. A commonly used pneumonic is PQRST (Table 5-2).

TREATMENT

Table 5-3 lists the treatments of the eight most common high-yield causes of CPP. Symptoms are typically managed in one of three ways: Using medications to control the pain, using interventional nerve blocks to control the pain, or removing the pelvic organs that may be the pain generators.

Medications

Medications can be used to combat the symptoms of CPP. If the pain is thought to be somatic or visceral in nature, NSAIDs would be a first-line option. If the pain has a neuropathic quality—described as electric or burning—a neuropathic medication should be used. Pelvic pain can often be described as squeezing and spasmodic. If this is the case, a muscle relaxant is appropriate. If conservative medical management options fail, opioid medications are the next option. Opioid therapy may allow the return of normal function. To read about specific medication choices and how to properly dose and titrate them, please see the specific medication chapters.

If the patient with CPP reports that symptoms are worse at the time of menstruation, a valid option would be either a combination or a progesterone-only–based birth control.

Leuprolide (Lupron) is an agonist of the pituitary gonadotropin-releasing hormone, which downregulates luteinizing hormone (LH) and follicle-stimulating hormone (FSH), leading to a hypogonadal state—a reduction in both estrogen and testosterone. If the patient's pain is worse at the time of menstruation and she does not respond to oral contraceptives, a lupron-induced hypogonadal state may be helpful. Hormonal manipulating formulations may be best prescribed by a gynecologist.

Injections

Interventionally, there are minimally invasive procedures that can be used to help control pelvic pain. The superior hypogastric plexus is the relay station for sending pelvic pain to the brain, where as the ganglion impar

TABLE 5-3 Treatment of the Most Common High-yield Causes of CPP

Diagnosis	Treatment
Postoperative pelvic adhesions	Laparoscopy is commonly used for adhesiolysis because of the elective nature of the procedure and shorter recovery time. The value of adhesiolysis for pain is unclear. It has been shown that patients have had resolution of their pain after a laparoscopy where no adhesions were found. In addition, some patients who have undergone a successful adhesiolysis reported no change or worsening of their pain.
Endometriosis	Oral contraceptives which have been shown to reduce menstrual pain associated with endometriosis. Progesterone counteracts estrogen and inhibits the growth of the endometrium. NSAIDs can also be very helpful. Surgery for endometriosis-associated pain is a more invasive option but is used for both diagnosis and treatment.
Pelvic congestion syndrome (pelvic varices)	Estrogen which is a venous dilator. In cases of venous congestion, pelvic varices, a hypoestrogenic state may result in resolution of symptoms. In a study in which patients with lower abdominal pain caused by pelvic congestion received either a GnRH agonist or placebo, 73% of subjects reported at least a 50% improvement compared to placebo.[6] Interventional radiologic techniques can be used for pelvic congestion syndrome. A percutaneous catheter is placed into the vein and the vein is embolized. This has shown to provide relief of pain in 50–80% of patients.[7]
Leiomyoma (fibroid)	Medications that help to regulate the menstrual cycle as well as medications that create a hypogonadal state (Lupron) can be of benefit. They help control menstrual bleeding, but they do not reduce fibroid size. In a myomectomy the fibroid is removed, leaving the uterus in place. The removal of the uterus remains the only proven permanent solution for uterine fibroids.
Interstitial cystitis (IC)	Elmiron which is specifically approved for treating IC. It is taken orally. Elmiron is similar to a class of medications called low-molecular-weight heparins. It works by preventing irritation of the bladder walls. Of note: Although the cause of interstitial cystitis is not known, the neuropathic pain medication amitriptyline can lead to improvement of symptoms in about two-thirds of subjects treated with 25–75 mg a day.[8]
Chronic prostatitis	Although there is no evidence of it being associated with infection, it is usually treated with oral antibiotics.
Irritable bowel syndrome	No specific treatment. Fiber supplementation may improve symptoms of constipation and diarrhea. There is no specific treatment. Reassurance can be beneficial.
Extra-pelvic referred pain	Treatment is determined by the cause.

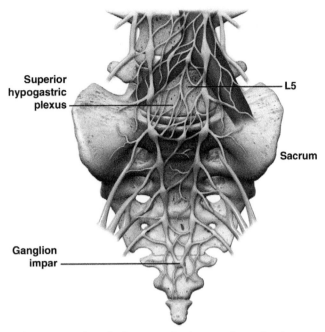

Figure 5-1 Superior hypogastric plexus and ganglion impar.

is the relay station for sending perineal pain to the brain. The superior hypogastric plexus lies at the interspace between the fifth lumbar vertebra and the sacrum. The ganglion impar (Ganglion of Walther) is located at the junction of the sacrum and the coccyx (Fig. 5-1). A needle can be advanced under fluoroscopic guidance to both of these locations. There is evidence to support the use of performing these blocks using a local anesthetic rather than a neurolytic substance (generally reserved for cancer pain) to help relieve nononcologic pelvic and perineal pain.[9] To learn more about how these procedures are done, refer to the chapter on sympathetic blocks, Chapter 24.[10,11]

Pelvic wall injections can be beneficial for suspected pelvic wall pain, somatic pain, of unclear etiology or pelvic wall pain from a neuroma. An injection into the area using a local anesthetic coupled with a steroid can be effective. For reasons that are not clearly understood, this type of injection may provide long-term pain relief. The theory is that the anesthetic breaks a chronic pain cycle and the steroids enhance the anesthetic effect by leading to neuronal membrane stabilization. Experimental modals have shown that these injections reduce ectopic neural discharge from neuromas.[12] The analogy I give to my patients is if something that requires electricity is not working correctly, like your computer, the first thing you do to fix it is turn off the power and then turn it back on. This is what the injection is doing. To see how these injections are performed, please see the common nerve block chapter.

Surgery

For pain thought to be visceral in nature, removing the offending agent has been explored as a treatment modality. Removing the pelvic organs that may be the pain generators remains a very controversial topic in obstetrics and gynecology. Some 10% to 19% of hysterectomies and 40% of laparoscopies are done for nononcologic CPP.[13] Overall, the expected probability of success in the absence of obvious pathology is 60%. The success rate rises to 80% to 90% when pelvic lesions are present.[6] The most common findings after hysterectomy and bilateral salpingo-oophorectomy are adhesions, endometriosis, and adnexal remnants.[14] A small percentage (3% to 5%) will experience worsening of pain or will develop new symptoms after surgery.[15]

Another surgical procedure presacral neurectomy has been shown to decrease midline pelvic pain. Presacral neurectomy is performed on the anterior aspects of vertebral body L5 and the sacrum. The procedure can be done via laparoscopy or laparotomy.

CASE STUDY

Case

A 23-year-old female who recently relocated to your state comes to see you. She states that she has been diagnosed with interstitial cystitis (IC). You review her workup and she has had imaging, blood work, and cystoscopy, all of which were negative. She complains of CPP associated with urinary frequency and urgency. She has tried Elmiron with only a minimal change in her symptoms. You start her on amitriptyline 25 mg at night. The patient returns to your office 2 weeks later; she is crying when you walk in the room, stating that she cannot live like this. You provide emotional support and explain that the medication needs to be titrated to a therapeutic level. You titrate the medication to 50 mg qhs. Unfortunately, the patient never returns for a follow-up.

REFERENCES

1. Zondervan KT, Yudkin PL, Vessey MP, et al. Prevalence and incidence in primary care of chronic pelvic pain in women: Evidence from a national general practice database. *Br J Obstet Gynaecol.* 1999;106(11):1149–1155.

2. Howard FM. Laparoscopic evaluation and treatment of women with chronic pelvic pain. *J Am Assoc Gynecol Laparosc.* 1994;1 (4 Pt 1):325–331.

3. Reiter RC, Gambone JC. Nongynecologic somatic pathology in women with chronic pelvic pain and negative laparoscopy. *J Reprod Med.* 1991;36(4):253–259.

4. Toomey TC, Hernandez JT, Gittelman DF, et al. Relationship of physical and sexual abuse to pain and psychological assessment variables in chronic pelvic pain patients. *Pain.* 1993;53(1): 105–109.

5. Lower AM, Hawthorn RJ, Ellis H, et al. The impact of adhesions on hospital readmissions over ten years after 8849 open gynaecological operations: An assessment from the Surgical and Clinical Adhesions Research Study. *BJOG.* 2000;107(7):855–862.

6. Vercellini P, Daguati R, Abbiati A. Chronic pelvic pain. In: Arici A, Seli E, eds. *Non-invasive Management of Gynecologic Disorders.* London: Informa Healthcare; 2008:33–51.

7. Kim HS, Malhorta AD, Rowe PC, et al. Embolotherapy for pelvic congestion syndrome: Long-term results. *J Vasc Interv Radiol.* 2006;17(2 Pt 1):289–297.

8. Hanno PM, Buehler J, Wein AJ. Use of amitriptyline in the treatment of interstitial cystitis. *J Urol.* 1989;141(4):846–848.

9. Lee RB, Stone K, Magelseen D, et al. Presacral neurectomy for chronic pelvic pain. *Obstet Gynecol.* 1986;68:517–521.

10. Pratt RB, Plancarte R. Superior hypogastric plexus block: A new therapeutic approach for pelvic pain. In: Waldman SD, Winne A, eds. *Interventional Pain Management.* Philadelphia, PA: Saunders; 1996:387–391.

11. de Leon-Casasola OA, Kent E, Lema MJ. Neurolytic superior hypogastric plexus block for chronic pain associated with cancer. *Pain.* 1993;54(2):145–151.

12. Devor M, Govrin-Lipmann R, Raber P. Corticosteroids suppress ectopic neural discharge originating in experimental neuromas. *Pain.* 1985;22(2):127–137.

13. Peterson HB, Hulka JF, Phillips JM. American Association of Gynecologic Laparoscopists' 1988 membership survey on operative laparoscopy. *J Reprod Med.* 1990;35:587–589.

14. Behera M, Vilos GA, Hollett-Caines J, et al. Laparoscopic findings, histopathologic evaluation, and clinical outcomes in women with chronic pelvic pain after hysterectomy and bilateral salpingo-oophorectomy. *J Minim Invasive Gynecol.* 2006;13:431–435.

15. Hillis SD, Marchbanks PA, Peterson HB. The effectiveness of hysterectomy for chronic pelvic pain. *Obstet Gynecol.* 1995:86(6): 941–945.

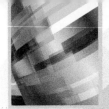

CHAPTER 6

Podiatric (Foot and Ankle) Pain

PAIN IN THE HEAL AND BOTTOM OF THE FOOT
▸ Plantar Fasciitis

PAIN ON THE SIDE OF THE BIG TOE
▸ Hallux Valgus (Bunion)

PAIN BETWEEN 3RD & 4TH TOE
▸ Morton's Neuroma

PAIN FROM THE MEDIAL MALLEOLUS INTO THE FOOT
▸ Tarsal Tunnel Syndrome

PAIN IN BOTH FEET
▸ Diabetic Peripheral Neuropathy

This chapter presents the most common clinical causes of chronic pain in the foot and ankle. They include plantar fasciitis, hallux valgus (bunion), Morton's neuroma, tarsal tunnel syndrome, and diabetic peripheral neuropathy. The focus of this chapter will be on pain that originates from the foot and ankle. Note, however, that pain originating from the lumbar spine can present as foot-and-ankle pain. Nerves come out of the lumbar spine and down into the legs, acting as the control center for both sensation and movement of the lower extremities. In the case of concurrent back and leg pain, it is important to image the lumbar spine with an MRI. This is covered in Chapter 2, Neuropathic Pain, in the section Lumbar Radiculopathy.

If the pain is located solely at the foot (pardon the pun) or ankle, then a proper history and examination will be key in securing a diagnosis.

PAIN IN THE HEAL AND BOTTOM OF THE FOOT

Plantar Fasciitis

The plantar fascia is a thick, fibrous tissue that runs along the plantar surface of the foot. Its function is to provide support for the longitudinal arch of the foot and act as a shock absorber. Pain is caused by inflammation of the plantar fascia at its insertion site on the medial aspect of the calcaneal tuberosity (heel; Fig. 6-1). Patients with pes

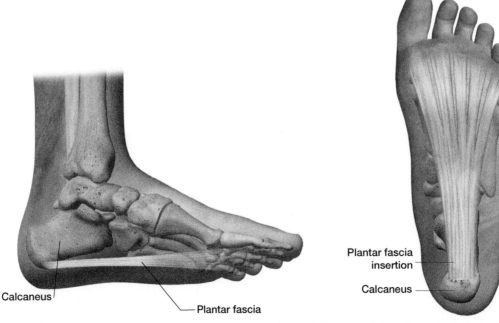

Calcaneus

Plantar fascia

Plantar fascia insertion

Calcaneus

Figure 6-1 The plantar fascia at its insertion site on the medial aspect of the calcaneal tuberosity (heel).

planus (low arch) or pes cavus (high arch) feet have an increased stress placed on the plantar fascia. There is a high incidence of plantar fasciitis in runners, which is possibly caused by repeated microtrauma. Pain is often most severe at the anterior aspect of the heel. It has been estimated that 1,000,000 patient visits per year are because of plantar fasciitis.

In plantar fasciitis there is an intensely sharp heel pain with the first few steps of the morning. Early in the morning the plantar fascia is constricted and tight—this is intensified in plantar fasciitis. The pain will decrease during the day as the plantar fascia becomes more flexible.

On physical examination, you can usually reproduce the pain by palpation of the medial anterior aspect of the heel (Fig. 6-2). In the windlass test, the patient puts weight on the heel while the examiner dorsiflexes the toes to reproduce the pain. Clinically, if there is more pain on the lateral aspect of the heel versus the medial aspect, a calcaneal stress fracture should be ruled out. If you suspect plantar fasciitis and the symptoms do not resolve with conservative treatment, an x-ray is warranted. Radiographs may show a plantar heel spur in 50% of patients with plantar fasciitis, but it is important to remember that many asymptomatic patients have heel spurs.

First-line treatment includes physical therapy (calf and Achilles tendon stretching), ice, and an anti-inflammatory medication (e.g., nonsteroidal anti-inflammatory drugs, NSAIDs). A patient's shoes should also be replaced and proper arch support provided to match the patient's feet.

Night splints may be very effective in treating plantar fasciitis. People naturally sleep with their feet in a plantar-flexed position, which causes the plantar fascia to be shortened. Night splints keep the ankles in a

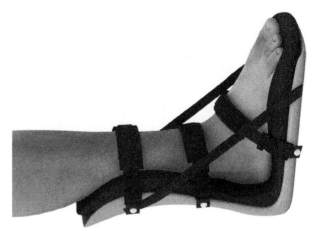

Figure 6-3 Night splints allow for the lengthening of the plantar fascia at night which can help alleviate plantar fasciitis.

neutral position, which causes passive stretching of the plantar fascia overnight (Fig. 6-3). This allows the plantar fascia to heal in the elongated position, decreasing tension on the fascia with the first step in the morning. Studies have shown that 80% of patients using night splints had improvement of their plantar fasciitis.[3]

A cortisone injection to decrease inflammation can be very helpful (Fig. 6-4). The physician identifies the medial aspect of the calcaneal bone and palpates the soft tissue, locating the point of maximal tenderness or swelling. This area is marked with a felt-tip marking pen. The area is prepped in standard sterile fashion. As a therapeutic agent I use 40 mg of Kenalog mixed with 3 mL of 0.25% bupivacaine in a 5-mL syringe. The needle is a 1.5-in, 22 gauge needle. The needle angle is perpendicular to the skin and introduced through the skin to the tendon sheath. The medication is then

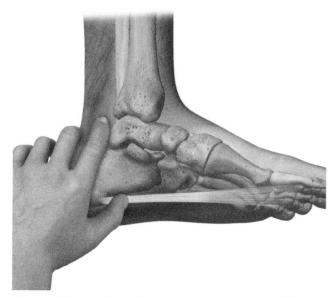

Figure 6-2 Palpation of the medial anterior aspect of the heel reproduces the pain of plantar fasciitis.

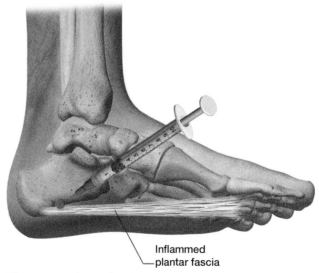

Inflammed plantar fascia

Figure 6-4 Plantar fasciitis injection at the incretion site of the plantar fascia to the medial aspect of the calcaneus bone.

injected at the heel. A cortisone injection can slightly increase the risk of plantar fascia rupture. In 95% of patients with plantar fasciitis, symptoms resolve within 12 to 18 months. In cases that are refractory to conservative treatment, a surgical release of the plantar fascia can be performed.

PAIN ON THE SIDE OF THE BIG TOE

Hallux Valgus (Bunion)

Hallux is the big toe and valgus is an abnormal displacement of a body part away from the midline of the body. The distal aspect of the first metatarsal deviates away from the midline of the body, away from the second toe so that it causes an outward bump (Fig. 6-5). The medial eminence of the first metatarsophalangeal joint becomes prominent, often referred to as a bunion. *Bunion* is the Greek word for turnip. The most common cause of hallux valgus is biomechanical instability. When we walk or run, roughly 65% of dorsiflexion is focused on the first metatarsophalangeal joint. This intense force makes the first metatarsal vulnerable for the development of hallux valgus. The more the big toe shifts into a valgus position the greater mechanical advantage it has, to a point. Patients present with complaints of pain over the medial eminence, made worse with tight shoes.

This condition affects roughly 1% of the North American population, but the incidence has been shown to be as high as 15% in those older than 60 years of age. Tight dress shoes worn by many women are more constraining than the shoes worn by men and are believed by many podiatrists to be a common factor in many cases of hallux valgus. This could explain the 10:1 female to male ratio seen with this disorder.

In hallux valgus (bunion), patients often present with pain at the first metatarsophalangeal joint during ambulation. Often the pain is relieved with removal of tight-fitting shoes. If the patient notes a burning pain in this area along with deep, achy pain, there may also be entrapment of the medial dorsal cutaneous nerve (Fig. 6-6). Medial dorsal cutaneous nerve pain is often described as burning and electric. While taking a history, determine how the pain affects the patient's quality of life. Some patients with larger deformities have mild discomfort and are not particularly affected, whereas some patients with smaller deformities are severely affected. On examination evaluate: (1) Hallux (big toe) position, (2) medial prominence (how big the bump is), and (3) range of motion of the metatarsophalangeal joint. Normal range of motion is 65 degrees with dorsiflexion and 15 degrees with plantar flexion. Obtain x-rays of weight-bearing feet, including anteroposterior, lateral oblique, and lateral views.

Treatment for hallux valgus is based on the extent of the deformity and the severity of the symptoms. Conservative medical treatment can help with the painful symptoms and slow the progression but it cannot change the irreversible cartilage, bone, and soft tissue deformity. Anti-inflammatory drugs and/or a

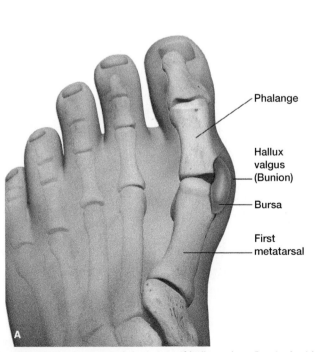

Phalange

Hallux valgus (Bunion)

Bursa

First metatarsal

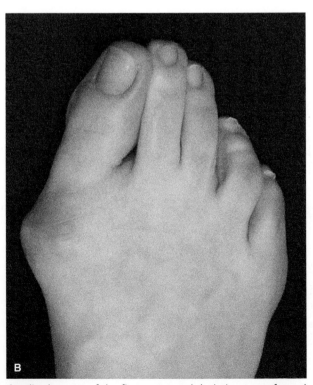

Figure 6-5 A. Anatomical depiction of hallux valgus (bunion) with the distal aspect of the first metatarsal deviating away from the second toe. **B.** Photograph of a patient with a right foot hallux valgus (bunion).

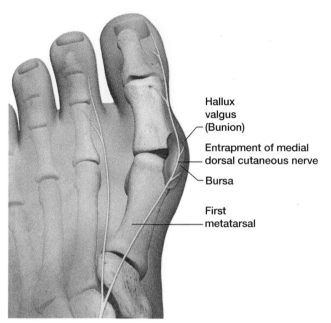

Figure 6-6 Entrapment of the medial dorsal cutaneous nerve at the hallux valgus (bunion). Patients report not just an achy sharp pain from destruction of the joint but a burning electric pain from medial dorsal cutaneous nerve irritation.

cortisone injection can help to decrease the pain. For the injection a local anesthetic with a steroid (e.g., I use 1 mL of bupivacaine 0.25% with 20 mg of Kenalog) can be injected into the area (Fig. 6-7). Currently, there is no evidence to support prolonged physical therapy.

If pain persists despite conservative treatment, an osteotomy is commonly performed. An osteotomy is surgery to cut away a portion of the bone. Depending on the type of surgery and degree of correction, recovery time is 6 weeks to 6 months. The foot is immobilized in a waking boot for about 6 weeks. Walking is then transitioned to a stiff shoe for a month.

PAIN BETWEEN 3ᴿᴰ & 4ᵀᴴ TOE

Morton's Neuroma

Morton's neuroma is a benign interdigital growth of tissue that surrounds the digital nerve of the toes. It most commonly presents in between the third and fourth metatarsal web space (Fig. 6-8). Females are five times more likely to have Morton's neuroma—again, which may be a function of the tendency for women to wear tight-fitting shoes more than men.

In Morton's neuroma, the pain is described as being intermittent. The most common location is between the third and fourth metatarsal web space. The examination commonly reveals no problems and often the neuroma cannot be palpated. Lateral pressure on the metatarsophalangeal joints can be applied while the interspace is palpated, which can reproduce the symptoms. Metatarsophalangeal joint synovitis can present like Morton's neuroma, but there is subtle swelling around the joint and pain elicited with toe flexion for this condition.

The range of treatment options for Morton's neuroma is vast. The first line of treatment is a change of shoes.

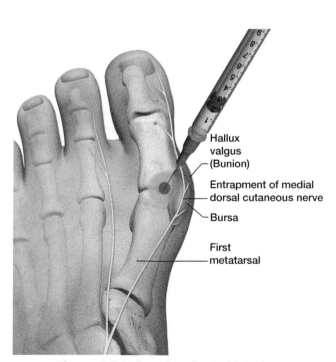

Figure 6-7 Hallux valgus (bunion) injection.

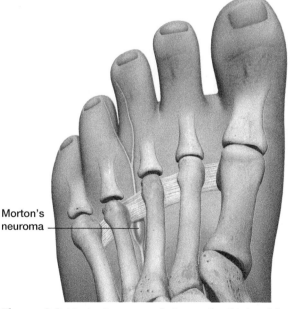

Figure 6-8 Morton's neuroma between the third and fourth metatarsal web space.

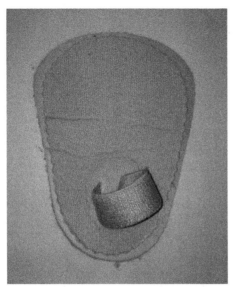
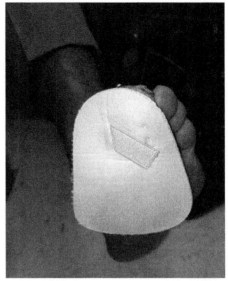

Figure 6-9 Metatarsal support pad.

The use of a metatarsal support pad (Fig. 6-9) may relieve pressure from the area by distributing force throughout the mid-arch and metatarsals. Medical treatment is based on medications used for neuropathic pain (see the chapters on antidepressant and antiseizure medications used for neuropathic pain, Chapters 13 and 14, for proper dosing and titration). An injection of cortisone and a local anesthetic can be helpful (e.g., I use 2 mL of 0.25% bupivacaine and 20 mg of Kenalog, Fig. 6-10). If conservative options fail, the neuroma can be removed surgically.

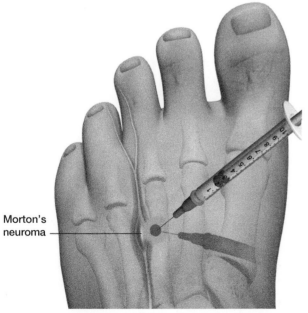

Morton's neuroma

Figure 6-10 Morton's neuroma injection.

PAIN FROM THE MEDIAL MALLEOLUS INTO THE FOOT

Tarsal Tunnel Syndrome

Tarsal tunnel syndrome is an entrapment neuropathy of the posterior tibial nerve in the tarsal tunnel. The tarsal tunnel is made up of bone on the inside and the flexor retinaculum on the outside. The posterior tibial nerve passes into the foot through the tarsal tunnel, which is located posterior and inferior to the medial malleolus (Fig. 6-11). In the tunnel, the posterior tibial nerve splits into three separate nerves. One nerve continues to the heel; the other two (medial and lateral plantar nerves) continue to the bottom of the foot. In tarsal tunnel syndrome, the nerve becomes trapped as the area under the flexor retinaculum becomes too small. This is analogous to carpal tunnel syndrome of the wrist.

The main cause of this syndrome is idiopathic, but it may be post-traumatic or a result of a space-occupying lesion. Pain radiates from the tarsal tunnel into the foot. Nerve conduction studies can be helpful to confirm the diagnosis, but a negative study does not rule out tarsal tunnel syndrome.

In tarsal tunnel syndrome, pain is often described as shooting, electric, and radiating from the medial malleolus into the big toe and first three toes. Pain is worse with prolonged standing, worse with activity, and relieved with rest. On examination, pain in some instances can be induced by tapping on the tarsal tunnel (Fig. 6-12, Tinel sign). In severe cases, there is atrophy of the intrinsic foot muscles.

In tarsal tunnel syndrome, the basis of treatment is to increase the amount of room for the posterior tibial nerve. A conservative option includes the injection of a local anesthetic and cortisone. To perform the injection,

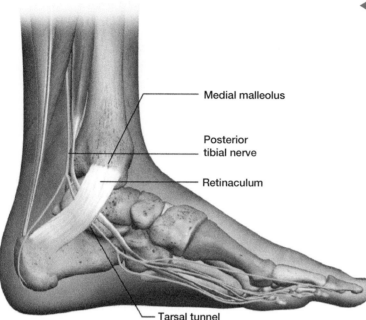

◄ **Figure 6-11** The posterior tibial nerve travels in the posterior leg with the posterior tibial artery, in the fascial plane between the superficial and deep muscle groups. It is a mixed sensory and motor nerve. Further distally, it passes posterior to the medial malleolus at the ankle.

Medial malleolus

Posterior tibial nerve

Retinaculum

Tarsal tunnel

the ankle is rested on the examination table with the medial malleolus facing up. The ankle is prepped in standard sterile fashion. The needle enters the superior posterior aspect of the medial malleolus at a 30-degree angle. I use a mixture of 2 mL of 0.25% bupivacaine, and 20 mg of Kenalog. This injection can be done in the office (Fig. 6-13). Because the nerve is irritated, medications that target nerve pain can be helpful (see the chapters on antiseizure and antidepressant medications used for neuropathic pain, Chapters 13 and 14, for information on dosing and titration). A foot orthotic, or orthopedic apparatus, may reduce tension on the tibial nerve by decreasing the load on the medial column.

If conservative options fail, the nerve needs to be surgically released. After surgical release of the posterior tibial nerve, the patient should be non–weight-bearing for 3 weeks.

PAIN IN BOTH FEET

Diabetic Peripheral Neuropathy

Also known as distal axonopathy, diabetic peripheral neuropathy is a dysfunction of the small nerves. The small nerves of the feet are the most susceptible to damage from diabetes as they are the farthest nerve fibers away from the heart. Peripheral neuropathy starts in the toes and ascends toward the ankle. Patients complain of a symmetric pain in their feet that is often described as burning or a feeling of pins and needles. About 7.5% of patients at the

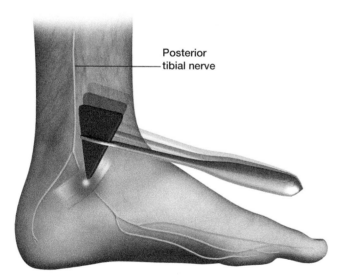

Posterior tibial nerve

Figure 6-12 Tinel sign. Tapping on the posterior tibial nerve as it passes through the tarsal tunnel, Tinel test, may re-create the symptoms and indicate tarsal tunnel syndrome.

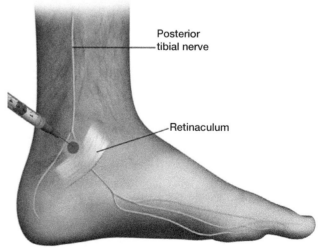

Posterior tibial nerve

Retinaculum

Figure 6-13 Tarsal tunnel syndrome injection.

time of diabetes diagnosis have neuropathy.[1] Eventually, 47% of patients with diabetes have some peripheral neuropathy.[2] Diabetic neuropathy occurs at any age but is more common with increasing age and severity of diabetes. Patients with diabetic peripheral neuropathy are prone to foot ulcers. Fifteen percent of diabetics develop foot ulcers during their lifetime. Neuropathy deprives the patient of early warning signs of pain or pressure on the foot, making them vulnerable to developing foot ulcers. Other prevalent causes of peripheral neuropathy include alcohol abuse, HIV, vitamin deficiencies (including E, B_1, B_6, B_{12}, and niacin), and Lyme disease.

The presentation of diabetic peripheral neuropathy is usually symmetrical, and the patient may have sensory loss and paresthesia (an abnormal sensation of the skin, such as numbness, tingling, pricking, or burning). Walking may provoke symptoms. The pain is typically of slow onset and progressive. On examination, patients may have no clinical findings. As the disease progresses, patients develop sensory deficits to light touch. It is important to examine the feet for abnormal skin breakdown in patients with deep sensory deficits. Ulceration followed by infection, and finally amputation, is a known sequela.

Management of the painful burning symptoms of diabetic peripheral neuropathy can be achieved by both the antiseizure and antidepressant medications used to treat neuropathic pain. A topical anesthetic is another option for treating the pain of peripheral neuropathy. Interventionally, a spinal cord stimulator (SCS) is FDA approved for the treatment of pain from peripheral neuropathy. A SCS trial is often done in the interventional pain doctor's office using a local anesthetic for comfort. The patient wears the device for 3 to 5 days during the trial period to see if there is a significant decrease in pain during activities of daily living. Along with pain control, small studies have shown that patients with good outcomes from SCS have an increase in their microcirculatory blood flow as measured by Doppler laser flow in the symptomatic legs. SCS is worth considering if neuropathic pain medications are not controlling the symptoms (see the chapter on spinal cord stimulation, Chapter 29, for more on this procedure).

CASE STUDIES

Case 1

A 24-year-old male presents with complaints of pain in his feet. The right foot bothers him more significantly that the left. He has tried over-the-counter ibuprofen but the pain seems to be getting worse and affects his activities of daily living. He states that he used to run daily in the morning before work but now sometimes runs after work when the pain is not as bad. You examine the feet and he has full strength, his reflexes are 2+, and sensation is intact to light touch. He has increased pain with palpation of the medial aspect of the heel on both feet, but more so on the right. You push on this area, he states that this is where the pain bothers him most.

You diagnose plantar fasciitis and prescribe night splints, explaining how they work. You also prescribe Celebrex 200 mg once a day as needed, and ice treatments over the area. The patient then asks you, "Is there some sort of injection you can do today?" Although this may be a possibility in the future, you ask your patient to try conservative treatment for 2 weeks first. On return visit the pain level has decreased 50% and you both agree to continue the current plan.

Case 2

A 35-year-old man presents with a chief complaint of pain in the left foot. He has no past medical or surgical history. The patient states that the symptoms have been slowly progressive and started about 3 years ago. The patient notes that the pain started after a 2-week trip to Europe, where he did an excessive amount of walking wearing an old pair of sandals. The pain is described as burning and electric in nature. It is not affected by the time of day. The pain starts at the medial ankle and radiates into the sole of the foot. The patient has been taking ibuprofen daily for the pain. On examination, the pain can be reproduced by pushing on the tarsal tunnel. You diagnose the patient with tarsal tunnel syndrome. After treatment options are reviewed with the patient, he decides to go forward with tarsal tunnel injections. He also makes a change in his footwear to a more comfortable supportive show. At 1 month follow-up, the patient reports a 70% reduction in his pain; the injection is repeated to see if further pain reduction can be achieved.

REFERENCES

1. Pirart J. Diabetes mellitus and its degenerative complications: A prospective study of 4,400 patients observed between 1947 and 1973. *Diabetes Care.* 1978;1:168–188.
2. Dyck PJ, Kratz KM, Karnes JL, et al. The prevalence by staged severity of various types of diabetic neuropathy, retinopathy, and nephropathy in a population-based cohort: The Rochester Diabetic Neuropathy Study. *Neurology.* 1993;43(4):817–824.
3. Batt ME, Tanji JL, Skattum N. Plantar fasciitis: A prospective randomized clinical trial of the tension night splint. *Clin J Sport Med.* 1996;6(3):158–162.

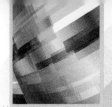

CHAPTER 7

Miscellaneous Pain Disorders that Affect Multiple Areas of the Body

COMPLEX REGIONAL PAIN SYNDROME
   (FORMERLY KNOWN AS REFLEX SYMPATHETIC
   DYSTROPHY OR CAUSALGIA)

FIBROMYALGIA

SICKLE CELL ANEMIA

COMPLEX REGIONAL PAIN SYNDROME (FORMERLY KNOWN AS REFLEX SYMPATHETIC DYSTROPHY OR CAUSALGIA)

Complex regional pain syndrome (CRPS) is defined as a syndrome of diffuse limb pain, often burning in nature, usually a consequence of injury or painful stimulus. CRPS was first described in 1864 during the Civil War. Most soldiers went through a normal recovery period from superficial gunshot wounds, but for some a chronic pain syndrome developed. The pain was characterized by a severe burning sensation. These soldiers would go on to have painful limbs with marked dysfunction. The distribution of pain was inconsistent, not representing a single dermatome or peripheral nerve, distinguishing it from a single-nerve injury. Skin, hair, and nail changes developed in affected limbs.[1]

CRPS can occur after a major event such as knee surgery or after a minor event such as bumping your shoulder. Some common precursors include trauma, surgery, inflammation, nerve injury, stroke, and immobilization. CRPS is divided into two types: Types I and II. CRPS Type I, formerly known as reflex sympathetic dystrophy, occurs when there is no known preceding nerve damage—for example, an ankle sprain. No correlation exists between the severity of the injury and the resulting painful syndrome.[1] In 5% to 10% of patients, there is an absence of any painful event. Type I is more common than Type II. CPRS Type II, formerly known as causalgia (literally "hot pain"), occurs when there is apparent preceding nerve damage. The incidence after known peripheral nerve injury ranges from 1% to 14% in different series.

CRPS frequently occurs in young adults and is more common in females than males. No specific psychological factor or personality trait has been identified that predisposes individuals to the development of CRPS.

There is no definitive agreement among clinicians regarding the pathophysiology of CRPS. One of the main theories postulates that after a painful stimulus the body normally sends out a sympathetic discharge. If that discharge were to continue aberrantly without shutting down, this could lead to a sympathetic hyperdynamic state.[2] A continued sympathetic hyperdynamic state would cause peripheral tissue damage, generating further sympathetic discharge and perpetuating the vicious cycle (Fig. 7-1).

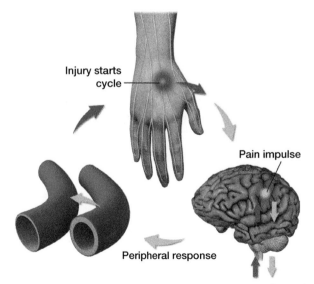

Figure 7-1 Complex regional pain syndrome (CRPS), formerly known as reflex sympathetic dystrophy. Suspected vicious pain cycle.

Eventually this leads to both peripheral and central nervous system (CNS) changes that exist independent of the sympathetic state. In recent years, the concept of a sympathetic cause has been challenged because a subset of patients with presumed CRPS do not respond at all to sympathetic block. This led to the name change from reflex sympathetic dystrophy to CRPS.

History and Examination

On history, CRPS sufferers often describe a constant burning pain in a limb, sometimes also described as an aching pain. Symptoms usually progress in a step-wise fashion, though not in every instance, with pain and decreased function always present. Hallmarks of CRPS are hyperalgesia (an exaggerated response to painful stimuli) and when the disease advances, allodynia (the sensation of pain to nonpainful stimuli, e.g., merely touching the skin). Initially there may be signs of increased sympathetic tone, such as increased sweating in the limb and temperature changes.[3] Vasomotor changes cause skin discoloration, including various hues of red and purple. Sudomotor changes in skin range from hyperhidrosis to bone-dry skin. It is important to note that vasomotor and sudomotor changes vary not only among individuals but also within individuals over time.[4] Later there may be physical trophic changes such as glossy skin, brittle nail growth, altered hair growth, and muscle atrophy. These changes usually develop months after the pain begins (Fig. 7-2).

CRPS may remain stable affecting the same area or may spread in three distinct patterns: Contiguous, independent, and mirror image. In contiguous spread, there is gradual enlargement of the area affected—from distal to proximal of the affected limb. In independent spread, there are signs and symptoms that develop at a site distant from the original symptoms, for example, symptoms spreading from the right leg to the left arm. In mirror image spread, symptoms appear in the opposite limb in a region similar to the site of initial presentation.

The physical examination varies greatly depending on when the patient is seen—in the early stages of CRPS or after the syndrome is full blown. Patients at all stages will tend to protect the painful limb—an arm will be folded in or a painful leg pulled back. Touching the affected limb will be very unpleasant for the patient. As the process becomes chronic, you may see the skin of the painful limb become glossy. There may be atrophy as well. The hair growth and nail beds are different between the painful and nonpainful limb. CRPS should be suspected if regional pain and sensory changes after a trauma exceed the duration or magnitude of the anticipated healing period. The key is not to wait for the chronic changes to develop before recognizing that this may be CRPS and administering treatment. If you have a reason to suspect CRPS, start treatment immediately.

CRPS is a diagnosis of exclusion, but in some cases, changes on a triple-phase bone scan may aid in confirmation. There is an increase in bone metabolism as shown by increased periarticular tracer uptake using a triple-phase bone scan. However, an abnormal bone scan is not required for the diagnosis of CRPS. These changes are not seen until at least 3 months after the symptoms start; treatment should begin before a triple-phase bone scan is performed to maximize the chance of effective treatment.

Treatment

Treatment is based on functional restoration. This often requires a multidisciplinary approach, including sympathetic nerve blocks, possibly a spinal cord stimulator, medication management, physical therapy, and control of any psychological dysfunction that may develop. Many patients with CRPS have anxiety, fear, depression, and other psychological symptoms. This is considered to be a result of and not a cause of CRPS.

Sympathetic Nerve Block: Treatment usually involves interventional sympathetic block of the region affected. The physician injects anesthetic solution under x-ray guidance onto the stellate ganglion (part of the sympathetic chain) for upper-extremity CRPS or the lumbar sympathetic chain for lower-extremity CRPS. Sympathetic nerve blocks can break the pain cycle. For years this was considered the gold standard of treatment. However, there are few well-controlled studies that have been conducted to determine the usefulness of

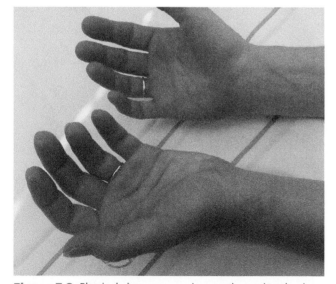

Figure 7-2 Physical changes seen in complex regional pain syndrome. The left hand has color changes and appears glossy.

sympathetic block. When grouped together, these studies show that 29% of patients obtain full pain relief whereas 41% obtain partial pain relief.[5] These numbers should be considered with caution as the studies are older & limited. Sympathetic blocks become less effective the more chronic the condition. In a study looking at sympathectomy (permanently cutting the sympathetic chain) the most important independent factor in predicting a positive response to sympathectomy is an interval of less than 12 months between the inciting event and the procedure.[6] Sympathetic nerve block is used in conjunction with physical therapy with the goal of allowing the patient to participate fully in the exercises with less pain. See the chapter on sympathetic blocks, Chapter 24, to learn how these procedures are performed.

Spinal Cord Stimulation: This procedure has been used with success for a number of neuropathic pain conditions. The medical device consists of polyurethane leads and a small battery analogous to a pacemaker—it has been called the pacemaker for pain. The flexible catheter style leads placed into the posterior epidural space never physically touch the spinal cord. Current is used to drive controlled electrical stimulation to the back of the spinal cord and stimulate the large myelinated fibers of the dorsal horn, which has been shown to inhibit pain. In a study by Taylor et al.,[7] patients with CRPS reported a statistically significant reduction in the visual analog pain scale at 24 months after a spinal cord stimulator implant. Almost two-thirds of patients reported at least a 50% improvement in their pain scores over a median follow-up period of 33 months. In another study looking at functional status of patients with sympathetically maintained CRPS Type I, spinal cord stimulation reduced deep pain and allodynia. Patients showed significant improvement in their motor strength over an average follow-up of about 3 years.[8] The advantage of spinal cord stimulation is that the patient gets to experience the device on a trial basis for 3 to 5 days to test its efficacy before deciding to permanently implant the leads and battery.

Medication: There are very few placebo-controlled trials on medication use for CRPS. Antiseizure and antidepressant medications used to treat neuropathic pain are often clinically applied in these cases. If an opioid is used, methadone—with its NMDA receptor antagonist properties—may be the most appropriate choice to treat if the pain is severe in this chronic painful condition.

Physical Therapy: Physical therapy helps facilitate functional recovery of the limb. The direct goals are desensitization of the affected region, mobilization, increasing strength and range of motion, and vocational and functional rehabilitation. The effect of physiotherapy on the natural course of the disease is unknown. However, it is important to remember that nearly all patients with advanced CRPS also have myofascial pain syndrome of the supporting joints because of their contracted state.

CASE STUDY

Case

A 47-year-old female presents with pain in her right lower extremity. The patient was at work and a clothing rack fell, hitting her shin. She was able to work the rest of the day. The next day she noticed a bruise on her shin. Over the last 3 months the pain in her right lower extremity has increased; she describes the pain as burning in nature. The patient has seen another primary care doctor, who prescribed Neurontin (gabapentin), which she states has not been very helpful for her pain at 300 mg qhs.

On examination, you elicit pain in her right leg with a simple touch. The pain is located circumferentially around her calf down to her feet. Previous x-rays were negative and the patient has no past medical history. At this point, you suspect CRPS Type I and send the patient to pain management for a series of lumbar sympathetic blocks. The patient returns to your office 10 months later. You notice that even though it is winter she is wearing sandals and she keeps her right leg pulled back. The patient reports that the pain has increased significantly and her leg has changed. She reveals that she was scared about having an injection and never went to pain management. The right foot clearly is atrophied and the skin looks glossy. The patient states that even her bedsheets touching her leg causes pain. The decision is made to start the patient on Lyrica with an aggressive titration schedule. You call the pain management group and negotiate a next-day appointment. The patient keeps this appointment; she undergoes a series of lumbar sympathetic blocks that helps alleviate the burning pain somewhat but overall provides only moderate relief. At this point it is agreed that the next step is to proceed with a spinal cord stimulator trial. The patient has pain relief with the trial and decides to proceed with full implantation, which is performed 2 weeks later. The patient currently is in physical therapy on Lyrica with the stimulator covering the area of her pain. There is a significant reduction in her pain; however, she has still not been able to return to work.

FIBROMYALGIA

In 1904, British physician Sir William Gowers described the symptoms of fibromyalgia and coined the term "fibrositis" based on his assumption that the syndrome was caused by inflamed muscle fibers. No evidence was found to support that notion, and in 1976 the name was changed to fibromyalgia. Fibromyalgia had no strict definition until 1990, when the American College of Rheumatology set formal diagnostic criteria: Fibromyalgia is defined as widespread pain lasting for at least 3 months. Pain is considered to be widespread when all of these conditions are present: Pain in both sides of the body, pain above and below the waistline, and axial skeletal pain. This occurs in combination with tenderness at 11 or more of 18 specific tender points (Fig. 7-3).

A clearer definition of fibromyalgia, allowed research to be more focused on better understanding its pathophysiology. Some experts believe that fibromyalgia is a central sensitivity syndrome with abnormalities in pain processing by the central nervous system (CNS).[9] Some studies have indicated an alteration of pain perception. Functional imaging in fibromyalgia patients as compared to controls shows an increase in CNS activity in response to lower pain stimuli. Control group patients required a 73% stronger stimulus to elicit the same subjective pain response as compared to patients with fibromyalgia.[10] However, the cause of fibromyalgia is not known—no gene, receptor, specific neurotransmitter, or alteration of tissue has been found to be associated with the condition. There is no specific laboratory test or imaging method for diagnosis.

The age of onset is typically between 25 and 40 years of age. It occurs predominantly in women, with a 10:1 female-to-male ratio. Genetic predisposition may play a role. First-degree relatives of patients with fibromyalgia display a more than eight-fold greater risk for developing fibromyalgia as compared with the general population.[10] Patients with the condition have a two- to seven-fold increased risk of depression, anxiety, headache, irritable bowel syndrome, systemic lupus erythematosus, and rheumatoid arthritis compared with healthy individuals.[11] Some $16 billion is spent annually on health care costs and disability claims related to this disorder in the United States.

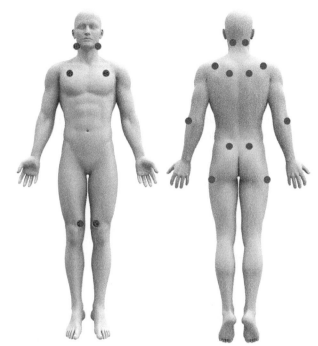

Figure 7-3 Diagnostic tender points for fibromyalgia. Eleven or more of these 18 specific tender points should be positive.

Patients commonly present with the chief complaint of pain all over. Competing diagnoses should be ruled out, the common ones being hypothyroidism, polymyalgia rheumatica, systemic lupus erythematosus, Lyme disease, and rheumatoid arthritis. It is important to remember that the patient may have one of these diseases along with fibromyalgia. See Table 7-1 for quick tips to help rule out these general medical conditions that mimic fibromyalgia.

History and Examination

Patients with fibromyalgia describe diffuse musculoskeletal aches. The pain is expressed as deep and tender. It should be located in at least three of the body's four quadrants. Often patients note fatigue and difficulty sleeping. Fatigue is seen in up to 80% of patients with fibromyalgia. Patients describe their sleep as nonrestorative. Nonrestorative or nonrefreshing sleep differs from insomnia. Whereas insomnia is characterized as difficulties in falling or staying asleep, nonrestorative sleep is essentially a qualitative phenomenon. Associated

TABLE 7-1 Differential Diagnosis for Fibromyalgia

Conditions to be Ruled out	Laboratory Test
Hypothyroidism	TSH (thyroid stimulating hormone)
Polymyalgia rheumatica	ESR (erythrocyte sedimentation rate)
Systemic lupus erythematosus	ANA (antinuclear antibody)
Lyme disease	Lyme titer
Rheumatoid arthritis	Rheumatoid factor

symptoms include anxiety, headaches, and irritable bowel syndrome. Fibromyalgia patients report difficulties in concentration and memory. Some clinicians refer to this as Fibro-fog.

The key to the physical examination is its normalcy, other than the presence of pain in at least 11 of the 18 predetermined tender points. The pain should affect at least three of the body's four quadrants. There should be no joint swelling. When testing the tender points with your thumb, just enough pressure is applied to dent the patient's skin and turn the tip of your fingernail white. Patients with fibromyalgia report pain at the following sites whereas controls do not.

Bilateral Fibromyalgia Tender Points

1. Low cervical region; anterior neck near transverse process of C5 to C7
2. Second rib, costochondral junctions
3. Occiput: Insertion of the suboccipital junctions
4. Trapezius muscles: Midpoint of the upper border
5. Supraspinatus muscles: Medial border of the scapular spine
6. Lateral epicondyle: 2 m distal
7. Gluteal muscle: Upper outer quadrant
8. Greater trochanter: Posterior to the trochanteric process
9. Knee: Medial fat pad

Treatment

Savella (milnacipran), Cymbalta (duloxetine), Lyrica (pregabalin), and Ultram (tramadol) have all been shown to be beneficial for fibromyalgia. Other than ultram (tramadol), which is an opiate-like substance but also increases serotonin and norepinephrine, no opioids (morphine-like substances) have been shown to be beneficial. Opioids thus are not recommended for treatment, nor are nonsteroidal anti-inflammatory agents based on lack of clear efficacy. Savella was approved by the FDA for the treatment of fibromyalgia in 2009, Cymbalta in 2008, and Lyrica in 2007.

Savella: In the study that helped Savella gain FDA approval for fibromyalgia, patients were divided into three groups. The first group received 200 mg of Savella per day, the second group received 100 mg/day, and the third group received a placebo. The proportion of patients reporting that their status very much improved at week 15 was 51% for those taking 200 mg, 48.3% for those taking 100 mg, and 32.9% for the placebo group. A significant reduction in pain was observed as early as 1 week, with maximal pain relief within 9 weeks.[12] Savella can be initiated by prescribing the starter pack.

Cymbalta: In the study that helped Cymbalta gain FDA approval for fibromyalgia, patients were randomized into two groups, one receiving Cymbalta 60 mg twice a day and the other receiving a placebo. All patients in the study were female. A 50% improvement from baseline function as measured by the Fibromyalgia Impact Questionnaire scores was seen in 30% of patients in the Cymbalta group as compared to 16% in the placebo group. The Cymbalta group reported fewer tender points on examination and less pain interference compared with the placebo group.[13] See the chapter on antidepressant medication used for neuropathic pain, Chapter 13, which reviews the starting doses of Cymbalta, titration schedule, and side effects.

Lyrica: In the study that helped Lyrica gain FDA approval for fibromyalgia, patients with fibromyalgia were randomized into four groups: Lyrica at 150 mg/day, 300 mg/day, or 450 mg/day, or placebo. A 50% pain reduction was reported in 29% of those treated with Lyrica 450 mg/day, 18.9% in the 300-mg/day group, and 13% in the 150-mg/day group. These values compared with 13% of patients in the placebo group. There was no difference in clinical response between patients in the 150-mg/day group and the placebo group.[14] Lyrica is ineffective for fibromyalgia if not titrated to therapeutic doses. The mean sleep quality scores improved significantly in the 300- and 450-mg/day Lyrica groups as compared to those on placebo.

Tramadol: Tramadol is not approved by the FDA for fibromyalgia. There are no clear and definitive studies showing its effectiveness. This may stem from the lack of private financial support to fund the magnitude of studies needed for the generic drug. Tramadol versus placebo in a double-blind study for 6 weeks showed that the tramadol patients were more likely to continue treatment as compared to placebo.[15] Tramadol can decrease uptake of both serotonin and norepinephrine, thus should be used with caution with medications that have a similar mechanism of action, such as Savella and Cymbalta.

There is a lack of formal studies evaluating the combination of two FDA-approved medications for fibromyalgia, but if one medication alone titrated to the therapeutic dose is not significantly effective, it may be beneficial to combine two. This is known as rational polypharmacy. I suggest administering one from the antiseizure medications used for neuropathic pain (Lyrica) and one from the antidepressants (Savella or Cymbalta) used for neuropathic pain.

Exercise has been shown to be beneficial for fibromyalgia. When comparing the effects of aerobic exercise versus simple flexibility exercises, aerobic exercises have been shown to more effective. Aerobic exercise has been demonstrated to improve tender-point thresholds. There is no strong evidence to support weight training. In patients with fibromyalgia, adherence to an exercise program can be problematic, because patients become sedentary and are often deconditioned.

CASE STUDY

Case

A 34-year-old female is referred to your practice. She says she has been diagnosed with fibromyalgia and nothing seems to help. In taking her history, you find that she has had widespread pain for at least the last 5 years. It is in all four quadrants of her body. When you examine the predetermined diagnostic fibromyalgia tender points, each is painful when you push with your thumb enough to cause the tip of your fingernail to go white. She has seen other doctors and tried a number of medications (Lyrica, naproxen, and baclofen) that have not worked. She is discouraged and depressed. She has seen a rheumatologist and all blood work was negative. Her cousin has similar symptoms and is on Percocet and still in pain.

You confirm the diagnosis of fibromyalgia and decide to start Lyrica. The patient states she already tried Lyrica

and it was not helpful. She is not sure of the dose but thinks it may have been 75 mg twice a day. After further discussion and explaining your rational, you advise trying Lyrica again at the FDA-approved dose that has been shown to be helpful. You titrate the patient to a dose of 225 mg po twice a day (450 mg/day). After 8 weeks the patient reports the higher dose of Lyrica is helping her sleep and her pain has reduced. However, she still has trouble concentrating at work and has pain every day. You decide to start a second medication for fibromyalgia. You add Savella, also approved by the FDA, to her Lyrica and titrate it to 50 mg twice a day. You also send the patient to physical therapy for aerobic exercises only. At her next visit, the patient reports that the combination of medications is helpful, she is participating in physical therapy, and she is doing much better at work.

SICKLE CELL ANEMIA

Sickle cell anemia is an inherited autosomal recessive disorder. Adult hemoglobin (hemoglobin A) consists of two α-globin chains and two β-globin chains. The cause of sickle cell anemia is a point mutation in the β-globin chains. It is a single amino acid substitution, a valine for a glutamic acid (Fig. 7-4). In sickle cell anemia both β-globin chains are altered, whereas in the asymptomatic sickle cell trait only one β-globin gene is affected (Fig. 7-5). In sickle cell anemia, red blood cells polymerize into long-fiber sickle cells when deoxygenated. This is because they are less soluble than normal hemoglobin.

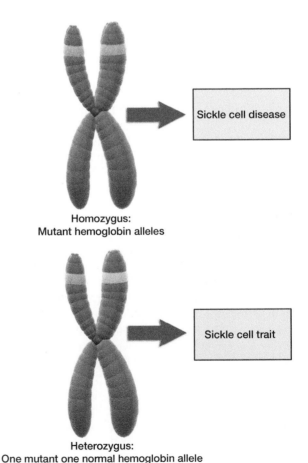

Homozygus:
Mutant hemoglobin alleles

Sickle cell disease

Heterozygus:
One mutant one normal hemoglobin allele

Sickle cell trait

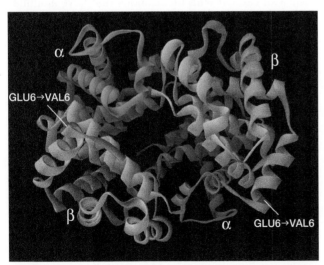

Figure 7-4 Sickle cell anemia is caused by a point mutation in both β-globin chains. There is a single amino acid substitution, a valine for a glutamic acid.

Figure 7-5 Sickle cell disease (anemia), is symptomatic and caused by a point mutation in both β-globin chains. Sickle cell trait, is asymptomatic and is caused by a point mutation in only one of the β-globin chains.

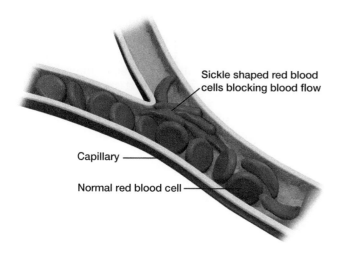

Figure 7-6 Vascular obstruction and ischemia seen in sickle cell disease.

Sickled hemoglobin leads to vascular obstruction and ischemia via three root mechanisms. The first is a physical block of the vessel by the sickled cell (Fig. 7-6). The second is an intravascular hemolysis that decreases the availability of nitric oxide (which allows blood vessels to dilate), which in turn increases vascular tone and pulmonary hypertension. The third is damage to the vascular endothelium itself by the sickled cell, a process that provokes a proliferative lesion involving white cells, smooth muscle cells, and platelets that underlie large vessel stroke. These episodes of sickling deprive tissues and organs of oxygen-rich blood; this can lead to organ damage especially in the lungs, kidneys, spleen, and brain.

Patients with sickle cell anemia have pain from acute vaso-occlusive crisis, which occurs when microcirculation is obstructed by sickled red blood cells. On top of these acute attacks, patients develop chronic pain as both the skeleton and end organs suffer the sequelae of repeated episodes of ischemia and infarction. Avascular necrosis (AVN) is a disease of bone death caused by interruption of blood supply. Clinically, AVN most commonly affects the end of long bones such as the femur.

About 300,000 children are born with sickle cell anemia each year. Males and females are affected equally. Sickle cell anemia is seen in African Americans. There was a benefit in having sickle cell trait (only one β gene affected) in regions such as Africa, where malaria was common. People with sickle cell trait are more tolerant of infection from malaria, giving them a survival benefit. About 1 in 500 African American children in the United States are born with sickle cell anemia. The severity of symptoms varies from person to person.

History and Examination

Sickle cell patients present with two types of pain complaints. One presentation is acute sickle crisis: Sudden tissue infarction in skeletal and soft tissue caused by obstruction in the microcirculation by sickled red blood cells. A pain crisis caused by sickle cell can involve the abdomen, joints, bone, and soft tissue. It can also involve the lungs, known as acute chest syndrome. Defined as a new infiltrate on chest radiograph associated with fever and respiratory problems, this is often preceded by infection, exposure to cold weather, hypoxia, or dehydration. Sickle cell crises usually require hospitalization. Patients report pain scores much higher than baseline; as the crisis resolves the pain usually stops.

The other presentation is chronic pain secondary to baseline destruction of tissue. Patients often complain of pain in the hips, shoulders, and ankles. This results from chronic infarction of the sensitive periosteum of bone. Interestingly, the knees are seldom involved. Pain also develops in the spine, causing chronic back pain. X-rays of the spine show a "fish mouth" appearance.

The examination of a sickle cell anemia patient should be no different than your typical examination. Patients with chronic pain from sickle cell anemia often have joint pain. It is of particular importance to test hip strength and range of motion, because the hips are most commonly affected. Both active and passive joint movements may be restricted and painful. An MRI is the most sensitive study and is the imaging modality of choice if AVN is suspected. The use of gadolinium is useful in early detection.

Treatment

Preventing the progression of the disease is key in helping with pain. Hydroxyurea, a cytotoxic drug, helps reduce the production of adult hemoglobin and therefore the number of circulation cells that can sickle. A small portion of hemoglobin comes from hemoglobin F, fetal hemoglobin, which does not have β chains. The production of hemoglobin F increases as the percentage of adult hemoglobin decreases. The use of hydroxyurea reduced the incidence of painful crises from a median of 5.5/yr to 2.5/yr in patients who had at least three painful crises in the previous year.

For an acute crisis, the goal is to combat the pain aggressively, knowing that the acute pain will dissipate as the crisis resolves. First-line treatment should be an opioid. There is no particular opioid that is more beneficial than others for a sickle cell crisis. Typically, patient-controlled anesthesia (PCA) should be used if the patient is in the hospital.

Most of the pain from sickle cell anemia is nociceptive. Nociceptive pain results from an injury that stimulates pain receptors, as compared to neuropathic pain, which is caused by nerve damage. Nonsteroidal anti-inflammatory drugs (NSAIDs) are the backbone of treating nociceptive pain. They can be very helpful in combating the pain of sickle cell but should be used with caution as they can alter kidney function. Patients with sickle cell anemia most likely have an underlying nephropathy from microvascular infarction in the kidneys. Treatment with an NSAID should last no longer than 1 week and sometimes less based on the patient's kidney status, which is monitored daily in the hospital.

Sickle cell anemia patients can have chronic pain from the progression of disease. Treatment is based on the severity and duration of pain. It is helpful to place patients into three treatment categories in this progression: Patients with mild pain; patients with more intense, but intermittent, pain; and patients with constant, severe pain. Tylenol should be administered for mild pain. A short-acting opioid used at most twice a day is the preferred treatment for more intense, intermittent pain. A long-acting opioid should be considered for constant, severe pain.

When joint pain becomes severe secondary to AVN and conservative options have failed, joint replacement should be considered. The average age for this surgery is roughly 32 years.[16] Bisphosphonates, a class of drugs that prevents the loss of bone mass, are helpful in delaying the collapse of the femoral head and thus delay the need for joint replacement. Common bisphosphonates include Fosamax (alendronate), Boniva (ibandronate), and Reclast (zoledronic acid).

CASE STUDY

Case

A 46-year-old man with sickle cell anemia has complaints of chronic pain in his right hip. His right hip generates constant pain, deep and achy. The pain is worse with walking. He takes Percocet 7.5/325 twice a day for this. He has not had any hospital admissions in the last year and is on hydroxyurea. His current pain intensity is a 7 out of 10 with Percocet.

You decide to add a long-acting pain medication. You start him on a fentanyl patch at 25 μg every 3 days and change the Percocet dose to once a day as needed. In addition, you order an MRI of the right hip because of suspected AVN. He had x-rays of his right hip 5 years ago. On follow-up, his pain is slightly better but it still affects him on a daily basis. The MRI reveals advanced AVN of his right hip. You advise a right hip replacement, but the patient does not agree to this. You increase the fentanyl patch to 50 μg every 3 days, keep him on Percocet once a day. You start him on a bisphosphonate to prevent progressive bone resorption, collapse of bone, and edema at the site of AVN.

REFERENCES

1. Raja SN, Grabow TS. Complex regional pain syndrome I (reflex sympathetic dystrophy). *Anesthesiology.* 2002;96: 1254–1260.
2. Bonica JJ. Causalgia and other reflex sympathetic dystrophies. *Postgrad Med.* 1973;53(6):143–148.
3. Harden RN. Complex regional pain syndrome. *Br J Anaesth.* 2001;87: 99–106.
4. Birklein F, Riedl B, Neudörfer B. Handwerker HO: Sympathetic vasoconstrictor reflex pattern in patients with complex regional pain syndrome. *Pain.* 1998;75:93–100.
5. Cepeda MS, Lau J, Carr DB. Defining the therapeutic role of local anesthetic sympathetic blockade in complex regional pain syndrome: A narrative and systematic review. *Clin J Pain.* 2002;18(4): 216–233.
6. AbuRahma AF, Robinson PA, Powell M, et al. Sympathectomy for reflex sympathetic dystrophy: Factors affecting outcome. *Ann Vasc Surg.* 1994;8(4):372–379.
7. Taylor RS, Van Buyten JP, Buchser E. Spinal cord stimulation for complex regional pain syndrome: A systematic review of the clinical and cost-effectiveness literature and assessment of prognostic factors. *Eur J Pain.* 2006;10(2):91–101.
8. Harke H, Gretenkort P, Ladleif HU, et al. Spinal cord stimulation in sympathetically maintained complex regional pain syndrome Type 1 with severe disability: A prospective clinical study. *Eur J Pain.* 2005;9(4):363–373.
9. Gracely RH, Petzke F, Wolf JM, et al. Functional magnetic resonance imaging evidence of augmented pain processing in fibromyalgia. *Arthritis Rheum.* 2002;46(5):1333–1343.
10. Arnold LM, Hudson JI, Hess EV, et al. Family study of fibromyalgia. *Arthritis Rheum.* 2004;50(3):944–952.
11. Weir PT, Harlan GA, Nkoy Fl, et al. The incidence of fibromyalgia and its associated comorbidities: A population-based retrospective cohort study based on International Classification of Diseases, 9th Revision codes. *J Clin Rheumatol.* 2006:12(3):124–128.
12. Clauw DJ, Mease P, Palmer RH, et al. Milnacipran for the treatment of fibromyalgia in adults: A 15 week, multicenter, randomized, double-blind, placebo-controlled, multiple-dose clinical trial. *Clin Ther.* 2008;30(11):1988–2004.
13. Arnold LM, Lu Y, Crofford LJ, et al. A double-blind, multicenter trial comparing duloxetine with placebo in the treatment of fibromyalgia patients with or without depressive disorder. *Arthritis Rheum.* 2004;50(9):2974–2984.
14. Crofford LJ, Rowbotham MC, Mease PJ, et al. Pregabalin for the treatment of fibromyalgia syndrome: Results of a randomized, double-blind, placebo-controlled trial. *Arthritis Rheum.* 2005;52(4):1264–1273.
15. Russell IJ, Kamin M, Bennett RM, et al. Efficacy of tramadol in treatment of pain in fibromyalgia. *J Clin Rheumatol.* 2000;6:250–257.
16. Hernigou P, Zilber S, Filippini P, et al. Total THA in adult osteonecrosis related to sickle cell disease. *Clin Orthop Relat Res.* 2008;466(2):300–308.

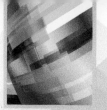

CHAPTER 8

Postoperative Pain

Pain after surgery is primarily derived from acute tissue manipulation. During surgery, inflammatory factors such as prostaglandins, bradykinin, and substance *p* are released. These increase the sensitivity of tissue pain receptors known as nociceptors (Fig. 8-1). Nociceptors are triggered by intense mechanical, chemical, or thermal noxious stimuli. For the most part, postsurgical pain is nociceptive.

In some cases, there can also be neuropathic pain, which occurs when a nerve is damaged. When a nerve is cut, it is engulfed by inflammatory molecules. Molecules such as tumor necrosis factor alpha act on injured nerve axons to pathologically increase their electrical activity until it becomes aberrant.[1] When an injured nerve fires spontaneously and irregularly, this is neuropathic pain. It is often felt as a burning, electric, shooting pain. Patients with nerve damage simultaneously experience increased pain, and sensory loss.

Pain is an individual, multifactorial experience influenced by culture, previous pain episodes, beliefs, mood, and ability to cope. Before surgery it is important to identify which patients are more likely to experience high levels of postoperative pain. Risk stratification preoperatively can be helpful. Some risk factors for higher postoperative pain levels include the following.

- Patients already taking opioids, have baseline pain requirements and higher tolerances.
- Smokers, who tend to metabolize analgesics considerably faster than nonsmokers.
- Men, as they require more analgesics than women (probably because of differences in the neuroendocrine mechanism of pain relief).
- The procedure, for example, a multilevel spine fusion, is more painful than an appendectomy.
- Anxiety, for example, patients with neurosis, suffer greater postoperative pain than those without neurosis.

Taking a history in which you gauge the patient's anxiety level before surgery is essential. In one study, 65 patients between 12 and 18 years of age reported their anxiety and expected levels of postoperative pain before surgery. Patient-controlled anesthesia use was then

Figure 8-1 Nociceptors are triggered by mechanical, chemical, or thermal noxious stimuli.

recorded through the end of the second postoperative day. Preoperative scores (anxiety and anticipated pain) predicted postoperative pain scores and number of PCA injections.[5]

In the postoperative period, you need to determine the patient's pain intensity. When possible, the visual analog pain scale from 0 to 10 should be used. The immediate postoperative examination may be limited based on the type of procedure the patient has undergone.

EFFECTS OF POSTOPERATIVE PAIN

It is critically important to control postoperative nociceptive pain and, when present, postoperative neuropathic pain. Uncontrolled postoperative pain can lead to many deleterious effects.

Physiologic Effects

Significant postoperative pain increases the catabolic demands of the body. This results in poor wound healing, weakness, and muscle breakdown. There is also increased sympathetic activity, leading to tachycardia and decreased intestinal motility. Patients with coronary artery disease are at higher risk because of uncontrolled sympathetic activity. Special care should be taken with these patients to prevent pain-induced tachycardia as well as hypertension, and emotional distress.

Functional Effects

Intense pain with any movement may cause an increased risk of postoperative deep vein thrombosis (DVT). Increased risk of atelectasis because of poor lung expansion secondary to pain is of particular worry in patients who have had procedures performed in the thoracic and upper abdominal regions. After surgery there is poor compliance with physical therapy with high pain levels.

Psychological Effects

Patients with high postoperative pain levels experience increased anxiety and depression. The best way to address anxiety is in the preprocedural office visit, where the practitioner can explain the questions and answers of the procedure and curb anxiety.

Chronic Pain Effects

Prolonged pain can lead to neuroplastic changes and the development of chronic pain when not properly treated during the acute postoperative period. Neuronal changes exist long after the offending stimulus has ended and the wound has healed. Chronic pain is pain lasting beyond what is typically expected based on the type of surgery. The intensity of acute postoperative

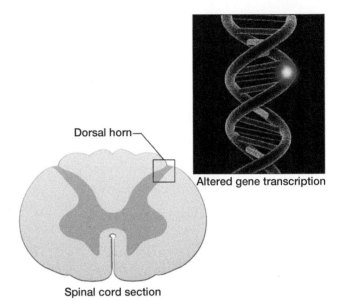

Figure 8-2 Alterations at the gene level occur in the spinal cord and brain after tissue injury from surgery.

pain correlates with the risk of developing a persistent pain state.[2] After surgery there is functional reorganization in the dorsal horn of the spinal cord. Altered gene transcription in sensory neurons and in the spinal cord occurs hours after tissue injury (Fig. 8-2). These alterations include the reduction of inhibitory pain neurotransmitters.[3,4] Further neuroplastic alteration takes place in the cortex. Maladaptive neuroplastic changes may cause a hyper-responsiveness to pain, with amplification of pain signaling. Unfortunately, if not controlled early, these neuroplastic changes can lead to chronic pain.

TREATMENT

Patients recovering from surgery can be broadly classified into two types: Ambulatory patients who are able to go home shortly after surgery and those who need to stay in the hospital for an extended period.

Patients who go home after surgery usually require a nonsteroidal anti-inflammatory drug (NSAID) for postoperative pain. NSAIDs are the backbone of treating nociceptive pain. These patients may also require a short-acting opioid such as Vicodin (hydrocodone and acetaminophen) or Percocet (oxycodone and acetaminophen) for a few days. Pain is very dynamic; therefore in the immediate postoperative period short-acting opiates are favored over long-acting ones. However, if the patient is on a long-acting opioid before surgery—for instance, for lumbar degenerative disc disease—and is going home after an anterior cruciate ligament repair, it is appropriate to continue the long-acting opioid and add the short-acting opioid to it.

Patients who remain in the hospital after surgery usually require a more advanced level of pain management. Often, these patients have decreased bowel function and can have nothing per mouth (nil per os [NPO]). Postoperative pain control for postsurgical hospitalized patients usually involves three routes of administration: Intravenous (IV) push medication, a patient-controlled analgesia (PCA), or epidural analgesia.

IV Bolus Medication

Morphine and Dilaudid are the most commonly prescribed IV opioids. They are given on an as-needed basis, usually every 2 to 4 hours. This is labor intensive for both the nurse and the patient. When the nurse-to-patient ratio is low, administration of medication at this rate is feasible. This becomes much more challenging for nurses in bigger institutions responsible for more patients and off-peak hours.

Patient-controlled Analgesia (PCA)

PCA is delivered through a programmable infusion device (Fig. 8-3). It is set up at the patient's bedside and connected to the patient's IV line. A bag of a premixed opioid solution is inserted into the machine. The patient can self-administer small doses of opioids—known as demand dose—by pushing a button connected to the PCA machine. After the patient presses the button, the machine delivers a set amount of medication. The machine will then lock for a predetermined amount of time before it can administer another demand dose (referred to as the lock-out period), to protect the patient from overmedicating.

The lock-out period is usually set at 6 minutes. The use of PCA helps to prevent the undertreatment of

pain, especially in the case of waiting for caregivers to administer dosing in large, overcrowded hospitals. PCA also helps to provide consistency in the plasma level of analgesics, decreasing the risk for side effects caused by plasma level fluctuation. There are few contraindications to PCA. Patients must be able to understand how to use the machine and must have the physical capacity to push the button. See the chapter on patient-controlled anesthesia, Chapter 16, to learn how to order a PCA.

Epidural Analgesia

Pain medication can also be delivered directly into the epidural space with the placement of an epidural catheter (Fig. 8-4). The epidural catheter is connected to a programmable infusion device, the same device that is used for PCA via an IV. The opioid solution is usually mixed with a local anesthetic, which cannot be done with a PCA. Placing the epidural catheter at the level of the nerve roots in the painful area provides a local sensory blockade. The local anesthetic blocks sympathetic output as well, allowing parasympathetic tone to dominate. Parasympathetic activity allows for intestinal peristalsis, which helps facilitate earlier bowel recovery. Because of the intimate nature of the catheter, less opioid is needed as compared to more systemic delivery; this also contributes to earlier postoperative bowel recovery.

Epidural analgesia is frequently used in patients who have had thoracic and upper abdominal operations that impair chest wall activity. The most common side effects of direct epidural opioids are urinary retention, pruritus, and nausea. Absolute contraindications include coagulopathy, septicemia, and local skin infection at the insertion site.

Patient-controlled Analgesia Versus Epidural Analgesia

An epidural catheter carries the insertional risk of dural puncture, postspinal headache, infection, hematoma, and paralysis. Another disadvantage is that it takes more time and skill to place an epidural catheter than to start a PCA or write a script for IV bolus medication. Anesthesiologists are primarily the only health professionals trained at properly placing the catheter. There can be problems with the catheter dislodging, migrating, and kinking. An epidural catheter cannot reach pain from head and neck surgery. In patients with respiratory problems, such as chronic bronchitis, epidural analgesia has the benefit of being able to use lower doses of an opiate as compared to PCA. For patients with cardiac problems, a thoracic epidural analgesia blocks cardiac sympathetic fibers, facilitating a slower heart rate, meaning less stress to the heart.

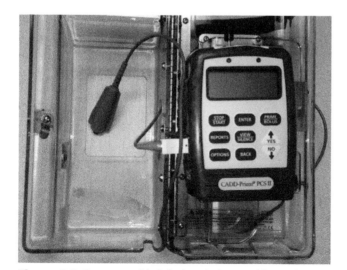

Figure 8-3 Programmable infusion device used for patient-controlled analgesia.

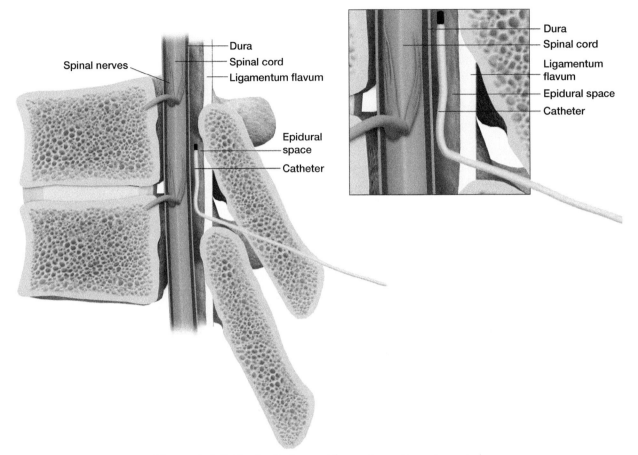

Figure 8-4 Epidural catheter used for postoperative pain control.

Some studies have shown better postoperative myocardial ischemia results with epidural analgesia, whereas others show no difference. Other outcomes of these analgesic delivery systems that have been evaluated include postoperative pain levels, bowel recovery, sedation, nausea and vomiting, and early discharge. The studies are mixed, some showing that an epidural catheter is better, whereas others show no difference. In general, early bowel recovery as well as less sedation was seen with epidural catheter placement as compared to IV PCA in most studies. Overall patient satisfaction is high with both epidural analgesia and PCA. There is no discernible difference in being able to discharge a patient earlier when comparing PCA and epidural analgesia.

NSAIDs in combination with opioids: NSAIDs are often used in combination with opioids for postoperative pain. Patients taking this combination have been shown to have lower pain scores and consume 31% fewer opioids with no difference in the incidence of adverse effects.[5] If the patient is NPO after surgery, the NSAID Toradol can be used via a IV or IM route. The typical dose is 15 mg or 30 mg IV or IM every 6 hours as needed.

If the patient complains of a burning, electric pain, or there is a high clinical suspicion of possible nerve damage, neuropathic pain medication should be administered. Symptomatic control for neuropathic pain is based on helping the nerves fire at a regular pattern. This can be accomplished by both antiseizure and antidepressant medication used for neuropathic pain. See the chapters on antiseizure and antidepressant medications used for neuropathic pain, Chapters 13 and 14, to learn the particulars of how to properly prescribe them.

It is critically important before surgery to address anxiety and catastrophizing by the patient. Presurgery is the appropriate time to provide education to families and set realistic expectations, which is especially important in elderly and pediatric populations.[6] This is also the time to formulate a plan for the best possible postoperative care for the patient.

CASE STUDIES

Case 1

A 65-year-old man with pancreatic cancer is scheduled for a Whipple procedure. A week before surgery you meet with the patient to discuss these issues in preparation for the upcoming surgery: Degree of pain he is currently feeling; the preoperative medications used for pain; his perception of the level of pain he will experience after surgery; and a review of the patient's social history including the use of alcohol, nicotine, and any previous history of dependence and abuse. You note that your patient is currently having a moderate amount of abdominal pain that he rated as a 5 out of 10 on a visual analog scale. The pain is helped by two tablets of Percocet 10/325, which he takes three to four times a day. The patient is excited to have the procedure done. He has a 30-year history of smoking but stopped 2 months ago when he was diagnosed.

You decide to use a PCA with Dilaudid for postoperative pain control. The patient is at high risk for significant postoperative pain because he is taking Percocet six to eight tablets a day, is male, has a long history of smoking, and is having a more invasive surgery known to be painful. The PCA is set at a continuous rate of 0, the demand dose is 0.4 mL, and a lock-out period of 6 minutes (see Chapter 16, The Patient-controlled Analgesia Device, for standard PCA settings and titration). You also decide to use Toradol, the IV anti-inflammatory, postoperatively to help with the pain and to reduce the amount of opioid needed.

After surgery, the patient remains on PCA and Toradol for 2 days; during this period, his pain is well controlled. He has some nausea, however, and is given an antiemetic. After 2 days, you begin the patient on a clear diet. The PCA is discontinued postop day 3. The patient is then switched back to Percocet. His bowel function returns completely and he is discharged with follow-up.

Case 2

A 32-year-old woman is seeing you for evaluation of a torn anterior cruciate ligament in the left knee. After you discuss the particulars of surgical repair, she decides to proceed with surgery. She is a nonsmoker with no history of opioid use. The surgery is uneventful. In the recovery room the patient is given IV Dilaudid 1.5 mg, which helps with the pain. The patient is discharged on Celebrex (celecoxib) 200 mg po bid and Percocet 7.5/325 one tablet every 6 hours as needed.

At a 10-day follow-up, the patient is doing well and is starting physical therapy. Two weeks later the patient calls the office for a refill of the Percocet, which you authorize. The patient reports no fever, chills, or night sweats. At a 6-week follow-up, the patient is complaining of knee pain and pain in the limb below the knee. The skin is sensitive as well. You examine the knee and there are no signs of infection or instability. At this point, you order an ultrasound, which is normal. Her laboratory work comes back normal as well. Unsure why the patient has pain, you order an MRI of the knee, which is also normal. You recommend further physical therapy. Four weeks later the patient comes back to see you and is depressed, stating that she was doing so well but now can hardly walk secondary to pain and that the skin of her leg is beginning to change color. These symptoms indicate that this is most likely complex regional pain syndrome (CRPS); you send her for a series of lumbar sympathetic blocks.

REFERENCES

1. Sorkin LS, Xiao WH, Wagner R, et al. Tumor necrosis factor-alpha induces ectopic activity in nociceptive primary afferent fibres. *Neuroscience.* 1997;81(1):255–262.
2. Kehlet H, Jensen TS, Woolf CJ. Persistent postsurgical pain: risk factors and prevention. *Lancet.* 2006;367(9522):1618–1625.
3. Samad TA, Moore KA, Sapirstein A, et al. Interleukin-1 beta-mediated induction of Cox-2 in the CNS contributes to inflammatory pain hypersensitivity. *Nature.* 2001;410(6827):471–475.
4. Harvey RJ, Depner UB, Wässle H, et al. GlyR alpha3: An essential target for spinal PGE2-mediated inflammatory pain sensitization. *Science.* 2004;304(5672):884–887.
5. Huang YM, Wang CM, Wang CT, et al. Perioperative celecoxib administration for pain management after total knee arthroplasty—a randomized, controlled study. *BMC Musculoskeletal Disorders.* 2008;9:77.
6. Logan DE, Rose JB. Is postoperative pain a self-fulfilling prophecy? Expectancy effects on postoperative pain and patient-controlled analgesia among adolescent surgical patients. *J Pediatr Psychol.* 2005;30(2):187–196.

PART II

Noninterventional Treatments

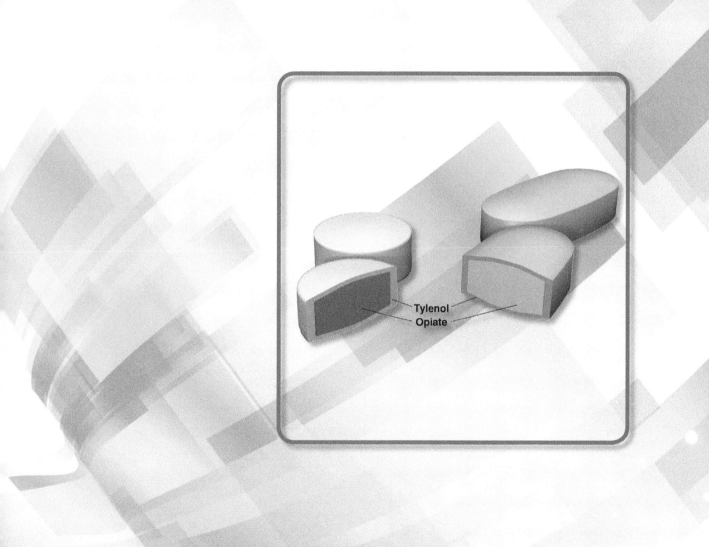

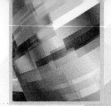

CHAPTER 9

Nonsteroidal Anti-inflammatory Drugs

WHEN TO USE	WHEN NOT TO USE AND POTENTIAL SIDE EFFECTS
HOW TO USE	▷ Gastrointestinal
	▷ Renal
	▷ Cardiovascular

Nonsteroidal anti-inflammatory drugs (NSAIDs) work by blocking inflammation at the site of pathology and by altering pain perception in the central nervous system (CNS). Peripherally, cyclooxygenase is an enzyme that converts arachidonic acid to a number of prostaglandins. Hormone-like substances, prostaglandins, participate in a wide range of body functions such as cell growth and the dilatation and constriction of blood vessels, as well as inflammation. The inflammatory prostaglandins sensitize nerve endings to the action of bradykinin, histamine, and other inflammatory factors, making them more likely to transmit pain. Peripherally, NSAIDs block the action of cyclooxygenase, halting the conversion of arachidonic acid into inflammatory prostaglandins, the key step in the inflammatory cascade (Fig. 9-1).

The cyclooxygenase enzyme has two isoforms: COX-1 and COX-2 (Fig. 9-2). Each isoform is responsible for the production of certain prostaglandins. The COX-1 isoform catalyzes the production of prostaglandins that help regulate normal physiologic function, especially in the gastrointestinal (GI) and renal tracts. The COX-2 isoform facilitates the production of

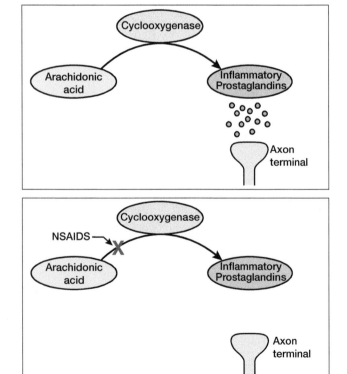

Figure 9-1 Cyclooxygenase, the enzyme blocked by NSAIDs, converts arachidonic acid to inflammatory prostaglandins.

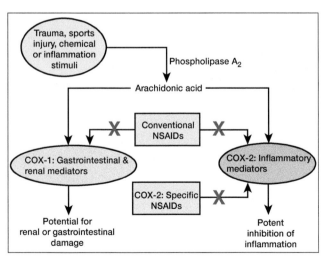

Figure 9-2 Cyclooxygenase cascade chart. Highlighting the difference between conventional NSAIDs & COX-2 specific NSAIDs.

inflammatory prostaglandins. Most NSAIDs block both the COX-1 and COX-2 isoforms of cyclooxygenase in a nonselective fashion.

The goal for treating pain has been to block the COX-2 isoform responsible for the production of inflammatory prostaglandins without blocking the COX-1 isoform responsible for the production of the homeostatic prostaglandins. Although no NSAID is completely selective for the COX-2 isoform, NSAIDs more selective for the COX-2 isoform (COX-2 inhibitors) were developed to block inflammation and pain selectively without adversely affecting the homeostatic prostaglandins regulating the GI and renal tracts. Several NSAIDs significantly more selective for COX-2 inhibitors came to market, each with a different affinity for the COX-2 isoform. Nonselective NSAIDs like ibuprofen demonstrate a seven-fold increased affinity for the COX-2 isoform; Celebrex (celecoxib), a more selective COX-2 inhibitor, shows a 30-fold increased affinity, whereas Vioxx (rofecoxib, no longer on the market) was 200 times more selective for the COX-2 isoform.

After coming to market, some COX-2 inhibitors were shown to increase the rate of adverse cardiovascular events. One such drug was Vioxx, which was taken off the market in 2004. Celebrex, the only selective COX-2 inhibitor currently on the market, has been shown to be no different in increasing the rate of adverse cardiovascular events than Naprosyn (naproxen), an older, over-the-counter, nonselective NSAID.[1] This could be explained by the fact that although Celebrex is more selective for the COX-2 isoform, it is not as potent as the previous COX-2 inhibitors. The severe imbalance in the prostaglandins produced because of Vioxx's 200-fold greater affinity for the COX-2 isoform likely led to a state in which thromboxane, a proaggregatory and vasoconstrictive prostaglandin produced from the COX-1 isoform, went unchecked.[2]

Centrally, NSAIDs work by direct action on the CNS, altering spinal nociceptive processing. As peripheral impulses reach the spinal cord, their signals can be altered before they are sent to higher centers. This modulates the perception of pain. The exact mechanism of action of NSAIDs in the CNS is not known at this point.

WHEN TO USE

NSAIDs are indicated as first-line treatment for acute or chronic conditions exhibiting pain and inflammation. They can alleviate swelling, stiffness, joint pain caused by osteoarthritis, rheumatoid arthritis, and other rheumatic conditions. NSAIDs work well for muscle strain, inflammation of a tendon or ligament, bursitis, gout, dental problems, dysmenorrhea (menstrual pain), and metastatic bone pain.

NSAIDs start to work in about 30 minutes, with a peak effect in 60 to 90 minutes. They can be used as the sole agent or in combination with other pain medications. When combined with an opioid, they have been shown to reduce the amount of opioid need by 20% to 35%.[3] The combination of an NSAID and opioid is known to have a synergistic effect—the whole is greater than the sum of its parts.

HOW TO USE

As previously discussed NSAIDs for practical application can be divided into three basic categories: Nonselective—those that block both the COX-1 and COX-2 isoforms; selective—Celebrex, which predominantly blocks the COX-2 isoform; and intravenous/intramuscular—Toradol (Ketorolac, a nonselective NSAID). Clinically, other than these three main categories, the difference between NSAIDs is minimal. There is no conclusive evidence supporting one nonselective NSAID over another for analgesia. There are over 25 different types of nonselective NSAIDs on the market. The scope of this book will focus on four of the most commonly used nonselective versions (see Table 9-1 for titration guidelines). Toradol is the only intravenous/intramuscular NSAID approved in the United States, and is nonselective (see Table 9-1 for titration guidelines). The bioavailability following administration of Toradol via IV or IM is equal but the time to

TABLE 9-1 Titration of Nonselective NSAIDs

Medication	Route	Starting Dose	Max Dose	Available Forms
Ibuprofen (Advil, Motrin)	po	200 po q6 p.r.n	800 q6 p.r.n	200, 400, 600, 800
Naproxen (Naprosyn)	po	250 po bid p.r.n	500 bid p.r.n	250, 375, 500
Meloxicam (Mobic)	po	7.5 po qd p.r.n	15 bid p.r.n	7.5, 15
Indomethacin (Indocin)	po	25 po bid p.r.n	50 tid p.r.n	25, 50
Toradol (Ketorolac)	IV or IM	15 IV or IM q6 p.r.n	30 IV or IM q6 p.r.n	15, 30

TABLE 9-2 Titration of COX-2 Selective NSAID

Medication	Route	Starting Dose	Max Dose	Available Forms
Celebrex (celecoxib)	po	100 po qd p.r.n	200 bid p.r.n	100, 200

peak plasma concentration is faster when administered via the IV route. Toradol (the intravenous NSAID) is most commonly used to control pain in patients after surgery or in those who cannot take oral medication. In a postoperative study, in which all patients received morphine by a patient-controlled analgesia (PCA) device, patients treated with Toradol at fixed intermittent boluses required 26% less morphine than the placebo group (PCA alone). Because of its potency, Toradol is limited to 5 days of use. Celebrex is the only selective COX-2 inhibitor available in the United States (see Table 9-2 for titration guidelines).

NSAIDs have a "ceiling effect"—the maximum amount of medication reached beyond which additional quantities no longer provide increased analgesia. Failure of NSAIDs to provide relief is often caused by lack of titration and a trial that lasts less than 2 weeks.

Topical NSAIDs are also available in gel and patch form, both of which last for roughly 12 hours. A topical application can be a very good option for patients who cannot tolerate oral NSAIDs, see Chapter 11, Topical Pain Medications.

WHEN NOT TO USE AND POTENTIAL SIDE EFFECTS

NSAIDs have a low abuse potential compared to other pain medication. The three main adverse effects of NSAIDs are GI, renal, and cardiovascular.

Gastrointestinal

The inhibition of the COX-1 isoform of cyclooxygenase reduces the levels of protective GI prostaglandins. These homeostatic gastric prostaglandins maintain blood flow to the gastric mucosa, promote the secretion of cytoprotective mucus, and decrease gastric acid

secretion. NSAIDs also cause direct irritation to the GI tract.

NSAIDs studied as a class are associated with a three- to five-fold increase in upper GI complications (peptic ulcer, bleeding, or perforation).[4] Generally, if oral NSAIDs are taken for at least 2 months on a regular basis, the risk of an endoscopically detectable ulcer is 1 in 5; for a symptomatic ulcer, about 1 in 70; for a bleeding ulcer, about 1 in 150; and for death from bleeding ulcer, about 1 in 1,300.[5] Risk for serious GI bleeding complications from an NSAID ranges from 1 in 2,100 in adults under age 45 to 1 in 110 for adults over age 75. Risk of GI complications increases with using NSAIDs at higher dose and with the duration of therapy. Therefore, it is essential that these medications should be used at the lowest effective dose for the shortest amount of time to treat pain. Commonly, it is possible to reduce adverse GI effects with the use of a proton pump inhibitor. NSAIDs should be avoided in people with a history of bowel disease, such as Crohn's disease and ulcerative colitis.

Renal

The inhibition of the COX-1 isoform of cyclooxygenase reduces the levels of prostaglandins that help mediate renal blood flow. Blocking these protective prostaglandins causes vasoconstriction of the afferent arterioles affecting normal glomerular perfusion. Typically, preexisting renal or systemic disease is a necessary precursor to analgesic-associated chronic renal failure.[6] Monitoring of patients on NSAIDs should include intermittent assessment of electrolytes and creatinine.

Cardiovascular

Patients taking any of the NSAIDs have an increased risk of heart problems. NSAIDs often cause salt retention and edema, putting more stress on the heart. Patients with a history of congestive heart failure have a two-fold increase in exacerbation of this condition.

NSAIDs are not recommended during the third trimester of pregnancy, as they may cause premature closure of the fetal ductus arteriosus. NSAIDs are contraindicated in individuals with Franklin triad (a syndrome of nasal polyps, angioedema, and urticaria) in whom anaphylactoid reactions have occurred.

CASE STUDY

Case
A 56-year-old female long-time patient of yours with a history of osteoarthritis states that over the last year she has had increasing pain in both her knees. The pain is dull achy and more significant in the right knee than the left. The pain is worse with movement and relieved with rest. This pain presents when she plays golf or goes for long walks. After examining both knees, you note no instability. X-rays show mild to moderate arthritis. You start an NSAID for pain control—Naproxen 250 mg po bid p.r.n. You educate the patient about side effects, especially GI, renal, and cardiovascular ones. The patient returns for follow-up stating that she uses the medication once or twice a week and that it really helps with the pain.

Five years pass and the patient reports that her knee pain over the last 4 months has increased. She finds she needs to take naproxen every day, usually twice a day. You send her for reimaging, which shows progression of her knee osteoarthritis. With the increased use of NSAIDs, you switch the patient to Celebrex 100 mg po bid p.r.n. In addition, you perform bilateral knee injections using the steroid Kenalog and the local anesthetic bupivacaine to help reduce pain and pain medication use.

REFERENCES

1. ADAPT Research Group. Cardiovascular and cerebrovascular events in the randomized, controlled Alzheimer's disease anti-inflammatory prevention trial (ADAPT). *PLoS Clin Trials.* 2006;1(7):e33.
2. Bennett JS, Daughtery A, Herrington D, et al. The use of nonsteroidal anti-inflammatory drugs (NSAIDs): A science advisory from the American Heart Association. *Circulation.* 2005;111(13):1713–1716.
3. Jirarattanaphochai K, Jung S. Nonsteroidal antiinflammatory drugs for postoperative pain management after lumbar spine surgery: A meta analysis of randomized controlled trials. *J Neurosurg Spine.* 2008;9(1):22–31.
4. Garcia Rodriguez LA, Hernandez-Diaz S. Relative risk of upper gastrointestinal complications among users of acetaminophen and nonsteroidal anti-inflammatory drugs. *Epidemiology.* 2001;12:570–576.
5. Tramer MR, Moore RA, Reynolds DJ, et al. Quantitative estimation of rare adverse events which follow a biological progression: A new model applied to chronic NSAID use. *Pain.* 2000;85(1–2):169–182.
6. Forced CM, Ejerblad E, Linblad P, et al. Acetaminophen, aspirin, and chronic renal failure. *N Eng J Med.* 2001;345:1801–1808.

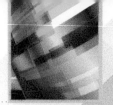

CHAPTER 10

Acetaminophen (Tylenol)

WHEN TO USE	WHEN NOT TO USE AND POTENTIAL SIDE EFFECTS
HOW TO USE	

Acetaminophen is commonly known as Tylenol in the United States and as Paracetamol in Europe. It is used to treat a variety of painful conditions. Its method of action is inhibition of prostaglandin synthesis in the central nervous system (CNS). Prostaglandins are hormone-like substances that participate in a wide range of body functions. The prostaglandins that acetaminophen inhibits in the CNS are responsible for pain transmission and fever; thus acetaminophen is useful as an analgesic and as an antipyretic (antifever) medication. Unlike ibuprofen and aspirin, acetaminophen is *not* an anti-inflammatory drug, an important distinction sometimes overlooked. Acetaminophen is a poor peripheral inhibitor of the enzyme cyclooxygenase, a key component of the inflammatory response, which is effectively inhibited by aspirin and ibuprofen. Acetaminophen also does not affect platelet function, like aspirin and ibuprofen, another important difference.

Acetaminophen can be given either orally or rectally. When taken orally, about 60% to 98% of the dose is absorbed; with rectal administration, only about 30% to 40% of the dose is absorbed. Acetaminophen is conjugated in the liver to its inactive form and excreted in the urine.

WHEN TO USE

Acetaminophen is useful as a first-line agent to relieve headache, muscle aches, and general pain. Because it lacks significant anti-inflammatory properties, it should not be used for inflammatory processes such as rheumatoid arthritis. Acetaminophen is useful when nonsteroidal anti-inflammatory drugs (NSAIDs) are contraindicated, such as in patients with a history of gastrointestinal or renal problems.

HOW TO USE

Over-the-counter Tylenol typically comes in 325-, 500-, and 625-mg pills. Maximal analgesic effects are achieved at 1,000-mg doses. Unlike other pain medication, Tylenol has a ceiling effect, that is, additional quantities do not provide additional analgesia. It is best to use the maximum dose every 4 to 6 hours as needed for pain, not to exceed a total of 4,000 mg during a 24-hour period.

WHEN NOT TO USE AND POTENTIAL SIDE EFFECTS

When used properly, acetaminophen is virtually free of any significant side effects. However, liver damage may occur with large doses. One should not exceed more than 4,000 mg in a 24-hour period. Hepatotoxicity may develop with the usual doses of acetaminophen in patients with significant alcohol intake.

Acetaminophen may be present in combination with other medications. For example, each pill of the analgesic Percocet contains 325 mg of acetaminophen as well as the opioid oxycodone, each tablet of Vicodin contains 325 mg of acetaminophen as well as the opioid hydrocodone, and Tylenol 3 contains 300 mg of acetaminophen as well as 30 mg of codeine. A careful inventory should be done of all medications patients are taking that may contain acetaminophen. Patients then should be made aware of their daily acetaminophen intake and the maximal safe daily dose of this drug. Patients should also be instructed to tell you when they start any new medications.

CASE STUDY

Case

A 58-year-old male presents with general complaints of knee pain that comes and goes. After evaluation, you determine that the patient has osteoarthritis. You prescribe Tylenol for the pain, two 500-mg tablets every 4 to 6 hours, not more than 6 tablets a day, and send the patient to physical therapy. He returns to your office stating he is having less pain and is able to function normally again. Later, during a routine annual check-up, the patient states that his knee pain began to increase 2 months ago. At that time, he went to another doctor who evaluated him for knee replacements. The patient states that the doctor determined he was not a candidate for knee replacements and instead prescribed Vicodin 5/325 one tablet every 6 hours as needed for pain. The patient says he has been taking the Vicodin 5/325 around the clock in combination with the Tylenol you prescribed, which helps with the pain. Each pill of Vicodin contains 5 mg of hydrocodone and 325 mg of Tylenol, thus four tablets a day equals 1,300 mg, added to the six tablets of acetaminophen 500 mg each, which equals 3,000 mg separately. With both medications, the patient is receiving a grand total of 4,300 mg of Tylenol a day, 300 mg over the 24-hour maximum of 4,000. You send the patient for liver enzymes, stop the Tylenol, and educate him about the presence of acetaminophen in multiple medications.

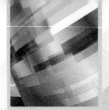

CHAPTER 11

Topical Pain Medications

WHEN TO USE

HOW TO USE

WHEN NOT TO USE AND POTENTIAL SIDE EFFECTS

Local anesthetics, nonsteroidal anti-inflammatory drugs (NSAIDs), and the neurolytic substance capsaicin are three commonly used topical pain medications. These topical medications provide localized relief, targeting tissue on which they are directly applied.[1]

The local anesthetic Lidocaine is approved by the Food and Drug Administration (FDA) in both patch and jelly form. When applied to the skin, it numbs the area underneath it. Lidocaine blocks sodium-gated channels, which have been shown to play a critical role in the initiation and maintenance of many types of pain. Pain models have demonstrated an upregulation of abnormal sodium channels in damaged peripheral sensory nerves.[2] In animal studies, inflammatory conditions such as osteoarthritis have also reported abnormal sodium channels that when antagonized reduce pain.[3] Roughly 1% to 5% of lidocaine from the patch (a very safe amount) has been shown to be systemically absorbed in healthy patients.[4]

The NSAID diclofenac was approved by the FDA in both patch and gel form. NSAIDs function peripherally by blocking the enzyme cyclooxygenase, which converts arachidonic acid to inflammatory prostaglandins. The inflammatory prostaglandins sensitize nerve endings to the action of bradykinin, histamine, and other inflammatory factors, making them more likely to transmit pain. Peripherally, NSAIDs halt this inflammatory cascade. After application directly to the knee nine times over a 5-day period, detectable concentrations of diclofenac are seen in the synovial fluid of the knee. Patients with osteoarthritis of the knee and hand treated with topical diclofenac gel reported pain reduction of 51% and 46%, respectively.[5] The amount of diclofenac systemically absorbed from the gel preparation is on average 93% less than that of the systemic exposure from oral diclofenac.[6]

Capsaicin, the last of the three topical pain medications covered in this book, is an active ingredient in chili pepper. It comes in both a cream form and a patch. Its method of action is to deplete—or "burn out"—small peptides in cutaneous nerves that are involved in sending pain transmissions to the brain. Capsaicin is thought to lead to the depletion of substance P in C fibers (C fibers are unmyelinated nerves that transmit pain), resulting in their reduced peripheral excitability. Although initial exposure excites these nociceptor terminals, prolonged exposure leads to their insensitivity to capsaicin as well as other noxious stimuli.

WHEN TO USE

Topical medications can be employed for pain in a focal area, when the patient has adverse effects with oral medication, when there is poor compliance with oral medication, or when patients are completely adverse to taking pills. Topical medications can be used with an oral medication or as a stand-alone pain medication.

Lidocaine patches are FDA approved for use in postherpetic neuralgia (PHN). Clinically, people have used the patch to treat a multitude of painful conditions including peripheral neuropathy, post-thoracotomy pain syndrome, postmastectomy pain syndrome, stump pain, and scar neuroma pain.

The topical forms of diclofenac are useful in both musculoskeletal pain (sprains, strains, and contusions) and osteoarthritis.[6,7]

Capsaicin is FDA approved for the treatment of PHN. Studies have shown it to be useful in osteoarthritis and diabetic neuropathy.[8] Clinically, capsaicin—like lidocaine—has been used to treat the above painful conditions.

TABLE 11-1 Topical Analgesics—Forms, Strengths, and Application

Medication	Form	Strength (%)	Application Instructions
Lidocaine	Patch	5	Apply once a day
Lidocaine	Jelly	2	Apply four times a day PRN
Diclofenac (Flector)	Patch	1.3	Apply once every 12 h PRN
Diclofenac (Voltaren)	Gel	1	Apply four times a day PRN
Capsaicin	Cream	0.025 and 0.075	Apply four times a day PRN
Capsaicin (Qutenza)	Patch	8	Applied once in the office

HOW TO USE

The standard strength of a lidocaine patch is 5% (Table 11-1). It is a 10- × 14-in patch with a sticky aqueous base on one side and a nonpolyester felt back on the other. The patient should apply a lidocaine patch directly over the area of pain. One can apply up to three lidocaine patches at a time if a broad area of coverage is needed. Directions accompanying the original lidocaine patches indicated that the patch should be applied 12 hours on and 12 hours off. Clinically, lidocaine patches can be applied safely for 12, 18, and 24 hours.[9] Lidocaine also comes in a 2% jelly form and is good for application to the hands, feet, and face.

The standard strength of a diclofenac patch is 1.3%. It too has a sticky aqueous base on one side and a nonpolyester felt back on the other. It works for roughly 12 hours. The patch should be applied directly over the area of pain and changed if needed, as it starts to wear out after 12 hours. The gel form of diclofenac is rubbed into the area of pain four times a day as needed. The recommended dosage is up to 4 g four times daily for the lower extremities (knees, ankles, and feet) and 2 g four times daily for the upper extremities (elbows, wrists, and hands).

Capsaicin cream is available in over-the-counter formulation (0.025% and 0.075%). It is applied directly to the area of pain four times a day. Although the other two topical pain medications work to relieve pain right away, capsaicin cream has an induction phase. During the induction phase the patient feels burning—remember that it has the same active ingredient as chili peppers. After repeated application, there is a functional desensitization over the area; the pain response is attenuated.[7] Remind the patient not to rub the eyes after applying capsaicin cream. The patch form is much stronger (8%) than the cream and must be applied at the doctor's office; this is a one-time application. The skin is prepped with topical lidocaine cream (2.5% lidocaine/prilocaine) amply applied to the area of pain and allowed to work in for 15 minutes until the skin is numb. The lidocaine cream is then removed, leaving the skin clean and dry. The capsaicin patch (8%) is applied to the skin and removed after an hour. Cooling packs and/or a shot of Toradol (30 mg IM) may be needed if the capsaicin causes a burning pain during the treatment. After the patch is removed a cleansing jelly, which comes in the pack, is applied to the area and neutralizes any capsaicin left on the skin. The jelly is then removed.

WHEN NOT TO USE AND POTENTIAL SIDE EFFECTS

The low systemic absorption and decreased side-effect profile is the clinical advantage of topical pain medication. Side effects appear to be limited to mild skin irritation at the site of application.[4] The major side effect of capsaicin cream is burning at the application site during the induction phase. The burning sensation diminishes with time but may take 3 days to 2 weeks of regular use before this happens.[10,11] Clinically, the use of capsaicin in cream is limited as some patients are unable to tolerate the induction phase.

CASE STUDIES

Case 1

A 75-year-old female is seeing you for the first time. She has significant osteoarthritis in both hands. The pain had been controlled for the most part with over-the-counter Motrin (an NSAID). Four months previously, the patient had a gastrointestinal bleed that has now resolved. Since that time, she has not been taking Motrin or any other NSAID, as per the instructions of the doctor at the hospital. The patient and her daughter want to know if it is OK for the patient to start taking Motrin again because it worked so well. You explain that there is a safer way that she can use an NSAID for the osteoarthritis of her hands. The NSAID, Voltaren gel is Prescribed to be applied four time a day as needed. The Voltaren should relieve the pain with only a minute amount of systemic absorption. This will minimize the risk of provoking a subsequent gastrointestinal bleed. The patient uses the gel on her hands with good pain relief.

Case 2

A 68-year-old male has been seeing you for PHN in roughly the T6 dermatome on the right. For this pain you prescribed tramadol, which caused nausea and the inability to think clearly. At a follow-up visit accompanied by his wife, the patient reports great difficulty tolerating any medication, the patient previously tried lyrica, and states that he does not want to be on any more pills. You explain to the patient that there are a number of options that can be used to treat the pain from PHN. You review the use of capsaicin cream, lidocaine patches, and a series of thoracic epidural steroid injections for the treatment of his PHN. After a full discussion, the patient decides to go with a series of thoracic epidural steroid injections and lidocaine patches. The patient does very well and goes from using the lidocaine patches around the clock to 2 to 3 days a week.

REFERENCES

1. Galer BS. Topical medications. In: Loesner JD, Butler SH, Chapman CR, Turk DC, eds. *Bonica's Management of Pain.* 3rd ed. Philadelphia, PA: Lippincott Williams & Wilkins; 2001:1736–1742.
2. Waxman SG. The molecular pathophysiology of pain: Abnormal expression of sodium channel genes and its contribution to hyperexcitability of primary sensory neurons. *Pain.* 1999;(Suppl 6):S133–S140.
3. Anand P. Capsaicin and menthol in the treatment of itch and pain: Recently cloned receptors provide the key. *Gut.* 2003;52(9):1233–1235.
4. Gammaitoni AR, Davis MW. Pharmacokinetics and tolerability of lidocaine patch 5% with extended dosing. *Ann Pharmacother.* 2002;36(2):236–240.
5. Endo Licenses US rights for Voltaren gel—The first FDA-approved topical treatment for relief of osteoarthritis pain. *Medical News Today* March 6, 2008.
6. Voltaren gel [prescription information. Parsippany, NJ: Novartis Consumer Health/Endo Pharmaceuticals; 2007].
7. Moore RA, Tramer MR, Carroll D, et al. Quantitative systemic review of topically applied non-steroidal anti-inflammatory drugs. *BMJ.* 1998;316(7128):333–338.
8. Recommendations for the medical management of osteoarthritis of the hip and knee: 2000 update. American College of Rheumatology Subcommittee on Osteoarthritis Guidelines. *Arthritis Rheum.* 2000:43(9):1905–1915.
9. Gammaitoni AR, Alvarez NA, Galer BS. Safety and tolerability of the lidocaine patch 5%, a targeted peripheral analgesic: A review of the literature. *J Clin Pharmacol.* 2003;43:111–117.
10. Bernstein JE, Korman NJ, Bickers DR, et al. Topical capsaicin treatment of chronic postherpetic neuralgia. *J Am Acad Dermatol.* 1989;21(2 Pt 1):265–270.
11. Watson CP, Evans RJ. The postmastectomy pain syndrome and topical capsaicin: A randomized trial. *Pain.* 1992;5(3):375–379.

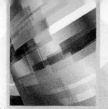

CHAPTER 12

Muscle Relaxants

WHEN TO USE

HOW TO USE

WHEN NOT TO USE AND POTENTIAL SIDE EFFECTS

Muscle relaxants are broadly classified into two categories: Those that act peripherally at the muscle itself and those that act in the central nervous system (CNS). Muscle relaxants that act peripherally work at the neuromuscular junction (where nerves and muscle fibers communicate) decreasing muscle tone and possibly causing paralysis. They are commonly used in surgery. An example of a peripherally acting muscle relaxant is succinylcholine. Peripherally acting muscle relaxants are beyond the scope of this book and rarely used in pain management.

Centrally acting muscle relaxants are used to reduce spasticity and alleviate pain caused by muscle spasm. Three of the most commonly used centrally acting muscle relaxants are Baclofen (Lioresal), Zanaflex (Tizanidine), and Flexeril (Cyclobenzaprine). Table 12-1 presents an overview of their methods of action.

- Baclofen acts like the inhibitory neurotransmitter γ-aminobutyric acid (GABA). It decreases activity from central neural outputs, primarily in the spinal cord, that control the contraction of skeletal muscle.

TABLE 12-1 Methods of Action of the Most Commonly Administered Centrally Acting Muscle Relaxants

Medication	Method of Action
Baclofen (Lioresal)	GABA agonist in the brain and spinal cord
Zanaflex (Tizanidine)	Centrally acting α_2 adrenergic agonist that inhibits excitatory amino acid release from spinal interneurons
Flexeril (Cyclobenzaprine)	Structurally related to tricyclic antidepressants (TCAs). The mechanism of action is unknown but thought to decrease α-motor neuron firing in the brain stem

Some studies have shown that baclofen also has analgesic effects by decreasing the responsiveness of nociceptive (pain) neurons (Fig. 12-1).[1]

- Zanaflex works as an agonist of the noradrenergic α_2 receptor. By stimulating the α_2 receptor, there is a

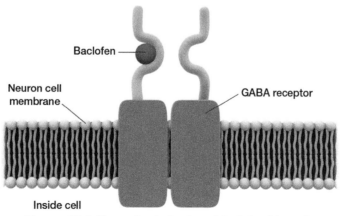

Figure 12-1 The method of action of Baclofen (Lioresal).

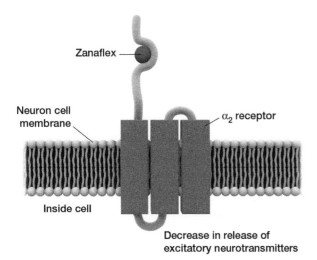

Figure 12-2 Method of action of Zanaflex (Tizanidine) is to decrease excitatory neurotransmitters.

decrease in the release of excitatory neurotransmitters. This increases the effects of inhibitory interneurons on skeletal muscle contraction (Fig. 12-2).

- Flexeril has an unknown mechanism of action. However, experts believe that the muscle relaxant works at the level of the brainstem, decreasing the firing of motor neurons.

WHEN TO USE

Practitioners use muscle relaxants as first-line agents to reduce spasticity in upper motor neuron syndromes such as multiple sclerosis, spinal cord injury, cerebral palsy, and poststroke syndrome. Spasticity is muscular hypertonicity with increased resistance to stretch. After an injury to the central nervous system (CNS), muscle tone is often flaccid with hyporeflexia. This precedes the spasticity that develops later. The interval between the CNS lesion and the appearance of spasticity varies from days to months. The most likely cause of spasticity is the removal of descending inhibitory influences on the spinal cord. These centrally acting muscle relaxants help to restore the natural inhibitory actions of the neural outputs from the spinal cord on skeletal muscle

contraction. The use of muscle relaxants may increase range of motion in a spastic limb which alone can improve both function and pain.

Muscle relaxants are also first-line agents for acute muscular pain or spasms from peripheral musculoskeletal conditions. Spasm is the sudden involuntary contraction of a muscle or a group of muscles. Conditions include myofascial pain syndrome and mechanical low back or neck pain. Muscle relaxants should be used in combination with physical therapy rather than in isolation. In clinical practice your patient might describe tight muscle spasms—for example, in the lower back—which can often respond nicely to a muscle relaxant. Procedures that involve manipulation of large skeletal muscles may also cause muscles to go into spasm; a muscle relaxant may be very helpful in this situation. Physicians routinely order muscle relaxants prophylactically after spinal surgery.

HOW TO USE

In 2001, a bill was passed by the Oregon state legislature requesting an evidence-based review of the state's most expensive drug classes, which included muscle relaxants. Work performed at the Oregon Health and Science University Center reviewed the available literature. Based on their work in comparing muscle relaxants[2] there is fair evidence that:

- Baclofen, Zanaflex, and Flexeril have consistently been found to be more effective than placebo in fair-quality clinical studies for relieving spasticity.
- Baclofen and Zanaflex may be better for spasticity.
- Flexeril and Zanaflex may be better for spasm caused by musculoskeletal painful conditions.

The use of muscle relaxants is usually limited to the treatment of spasticity from a CNS lesion or acute painful muscle spasms. Long-term use of muscle relaxants in chronic pain is controversial. In clinical practice they have been used for chronic pain, but studies of efficacy in this capacity are mixed. Table 12-2 presents dosing for the most commonly used muscle relaxants.

TABLE 12-2 Dosing Information for the Most Commonly Used Muscle Relaxants for Pain Management

Medication	Route	Starting Dose	Max Dose	Available Forms (mg)
Baclofen (Lioresal)	PO	5 mg tid p.r.n	20 mg tid	10, 20
Zanaflex (Tizanidine)	PO	2 mg tid p.r.n	8 mg qid	2, 4, 6
Flexeril (Cyclobenzaprine)	PO	5 mg tid p.r.n	20 mg tid	5, 10

There is an extended release form of Flexeril called Amrix (Cyclobenzaprine hydrochloride extended release). The recommended dose is 15 mg daily. It is usually given 4 hours before bedtime. Some patients may require up to 30 mg/day.

TABLE 12-3 Side Effects for the Most Common Muscle Relaxants

Medication	Side Effects
Baclofen (Lioresal)	Weakness
Zanaflex (Tizanidine)	Sedation
Flexeril (Cyclobenzaprine)	Dry mouth (anticholinergic effects)

WHEN NOT TO USE AND POTENTIAL SIDE EFFECTS

All muscle relaxants can cause dizziness, drowsiness, dry mouth, and weakness. Table 12-3 presents specific side effects for each of the muscle relaxants that go beyond the generalized potential side effects of all muscle relaxants.

Flexeril, as previously noted, is structurally related to tricyclic antidepressants (TCAs), which inhibit the reuptake of norepinephrine and serotonin. Flexeril should be used with caution with medications that also inhibit the uptake of norepinephrine and serotonin such as TCAs and Tramadol (which also goes by the name Ultram when combined with Tylenol). An example of a potentially dangerous medical regimen for pain would include a patient prescribed Flexeril, Elavil (Amitriptyline a TCA), and Tramadol together.

It is essential that these muscle relaxants should not be stopped abruptly unless the patient is on a starting dose. Hallucinations and seizures have resulted from abrupt withdrawal. A muscle relaxant can be tapered off over a 5-day period, but if the patient is on high doses for a prolonged period the medication should be tapered off over a 2-week period.

CASE STUDY

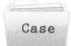

Case

A 27-year-old female with relapsing, remitting multiple sclerosis on β-interferon comes to see you. She has axial low back pain that she describes as a tight, squeezing pain that will wax and wane. MRI of her lumbar spine is normal. Her examination is normal except that increased muscle tone is palpable in the lumbar paraspinal muscles. You perform trigger point injections, send the patient to physical therapy (to learn proper low back stretching exercise), and prescribe Baclofen 10 mg one-half to one tablet three times a day as needed for muscle spasm. The patient has less pain and is performing at home the exercises she learned at physical therapy.

REFERENCES

1. Davidoff R. Antispasticity drugs: Mechanism of action. *Ann Neurol.* 1985;17(2):107–116.
2. Chou R, Peterson K, Helfand M. Comparative efficacy and safety of skeletal muscle relaxants for spasticity and musculoskeletal conditions: A systematic review. *J Pain Symptom Manage.* 2004; 28(2):140–175.

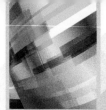

CHAPTER **13**

Antidepressant Medications Used for Neuropathic Pain

WHEN TO USE
▶ Neuropathic Pain
▶ Fibromyalgia

HOW TO USE

WHEN NOT TO USE AND POTENTIAL SIDE EFFECTS

Pain is transmitted through the nervous system. There are two main types of pain. Nociceptive pain and Neuropathic pain. Nociceptive pain is the natural consequence of tissue injury. Sensation from damaged tissue transmitted along well-functioning, healthy nerves to the brain for interpretation. An example of this is arthritis. The brain senses nociceptive pain as a sharp or achy type of pain.

In contrast, neuropathic pain involves nerve damage. When the nerves themselves become damaged, rather than their surrounding tissue (Fig. 13-1). Damaged nerves fire aberrantly and without provocation. A common example of neuropathic pain is diabetic peripheral neuropathy. The brain senses neuropathic pain as a burning, electric, tingling type of pain.

A stimulus with sufficient strength triggers the start of a neurotransmission. On a grand scale the impulses travel along the neural pathways from a small peripheral nerve, to a larger more centralized nerve, to the spinal cord, and then up to the brain for interpretation. At a local level a stimulus above the minimal threshold

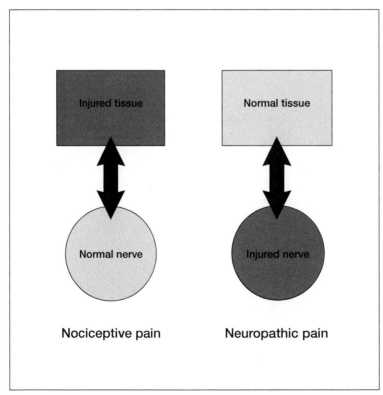

Figure 13-1 Neuropathic pain versus nociceptive pain.

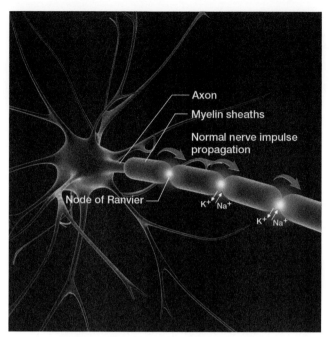

Figure 13-2 Normal nerve transmission.

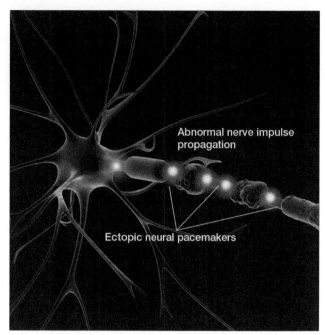

Figure 13-3 Ectopic neuronal pacemakers forming at various sites along the length of an injured nerve.

triggers the dendrites of a nerve to internalize the signal, propagate that action potential, in a well-controlled manner, along the axon as sodium rushes in and potassium rushes out between the nodes of Ranvier. Finally the nerve releases, via a calcium controlled–channel system, neurotransmitters across the synaptic cleft at the axon terminal to pass on the impulse on to the next nerve (Fig. 13-2). With nerve damage, ectopic neuronal pacemakers can form at various sites along the length of an injured nerve. In addition, there is an increased response to stimuli that would not normally be painful (Fig. 13-3).

The use of certain antidepressant medication for neuropathic pain occurred as the result of clinical observation. Patients were reporting back to their doctors that although the antidepressant medication may or may not have helped their depression, it reduced the burning pain in their feet. Doctors began to take note that a few of the antidepressant medications worked particularly well for their patients' neuropathy. At first, it was theorized that the antidepressants most likely helped with depression and pain reduction was a consequence of this. Then it was observed that the response occurred only with particular antidepressants and seemed to work irrespective of the drugs' effects on depression.[1] Further evidence showed that the antidepressants that worked on pain were found to work more rapidly on pain than depression and at doses significantly lower than have been shown to be therapeutic for depression.

The tricyclic antidepressants (TCAs), which work by blocking the reuptake of norepinephrine and serotonin,

were one of the first antidepressant medications found to be particularly helpful for neuropathic pain. The mechanism of action of TCAs in the prevention of neuropathic pain is not known. TCAs are divided into two classes: Tertiary amines and secondary amines. The tertiary amines typically work better but have a higher propensity for side effects. The two most commonly prescribed TCAs are amitriptyline (Elavil), a tertiary amine, and nortriptyline (Pamelor), a secondary amine.

Antidepressants that block both norepinephrine and serotonin, such as TCAs, can work well for neuropathic pain. Selective serotonin reuptake inhibitors (SSRIs) are not recommended for neuropathic pain.[2] In clinical trials, the efficacy of SSRIs for treating neuropathic pain in humans has been inconsistent.[3] SSRIs including Sertraline (Zoloft), Paroxetine (Paxil), and Fluoxetine (Prozac) are not recommended for the treatment of neuropathic pain.

Duloxetine (Cymbalta) is a serotonin and norepinephrine transport inhibitor. It is relatively balanced in its capacity for both serotonin and norepinephrine reuptake inhibition. Its method of action in pain relief is not known, but it is thought to modulate the descending inhibitory pain pathway in the brain and spinal cord, facilitating an endogenous analgesic mechanism. Pain messages travel like two-way traffic. One pathway, the ascending pathway sends the message to the brain whereas the other pathway, descending pathway, modulates its strength (Fig. 13-4). In 2004, the Food and Drug Administration (FDA) approved duloxetine (cymbalta) for the treatment

Figure 13-4 Descending inhibitory pain pathway. Certain antidepressants such as TCAs and cymbalta have been theorized to reduce neuropathic pain by working on the descending pathway.

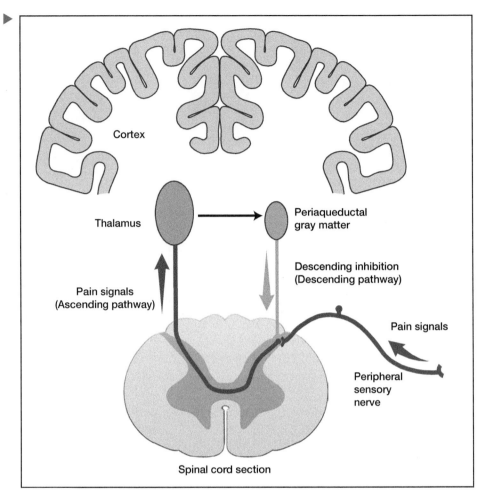

of diabetic peripheral neuropathy. It is a treatment for the same types of neuropathic pain for which TCAs are used.

WHEN TO USE

Neuropathic Pain

Nerve damage may occur in several ways. Uncontrolled diabetes, HIV, or alcohol abuse commonly injures distal peripheral nerves. The rate of diabetes, and thus diabetic peripheral neuropathy, in the United States is growing rapidly. One study looked at the rate of neuropathy in patients with newly diagnosed noninsulin-dependent diabetes who were followed for 10 years. On diagnosis, 8.3% of patients had neuropathy; at 10 years the rate of neuropathy grew to 41.9%.[4] Nerves can also be damaged by medications, such as ethambutol, which is used to treat tuberculosis. Nerves can be entrapped, such as in carpal tunnel syndrome, as well as entrapped by a herniated disc, such as in cervical and lumbar radiculopathy. Other common neuropathies include postherpetic neuralgia, trigeminal neuralgia, intercostal neuralgia, and stump neuromas. Sometimes a definitive

diagnosis is not possible, but if the patient describes the pain as electric and burning in nature it is reasonable to try a neuropathic pain medication.

The most common neuropathic conditions are covered in this book in Chapter 2, Neuropathic Pain. Always keep in mind that these medications are used for symptom control. Every effort should be made to detect and treat the underlying cause. Symptomatic treatment should begin while the underlying cause is being investigated. By curbing alcohol use, controlling blood glucose rates, and regulating thyroid level, further nerve damage can be prevented.

Fibromyalgia

One miscellaneous condition that responds to antidepressant medications used for neuropathic pain is fibromyalgia. Fibromyalgia is a disorder characterized by the presence of chronic widespread pain and tactile allodynia (pain caused by a nonpainful stimulus). The FDA has approved two medications: Cymbalta and Savella (milnacipran) for the treatment

TABLE 13-1 Recommendations for Use of Neuropathic Pain Medication

Drug	Starting Dose	Titration (days)	Usual Pain Range (mg/day)	Usual Depression Range (mg/day)	Available Forms (mg)
Amitriptyline (Elavil)	10 mg qhs (geriatrics) 25 mg qhs (adults)	3	10–150	50–300	10, 25, 50, 75, 100, 150
Nortriptyline (Pamelor)	10 mg qhs (geriatrics) 25 mg qhs (adults)	3	50–125	75–125	10, 25, 50, 75
Duloxetine (Cymbalta)	30 mg a day	3	60	20–60	20, 30, 60

of fibromyalgia. Although other medications may be helpful, the research to support their efficacy is insufficient.

Efficacy of Cymbalta and Savella for Fibromyalgia: Cymbalta: In the study that led to the approval of Cymbalta for fibromyalgia, researchers randomized patients into two groups. One received Cymbalta 60 mg twice a day, and the other received a placebo. All patients in the study were female. A 50% improvement from baseline function as measured by the Fibromyalgia Impact Questionnaire scores occurred in 30% of patients in the Cymbalta group compared with 16% in the placebo group. Patients in the Cymbalta group reported fewer tender points on examination and less pain interference compared with those in the placebo group.[5]

Savella: Savella is the newest medication approved by the FDA for fibromyalgia, the third in its class (joining pregabalin [Lyrica], an antiseizure medication used for neuropathic pain, and Cymbalta). Savella is a norepinephrine and serotonin reuptake inhibitor. In the study that led to the approval of Savella, researchers divided the patients into three groups. The first received 200 mg of Savella per day, the second received 100 mg per day, and the last received a placebo. The proportion of patients stating their status as very much improved at week 15 was 51% for those taking 200 mg, 48.3% for those taking 100 mg, and 32.9% for the placebo group. A significant reduction in pain was observed as early as 1 week, with maximal pain relief within 9 weeks.[6] Savella is primarily used to treat fibromyalgia and not other neuropathic pain conditions, unlike the other aforementioned antidepressants in wider use.

HOW TO USE

The starting doses and titration schedule of these medications for neuropathic pain are listed in Table 13-1.

One of the most common mistakes in using neuropathic medications is not titrating them. The medication dose for amitriptyline that works for pain is 10 to 150 mg per day. It has been shown that 73% of treated patients were prescribed 50 mg or less per day.[4] These medications can be effective only with proper titration. At 20 mg per day, the effectiveness of Cymbalta is questionable, but at 60 mg per day 51% of patients treated for diabetic peripheral neuropathy reported at least a 30% sustained reduction in pain.

These medications should be titrated for meaningful clinical pain relief. The medication should not be considered clinically ineffective if it is discontinued before the maximum dose is reached or the patient has side effects. A patient may report that Cymbalta was not effective for the pain; upon inquiry you may learn that the dosage was only 20 mg per day. If the patient has only partial pain relief, it may be necessary to add a second neuropathic pain medication.[1] This is referred to as rational polypharmacy. The second neuropathic pain medication added is usually from the other class of neuropathic pain medications; so an antiseizure medication used for neuropathic pain is added. Table 13-2 presents antidepressant dosage recommendations for treatment of fibromyalgia.

Savella is usually titrated over a 2-week period: 25 mg once a day for 4 days, followed by 25 mg twice a day for 4 days, then 25 mg in the morning and 50 mg at night for 4 days, and finally 50 mg twice a day.

TABLE 13-2 Recommendations for Use of Neuropathic Pain Medicaton in Fibromyalgia

Drug	Starting Dose (mg/day)	Titration (days)	Usual Pain Range (mg/day)	Usual Depression Range (mg/day)	Available Forms (mg)
Duloxetine (Cymbalta)	30	3	60–120	20–60	20, 30, 60
Milnacipran (Savella)	25	4	100–200	Not used for depression	12.5, 25, 50, 100

WHEN NOT TO USE AND POTENTIAL SIDE EFFECTS

There are very few contraindications to using this class of neuropathic pain medication. Table 13-3 lists possible side effects.

All of the medications mentioned in Table 13-3 inhibit the reuptake of serotonin and it is necessary that they be used with caution with other medications that also inhibit the reuptake of serotonin. These include the muscle relaxant Flexeril (Cyclobenzaprine), the analgesic Tramadol (Ultram), SSRIs for depression, and the triptan medications for migraine. Although rare, serotonin syndrome consists of agitation, diarrhea, tachycardia, increased body temperature, and mental status changes.

If it is necessary to discontinue any of these medications, it is recommended that they not be abruptly withdrawn but rather phased out gradually over a 1- to 2-week period. If you and your patient decide to switch to another medication of the same class, cross-tapering

TABLE 13-3 Possible Side Effects of Antidepressants in the Treatment of Neuropathic Pain

Drug	Most Common Side Effects
Amitriptyline (Elavil)	Anticholinergic effects (dry mouth, blurred vision, constipation, urinary retention). Contraindicated in people with cardiac conduction disturbances or arrhythmias.
Nortriptyline (Pamelor)	Anticholinergic effects (dry mouth, blurred vision, constipation, urinary retention). Contraindicated in people with cardiac conduction disturbances or arrhythmias.
Duloxetine (Cymbalta)	Nausea, somnolence, dizziness.

may be the best technique. In cross-tapering, the dose of the current medication is gradually reduced over a 1- to 2-week period, whereas the dose of the replacement medication is slowly increased simultaneously to a therapeutic range.

CASE STUDY

Case

A 55-year-old female presents for treatment of her diabetic peripheral neuropathy. You are working with her closely to help control her blood sugars. You prescribe Elavil for the painful symptoms of diabetic peripheral neuropathy. She returns to your office for routine follow-up a month later, stating that the medication did not help the burning, electric sensation she has in her feet. You had started her on 25 mg per day and allowed her to double the dose in a week if the medication was not helping. She never increased the dose past 25 mg once a day and stopped the medication 6 days before the appointment on her own because of its ineffectiveness.

You explain to the patient that this is a good medication for her neuropathic pain and that the dose may be too low. In this situation there is nothing wrong with starting at a conservative low dose. In these cases, I will often say to the patient: "I'm glad your body tolerated the medication and there were no side effects. I'm not surprised the medication was not helpful at this low dose—I just wanted to make sure your body could tolerate it." The medication should be restarted at 25 mg per day and increased by 25 mg per week for 4 weeks until the pain decreases or the patient experiences side effects. She returns for a follow-up 4 weeks later and you learn that the electric, burning pain in her feet did not subside until she reached the dose of 75 mg per day.

REFERENCES

1. Woolf CJ, Mannion RJ. Neuropathic pain: Aetiology, symptoms, mechanism, and management. *Lancet.* 1999;353(9168):1959–1964.
2. Mattia C, Paoletti F, Coluzzi F, et al. New antidepressants in the treatment of neuropathic pain: A review. *Minerva Anestesiol.* 2002;68(3):105–114.
3. Jung AC, Staiger T, Sullivan M. The efficacy of selective serotonin reuptake inhibitors for the management of chronic pain. *J Gen Intern Med.* 1997;12(6):384–389.
4. Partanen J, Niskanen L, Lehtinen J, et al. Natural history of peripheral neuropathy in patients with non-insulin dependent diabetes mellitus. *N Eng J Med.* 1995;333(2):89–94.
5. Arnold LM, Lu Y, Crofford LJ, et al. A double-blind, multicenter trial comparing duloxetine with placebo in the treatment of fibromyalgia patients with or without depressive disorder. *Arthritis Rheum.* 2004;50(9):2974–2984.
6. Clauw DJ, Mease P, Palmer RH, et al. Milnacipran for the treatment of fibromyalgia in adults: A 15-week, multicenter, randomized, double blind, placebo-controlled, multiple dose clinical trial. *Clin Ther.* 2008;30(11):1988–2004.

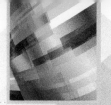

Antiseizure Medications Used for Neuropathic Pain

WHEN TO USE	**HOW TO USE**
▸ Neuropathic Pain	
▸ Fibromyalgia	**WHEN NOT TO USE AND POTENTIAL SIDE EFFECTS**

Neuropathic pain is a painful sensation from damaged nerves rather than damaged tissue (Fig. 14-1). A stimulus with sufficient strength triggers the start of a neurotransmission. On a grand scale the impulses travel along the neural pathways from a small peripheral nerve, to a larger more centralized nerve, to the spinal cord, and then up to the brain for interpretation. At a local level a stimulus above the minimal threshold triggers the dendrites of a nerve to internalize the signal, propagate that action potential, in a well-controlled manner, along its axon as sodium rushes in and potassium rushes out at the nodes of Ranvier. Finally the nerve via a calcium controlled–channel system releases neurotransmitters across the synaptic cleft at the axon terminal to pass the impulse on to the next nerve (Fig. 14-2). With damaged nerves, ectopic neuronal pacemakers can form at various sites along the length of the nerve. In addition, there is an increased response

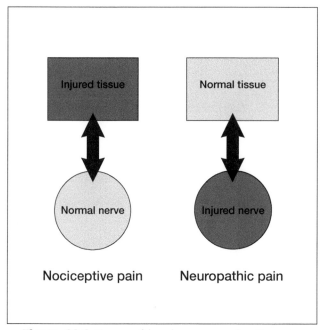

Figure 14-1 Neuropathic pain versus nociceptive pain.

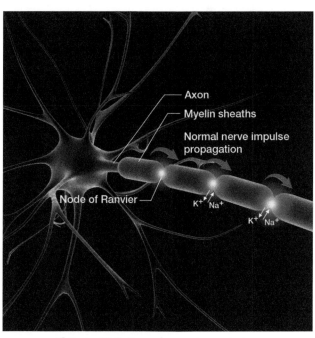

Figure 14-2 Normal nerve transmission.

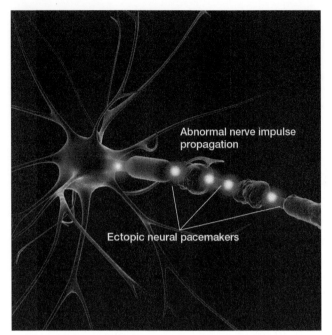

Figure 14-3 Ectopic neuronal pacemakers forming at various sites along the length of an injured nerve.

to stimuli that would not normally be painful (Fig. 14-3). This aberrant firing pattern of damaged nerves is transmitted to the brain and interpreted as neuropathic pain.

For years, physicians have been trying to control aberrant nerve firing that originates in the central nervous system (CNS) with antiepileptic (antiseizure) drugs. In seizure patients, the build-up of electrical charge from pathologic nerve firing provokes seizures. Most antiepileptic drugs work by desensitizing and decreasing the kindling of electrical charge produced by aberrant nerve firing. Although most of the antiepileptic medications function poorly in the peripheral nervous system, a few are effective. They help control pathologic nerve firing peripherally.

In clinical practice, three antiseizure medications are primarily used for neuropathic pain: Gabapentin (Neurontin), pregabalin (Lyrica), and carbamazepine (Tegretol). Ironically, gabapentin does not affect the neurotransmitter γ-aminobutyric acid (GABA). The drug received its name before its method of action was fully understood; developed to mimic GABA, gabapentin never did. Instead, it works by blocking the α_2/δ-calcium channel. When calcium enters a neuron through a voltage-gated calcium channel, the release of neurotransmitters into the synaptic cleft results, triggering an action potential. Experts think that blocking the calcium-dependent release of the neurotransmitters glutamate and substance P, reducing pathologic action potentials.

Lyrica is the newer form of gabapentin and also blocks the α_2/δ-calcium channel (Fig. 14-4). Lyrica has a higher affinity to hyperexcited neurons, selectively targeting aberrant nerve firing. Some experts believe it works faster. It is unclear if Lyrica has a clinical advantage over gabapentin, because the two drugs have not been vigorously compared in clinical trials. Gabapentin is also available as a time-release formula called Gralise.

Carbamazepine stabilizes neurons by blocking sodium channels, which decreases the likelihood of an

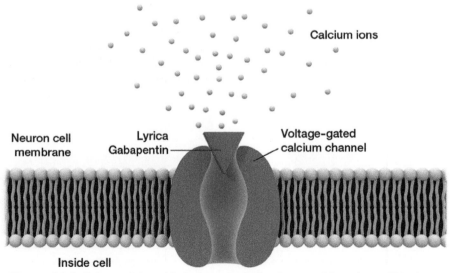

Figure 14-4 Gabapentin's and Lyrica's method of action as calcium channel blockers.

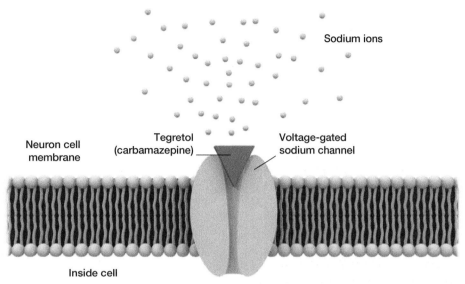

Figure 14-5 Carbamazepine method of action as a sodium channel blocker.

action potential (Fig. 14-5). An increased density of abnormal sodium channels occurs in damaged nerves. The sodium channels in damaged nerves differ pharmacologically and demonstrate different depolarization characteristics compared with ones in healthy nerves.[1] Tegretol is generally reserved for neuropathies of the facial region such as trigeminal neuralgia.

WHEN TO USE

Neuropathic Pain

Nerves can be damaged in multiple ways. The distal peripheral nerves are commonly damaged by uncontrolled diabetes, HIV, or alcohol abuse. The rate of diabetes, and thus diabetic peripheral neuropathy, in the United States is growing rapidly. One study looked at the rate of neuropathy in patients with newly diagnosed noninsulin-dependent diabetes who were followed for 10 years. On diagnosis, 8.3% of patients had neuropathy; at 10 years the rate of neuropathy grew to 41.9%.[2] Nerves can also be damaged by medications, such as Ethambutol, which is used to treat tuberculosis. Nerves can be entrapped, such as in carpal tunnel syndrome, as well as entrapped by a herniated disc, such as in cervical and lumbar radiculopathy. Other common neuropathies include postherpetic neuralgia, trigeminal neuralgia, intercostal neuralgia, and stump neuroma pain. Sometimes a definitive diagnosis is not possible, but if the patient describes the pain as electric and burning in nature, like a wire without the rubber wrapped around it, it is reasonable to try a neuropathic pain medication.

The most common neuropathic conditions are covered in this book in Chapter 2, Neuropathic Pain. Antiseizure medications that work for neuropathic pain are used for symptom control only—it is important to remember that every effort should be made to detect and treat the underlying cause—whereas symptomatic treatment is merely a stop-gap measure. For example, if your patient has diabetes, nerve damage will continue to worsen until blood sugars are controlled.

Fibromyalgia

One miscellaneous painful condition that responds well to an antiseizure medication used for neuropathic pain is fibromyalgia. Fibromyalgia is a disorder classified by the presence of chronic widespread pain and tactile allodynia (pain caused by a nonpainful stimulus). More on this condition can be found in Chapter 7, Miscellaneous Pain Disorders that Affect Multiple Areas of the Body. In 2007, Lyrica was approved by the FDA as the first medication for the treatment of fibromyalgia. Two double-blind, controlled clinical trials involving about 1,800 patients support approval for use of Lyrica in treating fibromyalgia with a dose of 300 to 450 mg per day. Doses higher than 450 mg per day have not been shown to offer any additional benefit. Although gabapentin may help in relieving the pain of fibromyalgia, the research to support its efficacy is insufficient.

HOW TO USE

Gabapentin is a generic drug that works well for neuropathic pain. The initial dose is commonly 300 bid, and the titration process involves increasing the morning

TABLE 14-1 Antiseizure Medication Used for Neuropathic Pain

Drug	Starting Dose	Titration	Max Daily Dose (mg/day)	Available Forms (mg)
Gabapentin (Neurontin)	300 mg bid	Every 5 days	3,600	100, 300, 400, 600, 800
Pregabalin (Lyrica)	25 mg (conservative) bid 50 mg (geriatric) bid 75 mg (standard) bid	Every 3 days	300 for PN 600 for PHN 450 for Fibro	25, 75, 100, 150, 200, 225, 300
Carbamazepine (Tegretol)	200 mg bid	Every 2 days	1,600	100, 200, 300, 400

PN, peripheral neuropathy; PHN, postherpetic neuralgia; Fibro, Fibromyalgia.

and evening dose by 300 mg every 5 days. Although there can be good clinical benefit as the dose is increased toward 1,800 mg per day, there is less of an efficacious response above 1,800 mg per day because of poor absorption. The maximum daily dose is 3,600 mg a day.

Lyrica, the newer form of gabapentin, is a drug that can be titrated more quickly, an advantage for people who need more rapid pain relief (e.g., hospitalized patients). Typically, practitioners start Lyrica at 25 mg bid in older patients with multiple medical comorbidities; at 50 mg bid in older, healthier patients; and at 75 mg bid in younger, healthy patients. In general, titration proceeds with the addition of 25 mg to the morning and evening dose every 3 days as needed. There is substantial variability between patients in dose response.

Carbamazepine remains the primary medical treatment for trigeminal neuralgia. It is usually second-line treatment for other painful neuropathic conditions. The usual effective dose ranges from 600 to 1,600 mg divided into two or three doses a day, but lower doses may lead to good pain relief. A typical starting dose for treating trigeminal neuralgia is 200 mg po bid.

These medications should be started individually and titrated for meaningful pain relief. The medication should not be considered clinically ineffective if it is discontinued before the maximum dose is reached or the patient has side effects. A patient may report having previously tried gabapentin and that it was not effective for the pain; upon inquiry you may learn that the dosage was 300 mg bid for a total of 600 mg a day when pain relief may not occur until a total daily dose of 1,800 mg is reached. If the patient has only partial pain relief after proper titration, a second neuropathic pain medication can be added to the first.[3] This is referred to as rational polypharmacy. The second neuropathic pain medication added is usually from the other class of neuropathic pain medications, so an antidepressant used for neuropathic pain is added.

The starting doses and titration schedule for antiseizure medications used for neuropathic pain are listed in Table 14-1. Although these medications are often studied with tid dosing, in everyday practice compliance with tid dosing is usually quite poor. In a clinical setting, giving the daily dose divided into bid dosing as compared to tid dosing may be more realistic and produce better results simply because of patient compliance.

WHEN NOT TO USE AND POTENTIAL SIDE EFFECTS

There are very few contraindications to using this class of neuropathic pain medication. Common side effects are listed in Table 14-2.

It should be noted that gabapentin and Lyrica may worsen vertigo in patients with a pre-existing condition; starting these two medications aggressively often leads to vertigo. Carbamazepine is not an option for patients with a history of bone marrow depression. A complete blood cell count is necessary before therapy to establish a baseline and after 3 weeks. Carbamazepine may inhibit the metabolism of tricyclic antidepressants and vice versa; thus using them together may elevate the levels of both drugs.

TABLE 14-2 Common Side Effects of Antiseizure Medications Used for Neuropathic Pain

Drug	Most Common Side Effects
Gabapentin (Neurontin)	Mild to moderate dizziness and sleepiness, edema
Pregabalin (Lyrica)	Mild to moderate dizziness and sleepiness, edema
Carbamazepine (Tegretol)	Drowsiness, headaches

CASE STUDY

A 48-year-old male presents with pain in both feet. The patient states that over the past 3 years he has had a slow progressive course of increased pain in his feet. He describes the pain as constant, with a burning, electric quality. He notes no pain in his back or legs. The pain is constant, symmetrical, and made worse when the patient laces up his shoes. He notes no trauma.

The patient has a long history of uncontrolled diabetes. He states that despite insulin treatment his blood sugar ranges from 150 to 350, and that he is working with his endocrinologist to better control his diabetes. The patient denies present or past use of alcohol, is on no medication besides his diabetes medication, and has a negative HIV test. At this point, it is more than reasonable to start symptomatic treatment for a painful diabetic peripheral neuropathy. You start the patient on gabapentin 300 bid, which he takes for a week and is only mildly helpful for his pain. As per your instructions he titrates the medication over time and at 1,200 bid, he finally feels pain relief. You inform the patient that although the medication helps with the pain it does not treat the underlying disease, and that it is key for him to more tightly regulate his blood sugar.

REFERENCES

1. Yaksh TL, Chaplin SR. Physiology and pharmacology of neuro-pathic pain. *Anesth Clin N Am.* 1997;15(2):335–352.
2. Partanen J, Niskanen L, Lehtinen J, et al. Natural history of peripheral neuropathy in patients with non-insulin dependent diabetes mellitus. *N Eng J Med.* 1995;333(2):89–94.
3. Sindrup SH, Jensen TS. Efficacy of pharmacological treatments of neuropathic pain: An update and effect related to mechanism of drug action. *Pain.* 1999;83(3):389–400.

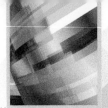

CHAPTER 15

Opioids

An opioid is a chemical substance that has a morphine-like action in the body. Opiates activate receptors that modulate our perception of painful stimuli (nociceptive pain). Opiates act within the brain and spinal cord to alter nociceptive transmission. There are three opioid receptors—μ, κ, and δ—but the primary analgesic effect is via the μ-receptor.

The scope of this book will focus on the seven main opiates used in clinical practice: Codeine, hydrocodone, oxycodone, morphine, Dilaudid (hydromorphone), fentanyl, and methadone. These are all direct agonists of the opioid receptor. Mixed opioid receptor agonist–antagonists such as Suboxone (buprenorphine and naloxone) are beyond the scope of this book.

WHEN TO USE

Opioids can be first-line medications for acute pain (a dislocated shoulder, postsurgical pain, an acute fracture) and typically are second-line drugs for chronic pain (lumbar spondylosis, diabetic peripheral neuropathy, osteoarthritis). After an acute pain state resolves, the patient should be taken off opioids. For chronic pain conditions, typically physicians use adjuvant medications (nonopioid pain medications) at therapeutic doses first. It is important to try nonopioid pain medication at clinically therapeutic doses before resorting to opioids. For example, 30 mg of Cymbalta for diabetic peripheral neuropathy has not been shown to be effective, whereas 60 mg has. Interventional pain management procedures may be used as well (joint injections, sympathetic nerve blocks, epidural steroid injections) to alleviate pain and can be a good option before prescribing opioids.

HOW TO USE

Physicians often struggle with which opiate to prescribe. It is important to remember that all of the opioids in this chapter have a similar method of action; thus morphine is not better for one type of pain as compared to oxycodone. None is disease or location specific—one is not better for orthopedic pain, whereas another better for pelvic pain. It often comes down to prescriber preference and comfort. Appropriate strength and frequency are more important than the choice of opioid itself. This chapter will focus on using opioids in both hospital and outpatient settings. A simple algorithm for prescribing opioids is as follows Table 15-1.

Hospital Setting: Intravenous Opioids

When in the hospital setting, determine if the opioid needs to be given intravenously (IV). If the IV route is needed, you only have three choices—morphine, Dilaudid, or fentanyl—as they are the only three of the primary seven opioids available in a common IV form (Table 15-1). If the patient does not need IV narcotics, please skip to the next section. Opioids given via the IV route are reserved for hospital patients who have an acute flare of pain. They are also warranted for patients with chronic pain hospitalized for other reasons who need to be nothing per mouth (nil per os [NPO]). These patients cannot receive their usual oral pain medication.

All IV medications are short acting by definition. At equal analgesic doses, no one opioid is stronger than another and none is better than another unless the patient has an allergy to one in particular. The medication is given via an IV push or via a patient-controlled

TABLE 15-1 The Seven Primary Opioids

Medication	Intravenous	Short Acting Form	Long Acting Form
Codeine		X	
Hydrocodone		X	
Oxycodone		X	X
Morphine	X	X	X
Dilaudid (hydomorphone)	X	X	X
Fentanyl	X		X
Methadone			X

analgesia ([PCA]; PCAs are covered in Chapter 16. Table 15-2 presents the equivalent doses for the three IV pain medications.

A common order would be 2 mg of IV morphine to be given every 4 hours as needed, or Dilaudid IV 0.4 mg every 4 hours as needed. Fentanyl 25 μg IV every 4 hours as needed can be used as well, but most hospitals typically have morphine and Dilaudid on the floor rather than fentanyl. If a patient does not respond to these doses, rather than switching between the different IV pain medications, you should increase the dose of the opioid you are currently using. I have been paged by the resident to be told that a patient did not respond to IV Dilaudid and asked what opioid would I like to try next. Upon inquiry, I discovered that the patient received a dose of 0.2 mg of Dilaudid. In a case such as this, if the patient does not respond to 0.2 mg IV Dilaudid every 4 hours as needed, increasing the dose to 0.4 mg every 4 hours as needed may be effective. If that does not work, the next step is 1 mg of Dilaudid every 3 hours as needed rather than giving up on Dilaudid and switching to another opioid. Patients who are opioid tolerant usually require more significant starting doses than opioid-naïve patients—for example, an opioid-tolerant patient should start with Dilaudid 1 mg rather than 0.4 mg.

Toradol (ketorolac)—the only nonsteroidal anti-inflammatory drug (NSAID) that can be given intravenous—is commonly used in combination with IV opioids. NSAIDs work by blocking inflammation at the site of pathology and by altering pain perception in the central nervous system (CNS). Toradol blocks inflammatory prostaglandins that sensitize nerve endings to the action of bradykinin, histamine, and other inflam-

matory factors, making them more likely to transmit pain. In a postoperative study, patients treated with Toradol IV at fixed intermittent boluses required 26% less morphine than the morphine-alone group. Because of its potency, Toradol is limited to 5 days of use. Typically prescribe this medication as 30 mg IV or intramuscular (IM) every 6 hours or every 6 hours as needed. It should be used with caution in patients with a history of gastrointestinal or renal disease. I will often add Toradol to the IV opioid I am using to lower the total amount of opioid needed to control the pain to enable better control of side effects, which include constipation, nausea, and pruritus.

Intravenous opioids are stronger than their oral counterparts. IV morphine is three times stronger than oral morphine; thus giving 5 mg of IV morphine is equivalent to 15 mg of oral morphine. IV Dilaudid is five times stronger than oral Dilaudid; thus giving 2 mg of IV Dilaudid is equivalent to 10 mg of oral Dilaudid. Caution should be taken when converting from IV to oral opioid medication and vice versa.

Hospital or Outpatient Setting

Determine whether the patient has an acute pain condition that will completely resolve, a chronic pain condition that does not require continuous narcotics or a chronic pain condition that needs continuous narcotic treatment.

Acute pain conditions are dynamic with large fluctuations of pain levels over time, even within 1 day. Short-acting oral pain medications are needed to match the quickly oscillating pain state. Short-acting oral pain

TABLE 15-2 Equal Analgesic Doses of Intravenous Pain Medications

Medication	Equivalent Dose	Starting Dose	Onset Time	Duration
Morphine	10 mg	2–3 mg	5–10 mins	3–5 h
Dilaudid	1.5 mg	0.2–0.4 mg	5–20 mins	3–4 h
Fentanyl	100 μg	25 g	Less than 1 min	1–2 h

TABLE 15-3 Short-acting Oral Opioids and Pain Levels for Which They are Most Useful

Level of Pain	Medication
Less severe pain	Codeine
Moderate to severe pain	Hydrocodone (hydrocodone + Tylenol = Vicodin) Oxycodone (Oxycodone + Tylenol = Percocet)
Severe pain	Morphine Dilaudid (hydromorphone)

medications have a quick onset and quick offset of action, lasting 4 to 6 hours. Of the seven primary opioids, there are five available in a short-acting oral form: Codeine, hydrocodone, oxycodone, Dilaudid, and morphine (Table 15-3). Again, none is disease specific. Methadone and fentanyl do not come in a short-acting oral form. Per the mission of this book, prescribing short-acting oral opioids will be broken down to the clinically most relevant pain states.

Short-acting Oral Opioid Medication Choices

For Less Severe Pain: Codeine: Tylenol with codeine (Tylenol 3) is typically prescribed. Tylenol 3 contains 30 mg of codeine and 300 mg of Tylenol (acetaminophen). It can be prescribed to take up to four times a day. Tylenol 3 may also be used for moderately severe pain in patients who cannot tolerate stronger opioids, for example, the elderly.

For Moderate to Severe Pain: Oxycodone or Hydrocodone: Oxycodone or hydrocodone is typically prescribed. Both of these medications are available as 5-, 7.5-, or 10-mg tablets. Typically a physician prescribes one tablet every 4 to 6 hours as needed. The

5-mg tablet is considered standard strength, the 7.5-mg tablet extra strength, and the 10-mg tablet extra-extra strength. Both oxycodone and hydrocodone usually come wrapped in a Tylenol coating. When oxycodone is wrapped in a Tylenol coating, it is know as Percocet (Fig. 15-1). When hydrocodone is wrapped in a Tylenol coating, it is known as Vicodin (Fig. 15-1). The standard Tylenol coating of Percocet and Vicodin is 325 mg. Thus if you prescribe Percocet 7.5/325 you are prescribing 7.5 mg of oxycodone wrapped in 325 mg of Tylenol. When you prescribe Vicodin 5/325 you are prescribing 5 mg of hydrocodone wrapped in 325 mg of Tylenol.

Overall, oxycodone is slightly stronger than hydrocodone. Tylenol, when used properly, is virtually free of any significant side effects. Large doses, however, may lead to liver damage. One should not exceed more than 4,000 mg of Tylenol in a 24-hour period. If you are prescribing Percocet 5/325 every 8 hours as needed and the patient takes the medication around the clock, you are prescribing less than 25% of the daily maximum Tylenol dose. Hepatotoxicity may develop with standard doses of acetaminophen in patients with significant alcohol intake. A careful history of the patient's medications should be taken to determine those that contain acetaminophen. The physician should make the patient aware of the maximal daily dose of acetaminophen and instruct him or her to inform you if other physicians prescribe medications.

For Severe Pain: Morphine or Dilaudid: Morphine or Dilaudid is typically necessary.

Morphine 15 mg is equal to 10 mg of oxycodone (an extra-extra strength Percocet 10/325). It is important to note that patients may process different medications differently even if the medications are mathematically equivalent. For a patient who does not respond to Percocet, morphine 15 mg po tid may be effective one 30-mg tablet of morphine sulfate immediate release every 8 hours as needed may be necessary.

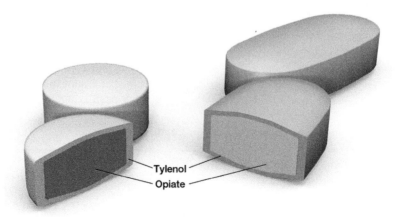
Tylenol
Opiate

Figure 15-1 Percocet and hydrocodone, respectively. Oxycodone wrapped in Tylenol = Percocet; hydrocodone wrapped in Tylenol = Vicodin.

Dilaudid 4 mg is equal to 10 mg of oxycodone (an extra-extra strength Percocet 10/325) or 15 mg of morphine. For patients in severe pain who do not respond to these doses, one 8-mg tablet of Dilaudid every 8 hours as needed may be necessary. For patients who still do not respond, the prescriber may need to decrease the time between doses to every 6 or every 4 hours.

Outpatient Setting

The best way to treat chronic pain is by keeping it under control at all times. Pain levels can climb very quickly—more opioid is required to bring the pain level down than to keep it at bay with a long-acting opioid. When using short-acting opioids around the clock, on the other hand, the patient is always chasing the pain, trying to knock the increasing level down rather than preventing it from reaching high levels. Chronic pain conditions strong enough to require opiates more than twice a day warrant treatment with long-acting opioids (time-release formulation). A switch from short-acting to long-acting oral pain medication may be necessary.

Of the seven basic opioids, you have five choices that come in a long-acting (time-release) formulation: Oxycodone, morphine, Dilaudid, fentanyl, and methadone. Codeine and hydrocodone do not come in a long-acting, time-release formulation. Long-acting opioids are given every 8 or 12 hours instead of every 4 or 6 hours, as are the short-acting oral opioids. The exception is a fentanyl patch, which lasts 72 hours (3 days; for some people the patch lasts only 2 days) and then needs to be changed. Like the previous section, which opioid you choose is a matter of prescriber preference and comfort. I typically switch the patient to the long-acting form of the short-acting medication currently prescribed. I may offer to switch the patient to a fentanyl patch to eliminate the need to take tablets.

Realistic expectations should be addressed from the start. Long-acting opioid treatment for chronic pain rarely eliminates a patient's pain, but rather it reduces it. An opioid-based treatment plan is doomed from the start if the patient expects to be completely pain free. The goal is to develop a meaningful degree of pain relief and thus improve quality of life. Rarely do patients become pain free—if this is the expectation then the development of a successful, nonabusive therapeutic treatment plan is unlikely.

Long-acting (Time-release) Opioid Medication Choices

Oxycodone: The long-acting (time-release) formulation of the short-acting oral pain medication oxycodone is OxyContin. Remember that oxycodone wrapped in Tylenol is Percocet; therefore if a patient is taking Percocet 10/325 around the clock every 6 hours, for a total of 40 mg of oxycodone a day, this is equivalent to 20 mg of OxyContin twice a day.

Morphine: The long-acting, time-release formulation of the short-acting oral pain medication immediate release (IR) morphine is MS-Contin (extended-release morphine). Morphine (IR) 15 mg is equal to 15 mg of MS-Contin (extended release). Thus if a patient is taking morphine 15 mg around the clock every 6 hours this would be 60 mg of morphine a day. Switching the patient to 30 mg of MS-Contin twice a day would be equivalent. Or if a patient is taking 30 mg of morphine around the clock every 6 hours, a total of 120 mg of morphine a day, this would be equivalent to 60 mg of MS-Contin every 12 hours.

Dilaudid: The long-acting, time-release formulation of the short-acting oral pain medication Dilaudid is Exalgo (Dilaudid-ER, extended release). Dilaudid 4 mg is equal to 4 mg of Exalgo. Thus if a patient is taking Dilaudid 4 mg every 6 hours, around the clock, a total of 16 mg of Dilaudid a day, this would be the equivalent of 8 mg of Exalgo twice a day or 16 mg of Exalgo once a day. Exalgo is marketed as a once-a-day medication.

Fentanyl: Fentanyl is the only option for administering a long-acting opioid transdermally (via skin patch). There are several reasons to choose a transdermal patch: Aversion to pill taking; cognitive inability to take multiple pills appropriately; or gastrointestinal issues (Crohn's disease, ulcerative colitis, previous gastrointestinal surgery) that prevent proper consistent absorption of oral medications. If the possible abuse of opioids is a concern, the fentanyl patch is the preferred choice over prescribing pills.

The medication in the patch absorbs into the body in a time-release fashion (Fig. 15-2). A rate-controlling membrane between the drug reservoir and the skin

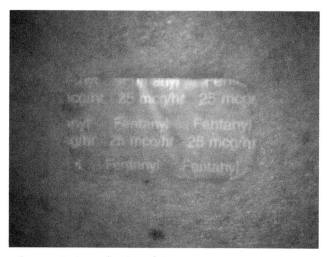

Figure 15-2 Application of the transdermal fentanyl patch.

controls delivery. The dose of drug delivered depends on the amount of drug held in the matrix and the area of the patch applied to the skin. Because the absorption of the medication from the patch is systemic, application directly to the painful area, as with a lidocaine or a diclofenac (NSAID) patch, is not necessary. The chest, back, or arms are appropriate sites. Typically, the patch lasts 48 to 72 hours (2 to 3 days—more often than not it lasts 3 days) before it needs to be reapplied.

The fentanyl patch is available in 12 μg and progressively higher strengths: 25 μg, 50 μg, 75 μg, and up to 100 μg. A 25-μg patch is equal to using 40 mg of oral oxycodone in a day (Percocet 10/325 every 6 hours around the clock) or 60 mg of oral morphine in a day (morphine 15 mg every 6 hours around the clock). Equianalgesic calculations vary among individuals. It is resonable to convert a person on four Percocet 10/325 four times a day to a 25-μg fentanyl patch every 72 hours. It is important to reassure a patient that if the fentanyl patch is not strong enough at this conservative starting dose, the dose will increase. However, a trial of at least 3 days, one patch cycle, to determine whether the current dose is truly helpful is necessary. It is important to note that the steady-state serum concentration, which is reached after 24 hours, is maintained as long as the patch is renewed.

Methadone: Methadone, the last of the long-acting opioids discussed here, works very well for treating pain. Though better known for treatment of addiction, its original use was to treat pain, as it binds directly to the opioid receptor, like the other seven primary opioids. Methadone is unique in that it also binds to the N-methyl D-aspartate receptor, also known as the NMDA receptor, which helps control synaptic plasticity. Two neurons form a synaptic connection; the structural and chemical changes that occur to strengthen that connection are reinforced if there is a significant transmission of impulses across the synapse, known as synaptic plasticity. Synaptic plasticity includes an alteration in the number of receptors located on a synapse. By blocking the NMDA receptor, the structural and chemical changes that strengthen the connection and transmission of pain over synaptic pathways is blocked in patients with chronic pain. Methadone is one of the most powerful medications used to break the development of negative CNS alterations that promote chronic pain.

For pain, methadone is prescribed twice a day or every 8 hours rather than once a day, as in addiction. People with painful conditions such as a vertebral fracture who were in a methadone clinic for addiction reported that approximately 8 to 12 hours after getting their morning methadone dose their craving for heroin was blocked but their spine pain returned.

The half-life for treating pain and addiction is different. Methadone should never be prescribed to an opioid-naïve patient.

Methadone is available in 2.5-mg, 5-mg and 10-mg tablets. Guidelines for prescribing methadone involve (1) determining the patient's total daily dose of opioid, (2) converting that number to the equivalent dose of morphine, and (3) starting at 25% total daily morphine dose. Here are three examples.

- Example 1: A patient takes morphine (IR) 30 mg every 6 hours around the clock (120 mg/d). Twenty-five percent of the total daily 120-mg morphine dose is 30 mg. Thus, the patient should start taking methadone at 10 mg every 8 hours.
- Example 2: A patient takes Percocet 10/325 every 6 hours (40 mg/d of oxycodone). Oxycodone 40 mg is equivalent to of oral morphine 60 mg (1 mg and 1.5 mg, respectively). Twenty-five percent of the total daily 60-mg morphine dose is 15 mg. Thus, the patient should start taking methadone at 7.5 mg twice a day (dispensing via a 2.5-mg tablet and 5-mg tablet) or 5 mg three times a day.
- Example 3: A patient takes Dilaudid 8 mg every 6 hours (32 mg/d). Dilaudid 32 mg daily is equivalent to that of oral morphine 128 mg (1 mg and 4 mg, respectively). Twenty-five percent of the total daily 128-mg morphine dose is roughly 30 mg. Thus, the patient should start taking methadone at 10 mg every 8 hours.

There are many good websites that have opioid analgesic converters, which allow you to plug in the medication and dose to obtain a conversion to the equal analgesic dose of a different medication. One such website is http://www.globalrph.com/narcoticonv.htm. There are apps as well that can be downloaded to your mobile phone. Here is a standard table (Table 15-4) of dose conversions.

The titration of methadone must proceed slowly. The metabolism of methadone occurs via the cytochrome P450 pathway (a superfamily of enzymes involved in the breaking down of medication). When methadone enters the bloodstream, it takes roughly

TABLE 15-4 Analgesic Dose Conversions

Codeine	100 mg
Hydrocodone	15 mg
Oxycodone	10 mg
Morphine (Oral)	15 mg
Morphine (IV)	5 mg
Dilaudid (Oral)	3.75 mg
Dilaudid (IV)	0.75 mg

22 hours for the blood plasma levels to be cut in half (half-life), whereas morphine's half-life is roughly 120 minutes. Thus when a patient takes the second scheduled dose of methadone 8 hours later, the first dose is still active; when the patient takes the third scheduled dose 8 hours after that, the first two doses are still being metabolized. This is known as stacking. It takes approximately 4.5 days for methadone to reach steady state, meaning that, the same amount of medication ingested is the same amount of medication being eliminated.

In addition, it is important to note that metabolism rates vary greatly between individuals; in some individuals the half-life of methadone may be 60 hours rather than the average 22 hours. At that rate, it would take 12.5 days for methadone to reach a steady state. A classic mistake is to prescribe methadone, for example, 5 mg twice a day. Two days later the patient may call back to report that the medication is not working and pain is still present, prompting the doctor to increase the dose to 10 mg twice a day. The 5-mg dose has not reached steady state; with the additional methadone, the patient becomes sedated and in severe cases has respiratory problems. In general, to avoid this you should wait about 7 days before increasing the methadone dose.

Breakthrough Pain Management

Patients who are on a stable regimen of long-acting (time-release) pain medications may have episodes of breakthrough pain, an unexpected increase of pain above a well-controlled baseline. For example, a woman controls her pain with long-acting pain medications, but shopping triggers a significant increase in back pain. This may require as-needed dosing of a short-acting oral pain medication.

When choosing a short-acting oral pain medication, it may be best to use the short-acting form of the long-acting medication prescribed to the patient (Table 15-5) because the patient's level of tolerance for the side effects of that particular medication is already known

and the possibility of drug–drug interaction is decreased. Although this is possible for most long-acting (time-release) formulations, for a fentanyl patch or methadone there is no short-acting form.

Patients should not be using their short-acting oral breakthrough pain medication around the clock but rather on an as-needed basis. This is why many physicians will not prescribe breakthrough short-acting pain medication more than once or twice a day. Some physicians do not resort to any short-acting pain medication when prescribing long-acting pain medication for chronic pain. If the patient is using breakthrough pain medication around the clock, an increase in the long-acting pain medication, an injection or surgery may be needed.

Patients on opiate treatment for chronic pain should be evaluated periodically to see if continuing opioid treatment is beneficial. If a patient does not report decreased pain levels and increased functionality, the utility of maintaining opioid treatment should be questioned. Although there is no ceiling dose for opioids that do not contain Tylenol, patients receiving opioid doses of significant magnitude rarely report satisfaction or improved function. Patients on increasing opioid doses with no increased analgesia and unimproved quality of life should have their treatment plan re-evaluated. Patients with chronic pain who are dissatisfied with their medications will occasionally voluntarily self-wean off large doses of narcotics and report no difference in their pain levels despite cessation of opioids. The utility of opioids in the treatment plan should be continuously evaluated.

Other Narcotics and Narcotic-like Pain Medications

Nucynta (Tapentadol): A commonly used opioid, Nucynta is relatively new to the market. It does not have the track record of the seven opioids previously mentioned but has a favorable response rate. It works as a direct agonist to the opioid receptor and also inhibits the reuptake of norepinephrine. It comes in both a

TABLE 15-5 Short-acting Forms of Long-acting Pain Medications

Long-acting Pain Medication	Duration of Action	Short-acting Form
Oxycodone extended release (OxyContin)	8–12 h	Oxycodone Oxycodone/Tylenol (Percocet)
Morphine extended release (MS-Contin)	8–12 h	Morphine (immediate release)
Exalgo (Dilaudid, extended release)	12–24 h	Dilaudid
Methadone	8–12 h	None
Fentanyl patch	48–72 h	None

TABLE 15-6 Conversion Doses—Nucynta to Oxycodone

Nucynta Dose	Equivalent Oxycodone Dose
50 mg	5 mg
75 mg	10 mg
100 mg	15 mg

short-acting and long-acting oral (extended-release) form. At present, there are three IR tablet formulations of Nucynta available in the United States: 50, 75, and 100 mg.

Unfortunately, no published data can clearly serve as a guide to converting doses between tapentadol and other opioids. When dosed every 4 to 6 hours for orthopedic (bunionectomy) surgical pain, tapentadol 50- and 75-mg dose groups appeared to experience about the same pain relief as the oxycodones 5 and 10-mg dose group respectively. In clinical practice, many practitioners are using the conversions in Table 15-6 but, again, conclusive data do not exist yet.

Tramadol: Tramadol, a synthetic version of codeine, works on receptors within the CNS but unlike the traditional seven opioids is only partially blocked by the opioid receptor antagonist naloxone. For this reason, it is not considered a true opioid. Its mode of action is not completely understood, but experts believe that it weakly binds to the μ-opioid receptor and simultaneously inhibits the reuptake of norepinephrine and serotonin.

Tramadol is a good option for patients with less severe pain or for those who cannot tolerate stronger medication. It offers analgesia with a reduced risk of abuse, sedation, and constipation. It comes in 50-mg tablets, Tramadol 37.5 mg wrapped in 325 mg of Tylenol is Ultracet 37.5/325. The peak effect occurs 2 hours after the initial dose, and the drug's effects lasts approximately 6 hours. Typical prescriptions are 50 mg or 100 mg three to four times a day as needed.

Contraindications to tramadol include a history of seizures, and coadministration of any medication that may lower the seizure threshold is not appropriate. Because tramadol inhibits the reuptake of serotonin and norepinephrine, it is necessary to completely evaluate its use with medications that have a similar method of action.

WHEN NOT TO USE AND POTENTIAL SIDE EFFECTS

Avoiding opioid abuse is covered in its own chapter, which reviews detecting drug-seeking behavior, narcotic agreements, urine drug screening, and the handling of a number of challenging situations so that opioids can be prescribed safely and monitored correctly.

The major side effects are the same for all opioids. The most common effect is constipation. Opioids lead to reduced peristalsis in the small intestine and colon, increased electrolyte and water absorption, and impaired defecation response. All patients given an opioid should be considered for a bowel regimen as well. Constipation does not dissipate as a patient becomes more tolerant to the side effects of opioids. Also, nausea, pruritus, and sedation may occur with use of any opioid. Respiratory depression is a rare but extremely important side effect. With slow, careful titration, it is easy to avoid this condition.

Low testosterone levels may occur in patients with chronic pain, for two reasons. The first reason is suppression of gonadotropin-releasing hormone (GnRH) from the hypothalamus by the opioid itself. Normally, GnRH production by the hypothalamus stimulates the pituitary gland to produce follicle-stimulating hormone (FSH) and luteinizing hormone (LH), which in turn stimulates the production of testosterone opioids are thought to inhibit this. The second reason is pituitary insufficiency caused not by the opioid but by the pain directly.

A lack of testosterone may result in poor pain control, depression, sleep disturbances, and lack of energy and motivation. Consequently, adequate testosterone levels are necessary for opioid receptor binding, transport across the blood–brain barrier, and activation of dopamine and norepinephrine activity. Although there is a steady decline in testosterone levels after the age of 40, the decline is relatively small. Only a small percentage of aging men have levels below those considered normal for their age.

To check testosterone levels, it is necessary to order a morning serum level. Two blood levels will come back: The free form (unbound component) and the total serum testosterone level. The free level may be more important for libido whereas the total serum testosterone level may be more critical for pain management, but this remains unclear. Treatment for low testosterone levels typically involves administration of the hormone as a topical gel or patch. The gel is available via a pump dispenser, a 1% concentration being the most common. A pump releases the required daily amount which is rubbed into the skin. The patch version, Androderm, comes in 2.5- and 5-mg strengths; normally, it is necessary to apply a new patch to the skin every night. Recommended follow-up serum concentrations should occur at 3 months, 6 months, and then annually. Other causes of low testosterone include cryptorchidism, hemochromatosis, craniopharyngioma, and alcohol abuse.

A side effect specific to methadone is cardiac QT prolongation. The QT interval represents the time involved in the electrical depolarization and repolarization of the heart's ventricles. This usually occurs only in patients with other cardiac risk factors. Recommended tests include a prescreening electrocardiogram (EKG), a follow-up EKG within 30 days, and an annual EKG. A QT interval greater than 450 msec is considered an indication to discontinue or reduce the methadone dose. In clinical practice, if a patient has no risk factors and the methadone dose is less than 20 mg, he or she may not always receive a prescreening EKG.

CASE STUDY

Three patients in the same car accident are taken to the hospital. At the hospital it is determined that all three patients have identical complicated fractures of the pelvis and must undergo surgery.

Patient 1 is opioid naïve and is prescribed 0.5 mg of Dilaudid IV every 3 hours as needed for postoperative pain. The first day he uses the Dilaudid around the clock. He is also prescribed Toradol 30 mg IV every 6 hours as needed. By the time he is ready for discharge, he is using 1.5 mg of IV Dilaudid a day. This is equivalent to roughly 20 mg of oxycodone a day. He is given Percocet 7.5/325 every 6 hours as needed as well as a prescription for Celebrex and is discharged. Within 3 weeks he is off all pain medication.

Patient 2 is not opioid naïve. He is taking MS-Contin 30 mg twice a day (60 mg total a day) for back pain from a previous lumbar fusion. He is prescribed 1.5 mg of Dilaudid IV every 3 hours as needed postoperatively. The first half a day he uses Dilaudid around the clock and is still in pain. His dose is then increased to 2.5 mg every 3 hours as needed and the pain abates. He is also prescribed Toradol 30 mg IV every 6 hours as needed. By the time he is ready for discharge, he is using 10 mg of IV Dilaudid a day. This is equivalent to roughly 200 mg of morphine a day, 140 mg above his baseline (0.75 mg of IV Dilaudid is equal to 15 mg of oral morphine, thus 10 mg is equivalent to 200 mg daily). He is given 60 mg of MS-Contin (long-acting morphine) twice a day and 30 mg of morphine (IR) (immediate-release morphine) three times a day for breakthrough pain for a total of 210 mg of oral morphine a day. He is also given a prescription for Celebrex and is discharged. His goal is to continue the MS-Contin and every day that his pain lessens, reduce his short-acting oral morphine. After 1 month he has weaned himself down to MS-Contin 60 mg twice a day. At that point he is given MS-Contin 30-mg tablets three times a day with a goal to get him back to his previous baseline dose of 30 mg MS-Contin twice a day.

Patient 3 is not opioid naïve. He takes MS-Contin 30 mg twice a day for his back pain (60 mg a day) from lumbar fusion. He is prescribed 1.5 mg of Dilaudid IV every 3 hours as needed. The first day he uses the Dilaudid around the clock and is still in pain. His *dose* is raised to 2.5 mg every 3 hours and the pain abates. He is also prescribed Toradol 30 mg IV every 6 hours as needed and uses it around the clock. During his hospital stay he develops a complication and must return to surgery. After his second trip to the operating room, his pain levels are increased and now he is on Dilaudid 3 mg IV every 2 hours as needed. By the time he is ready for discharge, he is using 15 mg of IV Dilaudid a day. This is equivalent to roughly 300 mg of morphine a day. This is 240 mg above his baseline. He is given 60 mg of MS-Contin every 8 hours and 30 mg of MSIR four times a day for breakthrough pain, for a total potential dose of 310 mg of morphine a day. He is also given a prescription for Celebrex and is transferred to a rehabilitation center. One month later he is still in pain daily and has not been able to reduce his pain medications. The decision is made to switch him to methadone. He is started on 25% of his daily morphine dose (25% of 300 mg is 75 mg). He is started on 25 mg of methadone every 8 hours and Percocet 10/325 twice a day for breakthrough pain. He does better on this regimen.

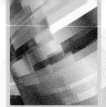

CHAPTER **16**

Patient-controlled Analgesia

Patient-controlled analgesia (PCA) was first used in 1971. PCA is a way of delivering pain medication via a programmable (IV) infusion device (Fig. 16-1). The PCA machine which is set up at the patient's bedside and connected directly via tubing to the IV line contains a bag of premixed opioid solution. The patient can self-administer small, physician-determined doses of analgesic medication on demand, referred to as demand dose, by pushing a button connected to the PCA machine (Fig. 16-2). The machine will then lock for a predetermined amount of time before it can administer another demand dose (referred to as the lock-out period), to protect the patient from overmedicating. It is also possible to program the machine to release the drug at a low-dose continuous infusion rate.

The advantages to using a PCA device are many: It is a painless route of delivering opioid medication, it provides prompt analgesia, decreases the burden on the nursing staff, gives patients an enhanced sense of control, and reduces fluctuations in medication level when

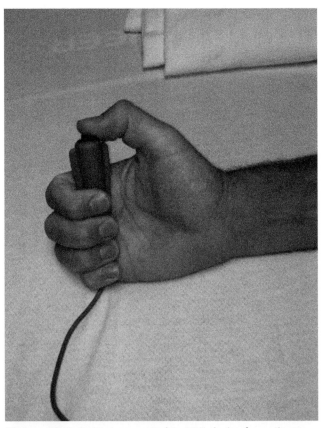

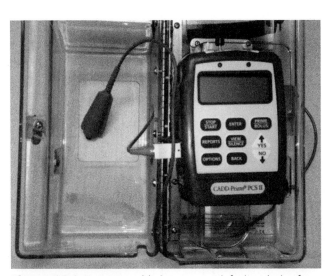

Figure 16-1 Programmable intravenous infusion device for PCA.

Figure 16-2 Button connected to PCA device for patient to self-administer analgesic medication.

compared to intermittent bolus administration. Comparing IV PCA to intramuscular opioid analgesia ordered every 3 to 4 hours as needed showed a significantly greater analgesia efficacy with PCA.[1,2] This is especially true in hospitals where the nursing staff has to cover a large amount of patients and cannot distribute medication as promptly as staff in hospitals whose nursing-to-patient ratio is 1:1.

WHEN TO USE

A PCA device is typically used when the patient cannot take pain medication orally. This situation may occur during the pre- or postoperative period when the patient is nil per os (NPO; nothing per mouth). It is also used when a patient has nausea and cannot hold down oral medication. PCA devices are frequently useful in cases of severe pain states such as acute pancreatitis, sickle cell crisis, and burn injuries.

HOW TO USE

Choosing the Opioid

Typically, one of three medications is used in a PCA device: Morphine, Dilaudid, or fentanyl. All three opiates activate receptors in the brain and spinal cord that modulate the perception of painful stimuli. These medications are available in standard premixed bags. For the scope of this book, the choice of which medication to use is a matter of personal preference. At equal analgesic doses, no medication is stronger than another or better than another unless the patient has an allergy to one of them. None of these three medications is disease specific—one is not better for orthopedic, pelvic, or other types of pain over the other medications. Renal failure may be the one situation in which the medication choice may make a difference: Fentanyl may be preferable because it has no active metabolites. Fentanyl is not typically kept on the hospital floor making morphine and dilaudid the more commonly used choices.

Choosing the Demand Dose

The next step is choosing the dose that the PCA device will deliver when the demand button is pressed—the demand dose. The starting dose for the three commonly prescribed opioids is listed in Table 16-1. It is necessary to double these starting demand doses for patients on chronic opioids. It is important to remember that the demand dose can be adjusted easily.

Choosing the Lock-out Period

The lock-out period is the interval during which the PCA device "ignores" further demands by a patient. It protects the patient from overmedicating. The standard lock-out period is usually 6 minutes. No matter how many times the patient pushes the button, the machine will not deliver medication. For patients who are potentially sensitive to medication, such as the elderly, a 10-minute lock is warranted. Like the demand dose, the lock-out period is also easy to change.

Choosing the Continuous Rate

A continuous rate is the amount of medication that is automatically administered every hour whether or not the patient self-administers the demand dose. For the scope of this book, the continuous rate should not be used; the continuous rate should be set at 0 on the PCA device. PCAs with a continuous rate as compared to PCAs without have been shown to provide no better pain relief or sleep, nor do they lessen the number of demand doses used.[3] That being said, a background infusion may be appropriate for some patients who have been on chronic high-dose opioids in select situations.[4]

Choosing the 4-hour Limit

The last of the four settings on the PCA device is the time-based cumulative dose limit, commonly referred to as the 4-hour limit, which restricts the total amount of medication a patient can receive in a 4-hour period. Generally, it is not necessary to use this feature when using a six minute look-out period. However, if the patient rarely needs the medication except when pain levels increase drastically (e.g., resulting from physical therapy or dressing changes) the 4-hour limit is a good option. It allows a burst of medication followed by a very short lock-out period with a restricted total amount of medication. You can set a 3-minute lock-out period (instead of the standard 6 minutes), but with a 4-hour

TABLE 16-1 Standard Starting Demand Doses for Patient-controlled Analgesia

Drug	Demand Dose	
	Little or No Previous Opioid Use	Chronic Opioid Use
Morphine	2 mg	4 mg
Dilaudid (Hydromorphone)	0.2 mg	0.4 mg
Fentanyl	25 µg	50 µg

limit of not more than, for example, 6 mg of morphine in a 4-hour period. This addresses the patient's particular pain medication needs in a safe manner.

Adjusting the Settings

The settings on the PCA device may require adjustment to provide optimal analgesia. The device indicates how many times the patient pushed the button and how many doses were received. If the patient consistently uses more than 4 demand doses per hour and the pain score remains high, titration of the PCA device settings is warranted.[3] To make the proper adjustments varying the amount delivered in the demand dose is the proper adjustment—varying the lock-out intervals has little effect on analgesia.[5] In one study, varying the lock-out interval from 11 minutes to 7 minutes made no difference in analgesia, anxiety, or side effects.[5] If the patient does not respond to the starting dose, rather than switching to a different opioid, I recommend increasing the demand dose of the opioid you are currently using, unless you have increased the demand dose three times. I am often paged by the resident when a patient is not responding to a Dilaudid PCA set at standard starting doses—a continuous rate of 0, a demand dose of 0.2 mg, and a lock-out of 6 minutes. The resident would like to know if we should switch to a morphine or fentanyl PCA, as the Dilaudid PCA does not seem to be working. It is not that the Dilaudid PCA is not working—it is that the demand dose is not strong enough. In this case, increase the demand dose on the Dilaudid PCA, for example, to 0.4 mg and leave the rest of the settings the same.

WHEN NOT TO USE AND POTENTIAL SIDE EFFECTS

Contraindications to PCA use include decreased cognitive ability of the patient, which would inhibit understanding how to operate the device, and physical impairment, which would prohibit use of the machine. It is important that only the patient pushes the PCA device button, not a family member who presumes that the patient is in pain. The machines are designed to be tamper proof, so that access to the medication requires a key.

Although respiratory depression remains a rare complication of opioid use, it is a serious concern. Data suggest that the overall incidence of respiratory depression in patients using a PCA without a continuous rate ranges from 0.1% to 0.8%. The incidence of respiratory depression with conventional methods of opioid administration ranges from 0.2% to 0.9%.[6]

All opioids can decrease bowel function. Opioids lead to reduced peristalsis in the small intestine and colon, increased electrolyte and water absorption, and impaired defecation response. Ballantyne et al. looked at studies evaluating bowel function (time to first flatus or stool) and pulmonary function. No differences were found between PCA and intramuscular analgesia.[1]

CASE STUDIES

Case 1 A 52-year-old female on the surgical floor who is opioid naïve is postoperative day 0 after removal of a pancreatic mass. You decide to start the patient on a PCA device using morphine. You order PCA morphine with a continuous rate of 0, a demand dose of 2 mg, and a lock-out of 6 minutes, with no 4-hour limit. When you check on the patient a few hours later, she is comfortable with minimal pain complaints. Her vitals are stable and mental status is clear.

Case 2 A 39-year-old male on the medicine service presents with an exacerbation of his chronic pancreatitis. The patient normally takes 4 to 6 pills of Percocet (5 mg oxycodone/325 mg acetaminophen) per day. You decide to start the patient on a PCA using Dilaudid. Based on the patient's history of opioid exposure, current opioid use, and pain level, you decide to start with a continuous rate of 0, a demand dose of 0.4 mg, and a lock-out of 6 minutes, with no 4-hour limit. When you check on the patient, he complains of a high pain level—he is pushing the demand button 15 times an hour and receiving 7 or 8 demand doses an hour on average. You give the patient a 2-mg dose of Dilaudid IV push to bring down the pain level and decide to titrate his PCA dose settings to a continuous rate of 0, a demand dose of 0.8 mg, and a lock-out of 6 minutes. You return and the patient states that he is still not comfortable, but the pain has decreased significantly. He has been using roughly 5 to 6 doses per hour over the last 4 hours. At this point, you change the settings to a continuous rate of 0, a demand dose of 1.2 mg, and a lock-out of 6 minutes. When you check on the patient later, he is comfortable.

REFERENCES

1. Ballantyne JC, Carr DB, Chalmers TC, et al. Postoperative patient-controlled analgesia: Meta-analyses of initial randomized control trials. *J Clin Anesth.* 1993;5(3):182–193.

2. Egbert AM, Parks LH, Short LM, et al. Randomized trial of postoperative patient-controlled analgesia vs. intramuscular narcotics in frail elderly men. *Arch Intern Med.* 1990;150(9):1897–1903.

3. Parker RK, Holtmann B, White PF. Effects of a nighttime opioid infusion with PCA therapy on patient comfort and analgesic requirements after abdominal hysterectomy. *Anesthesiology.* 1992;76(3):362–367.

4. Macintyre PE, Ready LB. *Acute Pain Management—A Practical Guide.* 2nd ed. London: WB Saunders; 2001.

5. Ginsberg B, Gil KM, Muir M, et al. The influence of lockout intervals and drug selection on patient-controlled analgesia following gynecological surgery. *Pain.* 1995;62(1):95–100.

6. Macintyre PE. Safety and efficacy of patient-controlled analgesia. *Br J Anaesth.* 2001;87:36–46.

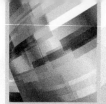

CHAPTER 17

Epidural Catheter Analgesia

WHEN TO USE	WHEN NOT TO USE AND POSSIBLE SIDE EFFECTS
▶ Surgical Setting	
▶ Childbirth Setting	
HOW TO USE	
▶ Surgical Setting	
▶ Childbirth Setting	

When most people hear the word *epidural* they think of what is administered to a woman for pain control before she delivers her baby. However, *epidural* simply refers to the epidural space. The outermost space in the spinal canal, the epidural space, lies outside the dura mater inside the surrounding vertebrae (Fig. 17-1). Its superior limit is the foramen magnum, where the spine meets the skull and its inferior limit is the end of the sacrum. The epidural space is important because it is possible to obtain access to the nerve roots to provide

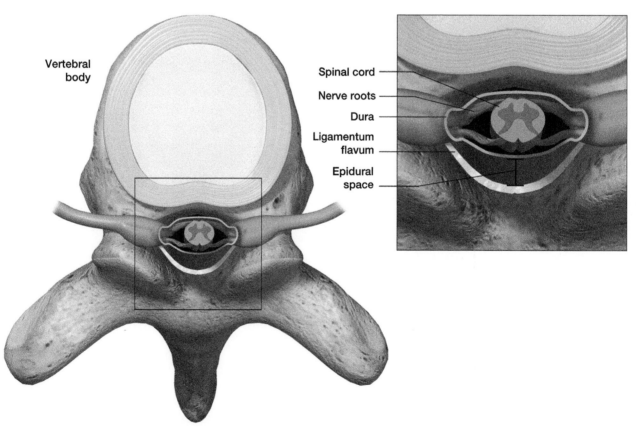

Vertebral body

Spinal cord

Nerve roots

Dura

Ligamentum flavum

Epidural space

Figure 17-1 The epidural space and surrounding anatomy. The epidural space lies outside the dura mater inside the surrounding vertebrae.

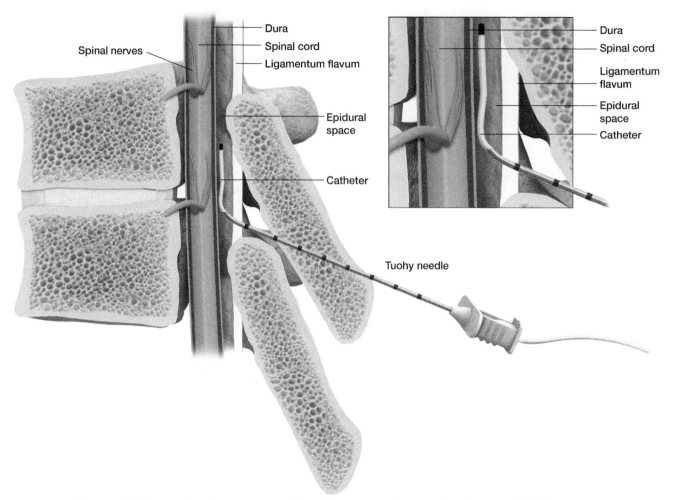

Figure 17-2 Epidural catheters are placed for pain control in the surgical setting and childbirth setting.

pain relief. There are several approaches to this space and different medications that can be injected into it. This chapter addresses the placement of a catheter into the epidural space to deliver pain medications (Fig. 17-2).

The first step in placing the catheter is choosing the proper location. The goal is to place the catheter at the spinal level most closely associated with the site of pain. Analgesia can be targeted best from five to seven continuous dermatomal regions. Table 17-1 presents

TABLE 17-1 Epidural Catheter Placement for Surgical Procedures

General Type of Surgery	Level of Epidural Placement
Thoracic	T2–T9
Upper abdominal	T4–L1
Lower abdominal	T10–L3
Lower extremity	T12–L3

information about proper epidural catheter placement location.

Without fluoroscopy the best way to determine the spinal level of interest is by palpating the spinous processes. These anatomic landmarks can help you locate an appropriate level to enter: The prominent cervical spinous process is C7, the bottom of the scapula is T7, and the last rib is T12. As long as the catheter is in the generalized area you are targeting, you can provide analgesia throughout the area by increasing the rate of infusion.

Once suitable location has been chosen the procedure can begin. With the patient sitting at the end of the bed and slightly leaning forward, the skin over and below the predetermined spinal level is prepped with betadine and drapes are placed over the area in standard sterile fashion. This procedure can also be done with the patient in the lateral decubitus position. When possible the space between two spinous processes is then palpated, and the skin and subcutaneous tissue is anesthetized with 2% lidocaine using a 1.5-in, 25G needle. In larger patients you may not be able to

Figure 17-3 **A.** Tuohy epidural needle. **B.** The ▶
slight curve at the end of the needle allows
the catheter passing through the needles
lumen to exit laterally at a 45 degree angle.
This safety feature makes it less likely the
dura will be punctured

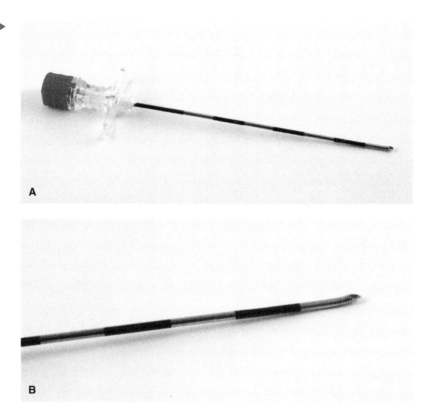

palpate the spinous process; in these cases, use the 25G needle after you have anesthetized the skin to locate the spinous process. After the skin is anesthetized and spinous process located, an 18G Tuohy epidural needle (Fig. 17-3) is placed in a perpendicular fashion to the skin. A small tilt of the needle tip in the cephalad direction may make catheter placement easier. Advance the needle through the skin, fascia, supraspinal ligament and interspinal ligament until it enters the ligamentum flavum, a typically thick ligament that "grabs" the needle as it enters. At this point, the stylet of the Tuohy needle is removed and a glass syringe is attached to the Tuohy needle (Fig. 17-4). I fill the glass syringe with 3 mL of saline; some doctors use air. When the needle is in the ligamentum flavum, the saline stays in the syringe despite application of light pressure to the plunger (Fig. 17-5). It is best to advance the needle in millimeter increments using the hand that is touching

both the needle and the patient's back. This technique will guard against any sudden movements by either patient or physician that could result in a sudden excessive needle depth.

As the needle advances, it eventually encounters the epidural space where the preservative free saline is sucked into the epidural space by negative pressure. This is known as the loss of resistance technique (Fig. 17-6). As long as the needle is in the process of being advanced, the syringe should be under continuous pressure or the physician should be checking intermittently for a loss of resistance. A novice may feel more comfortable attaching the syringe to the needle well before encountering the ligamentum flavum. The drawback to this is the hollow needle can pick up tissue as it is advanced over increasing distances. It is a good idea to disconnect the glass syringe and reinsert the stylet every couple of centimeters if a loss of resistance

Figure 17-4 Tuohy epidural needle with ▶
glass syringe attached.

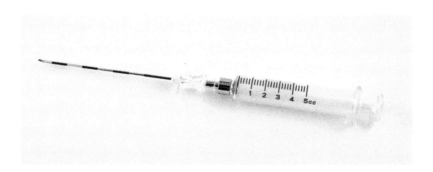

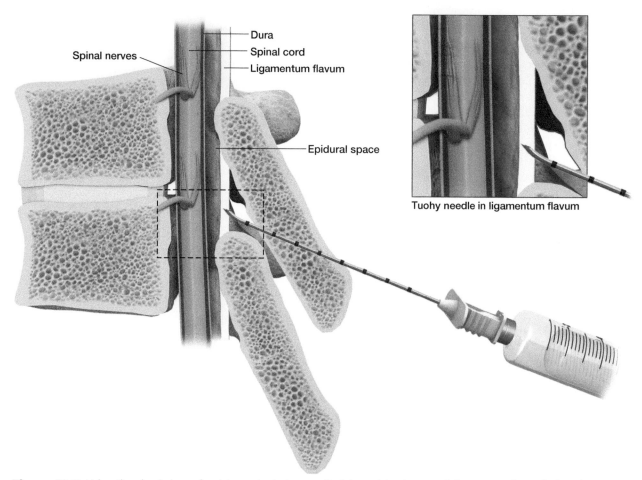

Tuohy needle in ligamentum flavum

Figure 17-5 Using the classic loss of resistance technique to find the epidural space, light pressure is applied to the glass syringe. While the needle is in the ligament flavum the tip of the needle is blocked by thick ligament tissue.

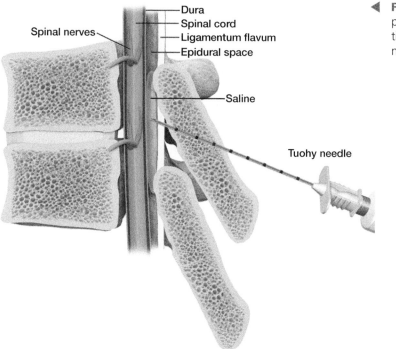

◀ **Figure 17-6** When the tip of the Tuohy needle pushes through the ligamentum flavum preservative free saline is sucked into the epidural space by negative pressure indicating proper needle position.

has not yet been obtained to ensure that the needle is not clogged. Then reattach the syringe and check for loss of resistance as you advance.

If you do not get a good loss of resistance, there are options to troubleshoot this. Detach your syringe and drain it of the normal saline. Fill it with 0.5 mL of air and check for loss of resistance this way. A second option is to redirect the needle more medially. You may be deep enough, but your needle is too lateral. If the needle is hitting bone before reaching the epidural space (usually very superficial), you are most likely hitting the spinous process and the needle should be redirected more cephalad or caudad. Pull the needle back a few centimeters and redirect. If the needle is contacting bone past the level expected of the spinous process, it is most likely touching lamina and needs to be directed cephalad or medial and cephalad.

After obtaining loss of resistance, the epidural catheter is then fed through the Tuohy needle into the epidural space (Fig. 17-7). Five centimeters of the catheter should be fed into the epidural space; the catheter has markings for every 1 cm for measurement purposes. To decide how much catheter will be needed, add the distance the needle had to transverse through tissue to reach the epidural space by counting the rungs on the needle still in view and subtracting it from 10. Then add 5 to that number. If the needle transverses 6 cm of tissue to reach the epidural space, 4 rungs on the needle will be still showing, the catheter should exit the skin at the

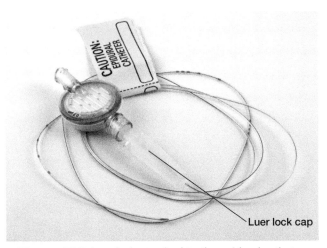

Figure 17-8 Luer lock attached to the epidural catheter.

11-cm mark, leaving 5 cm in the epidural space. There are special marks at 5, 10, and 15 cm on the catheter to help you determine your depth. The luer lock cap is then attached to the free end of the catheter (Fig. 17-8). Aspiration of the catheter is performed to rule out cerebral spinal fluid (CSF) or blood return, making sure that the catheter is neither intrathecal nor in a blood vessel. After confirming negative aspiration, the luer lock cap is removed and the needle is pulled out over the catheter. The luer lock cap is put back on the catheter.

The catheter should now be properly placed in the epidural space. However, there is a chance that even after negative aspiration the catheter could be in a blood vessel or that the catheter was advanced too deeply through the epidural space and directly into the intrathecal space. To further confirm proper catheter placement, it is necessary to give a "test dose." The kit is equipped with a vial containing a mixture of 1.5% lidocaine and 1/200,000 μg of epinephrine. Draw 3 mL of this solution into a 3-mL syringe. Attach the 3-mL syringe to the luer lock and inject the solution.

If the catheter is placed into a vessel, the epinephrine in the test dose will raise the heart rate at least 20 to 30 beats per minute, which will decrease shortly thereafter. If the catheter is intravascular patients may also have tinnitus or a metallic taste in their mouths. Intravenous placement is more common in pregnant patients because inferior vena cava compression by the enlarged uterus results in dilation of collateral veins in the epidural space ask patients to let you know if they experience either of these while giving the test dose. One clinical pearl to remember is that most of the vascularity of the epidural space is in the lateral region. This means that everything can go well from the loss of resistance to catheter threading, but test dosing will reveal an intravascular

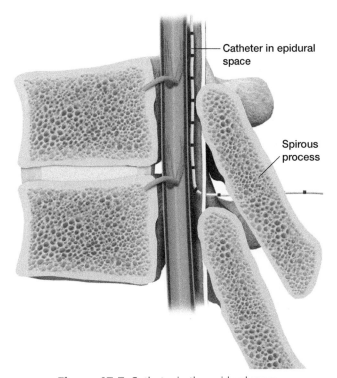

Catheter in epidural space

Spirous process

Figure 17-7 Catheter in the epidural space.

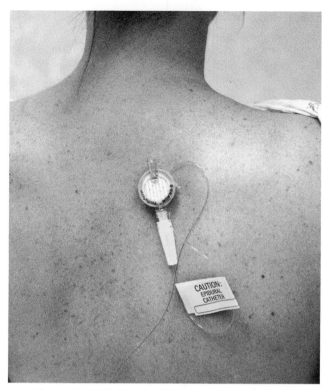

Figure 17-9 Epidural catheter secured to the back.

location. If this happens it is possible to make another attempt at threading the catheter, but often the needle will need to be redirected more medially. If the catheter is intrathecal, the patient will experience motor block below the level of the catheter from the test dose. If either occurs readjustment of the catheter is necessary.

Once proper catheter placement is confirmed the catheter is fully secured into place (Fig. 17-9). The

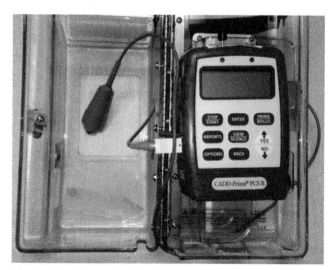

Figure 17-10 Patient-controlled epidural analgesia (PCEA) device.

epidural catheter is attached to the patient-controlled epidural analgesia (PCEA) device. PCEA is a way of delivering pain medication via a programmable intravenous infusion device (Fig. 17-10). The PCEA machine is set up at the patient's bedside and connected directly to the epidural catheter. A bag of premixed local anesthetic or local anesthetic–opioid combination is inserted into the machine.

WHEN TO USE

Surgical Setting

Epidural anesthesia via a catheter is typically used postoperatively to provide prolonged pain relief at the surgical site after intra-abdominal, thoracic, major orthopedic, or OB/GYN surgery.

The advantages to using an epidural catheter are that it administers medication painlessly and provides prompt analgesia. Epidural infusions with a local anesthetic reduce postoperative pain and may shorten the duration of a postoperative ileus after abdominal surgery. The disadvantage is that it takes more time and skill to place an epidural catheter and start a PCEA machine, then set up an intravenous (PCA) or write a order for IV opioids. Primarily only anesthesiologists are trained at properly placing the epidural catheter.

Multiple studies have examined whether intravenous PCA or epidural PCEA is better for postoperative pain management. Categories evaluated include postoperative pain levels, bowel recovery, sedation, nausea and vomiting, and early discharge. The studies are mixed, some showing that an epidural catheter is better, whereas others show no difference. In general, early bowel recovery as well as less sedation were seen with epidural analgesia as compared to intravenous PCA in most studies.

Childbirth Setting

Epidural anesthesia is chosen by some expectant mothers to provide pain relief during the birthing process. Roughly 60% of women choose to have epidural anesthesia but this number has been steadily increasing. Uterine contractions and cervical dilatation is relayed to the spine at the T11–L1 level and results in pain during the first part of delivery. This is the most intense and longest part of labor. The descent of the head and subsequent pressure on the pelvic floor and perineal structures is relayed via the sacral nerves S2–S4 and generates pain during the final phase of labor (Fig. 17-11) with the epidural catheter properly placed over the lowest thoracic levels. The medication tends to trickle down into the sacral region, but in some cases this does not occur. For this reason, even a well-placed lumbar epidural catheter may fail to produce

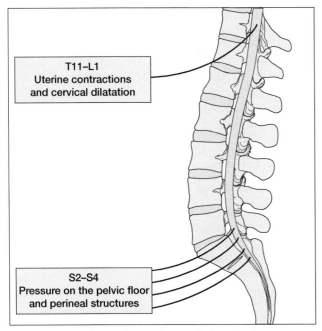

Figure 17-11 First and second part of labor. Uterine contractions and cervical dilatation is relayed to the spine at the T11–L1 level and results in pain during the first part of delivery. The descent of the head and subsequent pressure on the pelvic floor and perineal structures is relayed via the sacral nerves S2–S4 and generates pain during the final phase of labor.

good analgesia late in the delivery process. This phenomenon is known as "sacral sparing" and should be discussed in the informed consent process.

HOW TO USE

Surgical Setting

The first step is to choose what medication to administer. There are a good number of choices, most beyond the scope of this book. This chapter will focus on the single local anesthetic and three opioids most commonly used. The most frequently used local anesthetic is bupivacaine. It works in the epidural space at the dural cuff regions, where there is a relatively thin dural cover, as well as the spinal nerve roots. It comes in two premixed strengths: 0.0625% and 0.125%. For the most part, dosing should start at 0.125% with reduction to 0.0625% if the block is too strong. An opioid can be added to the local anesthetic to enhance efficacy. Adding an opioid allows for the lowest dose of each medication being used and maximizes the concentration of analgesia at the site where nociceptive fibers enter the spinal cord. There are three basic choices of opioid: Fentanyl, morphine, and hydromorphone (Dilaudid). All three opiates activate receptors in the brain and spinal cord that modulate our perception of painful stimuli. These medications come in standard premixed bags.

Epidural catheter analgesia without an opioid in the surgical setting has not gained wide use because of the failure rate resulting from the necessity of administering the local anesthetic at a level that causes hypotension from the sympathetic blockade as well as motor block.

It was formerly believed that lipid-soluble opioids such as fentanyl (approximately 800 times more lipid soluble than morphine) would be more likely to stay in the epidural space whereas morphine and hydromorphone would be more likely to gravitate toward the CSF. Fentanyl was thought to be safer because there was less risk of cephalad migration, reducing the risk of delayed respiratory depression. Studies have shown that the risk of clinically significant respiratory depression during epidural fentanyl infusion is 0.6%, whereas the incidence with patients receiving epidural morphine is 0.5% to 0.7%.[1,2] There does not appear to be a clinical advantage of using lipid-soluble opioids (fentanyl) over more water-soluble opioids (morphine and hydromorphone) in terms of lowering the risk of respiratory depression. Table 17-2 contains the standard strengths of all three opioids when used epidurally. The choice of which opioid to use is a matter of personal preference. At equal analgesic doses, no opioid is stronger or better than another for the patient unless the patient is allergic to one of them. None is disease or anatomy specific—for example, one is not better for orthopedic pain versus another more suited for pelvic pain.

The second step is to choose settings on the PCEA machine. Every PCEA should have a continuous rate—the amount of medication that automatically flows into the patient every hour. One major study reviewed patients recovering from gastrectomy (upper abdominal surgery) who had an epidural catheter. Patients on a continuous rate and a demand dose reported less postoperative pain than those who had no continuous rate and the same demand dosing.[3] Note to the reader: This is true for PCEA not PCA. In the lumbar region, the continuous rate is usually set to 10 mL/hr whereas in the thoracic region, the continuous rate is set to 8 mL/hr (see Table 17-3 for infusion ranges). Continuous rates for adult epidural analgesia may range between 3 and 20 mL/hr. These rates often require adjustment depending on how well the patient does clinically.

TABLE 17-2 Standard Opioid Strengths for Epidural Use

Opioid	Opioid Strength (%)	Local Anesthetic and Opioid Premixed Bag
Fentanyl	0.001	Bupivacaine 0.125% and fentanyl 0.001%
Morphine	0.01	Bupivacaine 0.125% and morphine 0.01%
Dilaudid	0.005	Bupivacaine 0.125% and hydromorphone 0.005%

TABLE 17-3 Common Continuous Infusion Rates for Epidural Analgesia

General Type of Surgery	Catheter Location	Continuous Infusion Rate (mL/hr)
Thoracic	T2–T9	4–10
Upper abdominal	T4–L1	4–10
Lower abdominal	T10–L3	8–18
Lower extremity	T12–L3	8–18
Childbirth	T10–L5	8–14

It is common practice to deliver epidural analgesia with a continuous rate and no demand dose. However, some practitioners prefer the addition of a demand dose. The demand dose is a bolus that the patient self-administers by pushing a button connected to the PCEA (Fig. 17-12) as with PCA. A lock-out period is used to prevent overdosing. The lock-out period is how long the machine will "lock" after a demand dose is delivered before it allows another demand dose, no matter how many times the patient pushes the button. The addition of a demand dose gives patients an enhanced sense of control. Patients who control their own level of pain by demand dosage have been shown to choose to administer less medication and accept higher pain levels rather than experience more side effects. The typical demand dose is 3 mL with a 20-minute lock. Common PCEA settings post-thoracic surgery are as follows: Premixed bag of bupivacaine 0.125% and morphine .01% with a continuous rate of 6 mL/hr, a demand dose of 3 mL, and a lock-out period of 20 minutes.

Childbirth Setting

The opioid of choice in the childbirth setting is fentanyl as it has a short half-life. Common settings for a labor and delivery PCEA are as follows: Fentanyl 2 mcg/mL and 0.125% bupivacaine set on a continuous rate of 10 mL/hr with a demand dose of 5 mL and a lock-out period of 10 minutes. Some doctors choose to have the nurse give a bolus dose rather than use the patient-controlled demand dose on the PCEA. A common bolus order is 5 mL every 10 minutes with a 4-dose lock-out per hour.

WHEN NOT TO USE AND POSSIBLE SIDE EFFECTS

Anticoagulation Guidelines

Guidelines on use of regional anesthesia in the presence of anticoagulants have been published by a number of societies throughout the world there are similarities and differences among them. In general epidural catheter placement can be performed on patients taking aspirin or NSAIDs. Plavix should be discontinued for 7 days before catheter placement. For patients on Warfarin (Coumadin) it is commonly believed that an INR value of ≤1.4 is acceptable for catheter placement. Low Molecular Weight Heparin (LMWH) at a therapeutic dose should be stopped 24 hours before placement. There is no usually no restrictions to performing the procedure with a patient on SC heparin (5,000 q12)

It is also generally accepted that an epidural catheter should only be removed for patients on Coumadin if the INR is ≤1.4. For patients in heparin the catheter should be removed 1 hour before subsequent heparin administration and 2 to 4 hours after the last heparin dose. In patients who are on LMWH, catheter removal should be performed at least 12 hours after the last dose.

Hypotension

A local anesthetic in the epidural space causes a sympathetic block. This can lead to unchecked parasympathetic activity causing vasodilation and hypotension. These effects are more pronounced if the patient is dehydrated. The sympathetic block is exacerbated if the block height reaches the cardiac acceleration fibers between T1 and T4, resulting in bradycardia. If this happens, it is necessary to lower the rate of infusion or temporarily stop it to address hypotension. Once the patient is hemodynamically stable, the infusion can restart.

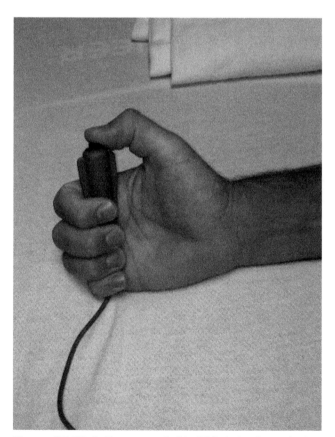

Figure 17-12 Button connected to PCA device for patient to self-administer analgesic medication.

Motor Block

The goal is to cause sensory blockade, not motor block. After the initiation of the infusion, a patient may temporarily lose the ability to move his or her legs. In these cases, it is necessary to reduce the infusion rate until a proper rate is found. Patients may also develop an asymetric block. Despite apparently proper placement roughly 5–8% of epidurals may provide incomplete analgesia of this sort. It is generally postulated that either an anatomic barrier to free flow of local anesthetic or unfavorable positioning of the tip of the catheter in responsible. In very rare cases, a patient who had a good epidural level and minimal weakness on a stable constant infusion rate develops new weakness. In these cases, it is important to lower the infusion rate; if that does not help, intrathecal migration of the catheter or epidural hematoma should be a consideration.

Headache

It is possible to advance the needle too far, causing dural puncture, which occurs in 0.32% to 1.23% of epidural placements.[5] This can result in the development of a postdural headache. This type of headache can be differentiated from other types such as tension, migraine, or cluster headache by a postural component, the headache is minimal in the supine position and becomes significant when the patient is sitting up. Postdural headaches can usually be managed conservatively with fluids and caffeine but may require a blood patch. Close monitoring in this situation is essential.

Other Effects

Also, there is a risk of infection as well as a risk of epidural hematoma with epidural analgesia, although the catheter is small. The risk of clinically significant epidural hematoma in the obstetric population is approximately 1 in 168,000.[4]

In addition, it is important to consider the analgesics used in PCEA. To a degree, all opioids have the ability to cause nausea, constipation, and pruritus. Although respiratory depression remains a rare complication of opioid use, it nonetheless is a significant concern. Data suggest that the overall incidence in patients using a PCEA is very small. If the epidural contains an opioid, the patient should be monitored for at least 12 hours after removal of the epidural catheter. (Catheter removal requires gentle traction.)

CASE STUDIES

Case 1

Nonchildbirth Surgical Case

A 52-year-old female who is opioid naïve has an epidural catheter placed preoperatively. The patient is scheduled to have a pancreatic mass removed. You order the PCEA machine to be set up as follows: Premixed bag of bupivacaine 0.125% and Dilaudid 0.005% with a continuous rate of 6 mL/hr, a demand dose of 3 mL, and a lock-out period of 20 minutes.

When you check on the patient postoperatively, her pain level is an 8 out of 10 and she feels uncomfortable. You increase the continuous rate to 10 mL/hr, the demand dose is kept at 3 mL, and the lock-out period is kept at 20 minutes. You check on her an hour later and she is comfortable, with minimal pain complaints. Her vitals and neurologic examination are stable and mental status is clear.

Case 2

Childbirth Case

A 32-year-old female has an epidural catheter placed in anticipation of a normal vaginal delivery. You order the PCEA machine to be set up as follows: Premixed bag containing fentanyl 2 μg/mL and 0.125% bupivacaine on a continuous rate of 10 mL/hr with a demand dose of 3 mL and a lock-out period of 20 minutes. The patient is comfortable with minimal pain complaints. Her vitals are stable and mental status is clear. The catheter is pulled 2 hours after the uncomplicated delivery.

REFERENCES

1. Weightman WM. Respiratory arrest during epidural infusion of bupivacaine and fentanyl. *Anaesth Intensive Care.* 1991;19:282–284.
2. de Leon-Casasola OA, Parker B, Lema MJ, et al. Postoperative epidural bupivacaine-morphine therapy: Experience with 4,227 surgical cancer patients. *Anesthesiology.* 1994;81(2):368–375.
3. Komatsu H, Matsumoto S, Mitsuhata H, et al. Comparison of patient-controlled epidural analgesia with and without background infusion after gastrectomy. *Anesth Analg.* 1998;87(4):907–910.
4. Ruppen W, Derry S, McQuay H, et al. Incidence of epidural hematoma, infection, and neurological injury in obstetric patients with epidural analgesia/anesthesia. *Anesthesiology.* 2006;105:394–399.
5. Giebler RM, Scherer RU, Peters J. Incidence of neurologic complications related to thoracic epidural catheterization. *Anesthesiology.* 1997;86:55–63.

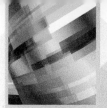

CHAPTER **18**

Radiation Therapy

Targeted radiation has become a valuable tool in treating both cancer and the pain caused by cancer. Roughly 50% of all cancer patients will receive radiotherapy at some stage during the course of their illness. Radiation therapy works by damaging the DNA of cancerous cells via both an indirect and direct action. The indirect action occurs as a result of ionizing water surrounding the cancer cells, which forms free radicals. These free radicals then damage the cellular DNA of both cancer and normal cells (Fig. 18-1). Cancer cells have a diminished ability to repair this sublethal damage compared to healthy differentiated cells, making them more prone for targeted cell death. Advanced solid tumors—whose blood supply is limited because of constriction of local blood vessels—often have less fluid to be ionized into free radicals, making the indirect action of radiation therapy less effective. The direct action occurs via a high linear energy transfer direct to cells in the path of the beam, causing a sublethal damage to cellular DNA (Fig. 18-2).

Patients most commonly receive radiation through an external linear accelerator (Fig. 18-3). The linear accelerator uses electricity to form a stream of fast moving subatomic particles. By subjecting charged particles to a series of oscillating electric potentials along a linear beam line. In microseconds, the device moves stationary electrons to nearly the speed of light —186,000 miles a second. When these high speed electrons are fired they release a stream of photons that can be aimed to a specific part of the body. It is possible to change the radiation beam to different amounts to provide the desired tissue penetration. The amount of radiation used is measured in gray units (Gy) and the total dose varies depending on the type and stage of cancer being treated. Treatment often lasts less than 5 minutes and is not painful.

Each type of tumor carries its own sensitivity to radiation therapy. Tumors known to be especially radiosensitive include leukemias, most lymphomas, and germ cell tumors. Tumors known to be especially radioresistant

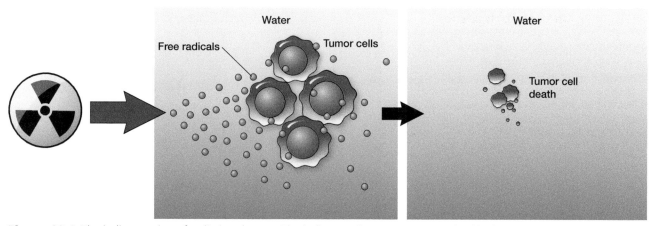

Figure 18-1 The indirect action of radiation therapy. The indirect action occurs as a result of ionizing water surrounding the cancer cells, which forms free radicals. These free radicals then damage the cellular DNA of both cancer and normal cells.

Figure 18-2 The direct action of radiation therapy. A high linear energy transfer occurs to cells in the path of the beam, causing sublethal damage to cellular DNA. ▶

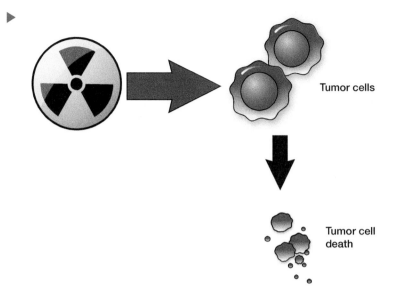

Tumor cells

Tumor cell death

are renal cell cancer and melanoma. Size is also a significant factor, as very large tumors do not respond as well as smaller tumors to radiation therapy.

WHEN TO USE

Pain from a Solid Tumor

Solid tumors cause pain by invasion, obstruction, distension, or compression of surrounding tissue or nerves. They also can cause pain by secreting inflammatory mediators. Radiation therapy is used to treat localized solid tumors, such as cancers of the brain, breast, or cervix. One challenge in treating solid tumors with radiation is that the microenvironment of solid tumors is hypoxic compared to normal tissue, and this hypoxia is associated with decreased radiosensitivity. Lack of hydration decreases the indirect action of radiation therapy.

Pain from Bone Metastases

The most common cause of pain in cancer patients is bone metastasis. Seventy percent of patients with bone metastasis have bone pain, which is caused by the tumor stretching the periosteum (membrane that lines the outer surface of all bones). Pain is also caused by nerve irritation in the endosteum (tissue lining the medullary cavity of the bone). Understanding of the mechanism of metastatic bone lesion pain is limited, because more than 25% of patients with bone metastasis are pain free and patients with multiple bone metastases typically report pain in only a few of the areas where they have lesions. Cancers that tend to metastasize to bone originate from the breast, lung, thyroid, kidney, and prostate. The ribs, pelvis, and spine are normally the first bones to which cancer metastasizes. Pathologic fractures are common in breast cancer because of the lytic nature of the lesions.

Figure 18-3 External linear accelerator. The Elekta Synergy combines x-ray imaging and treatment delivery into one integrated gantry-mounted system. Both planar images and cone-beam computed tomography three-dimensional volume reconstruction images can be obtained for position verification. (Courtesy of Elekta, from Kavanagh BD, Timmerman RD. *Stereotactic Body Radiation Therapy*. Lippincott Williams & Wilkins, 2005, p 82.). ▶

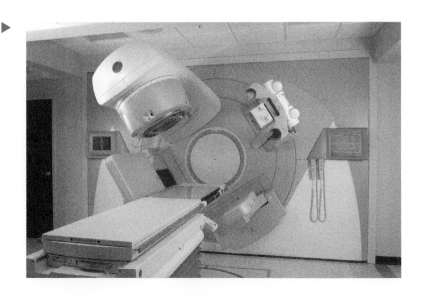

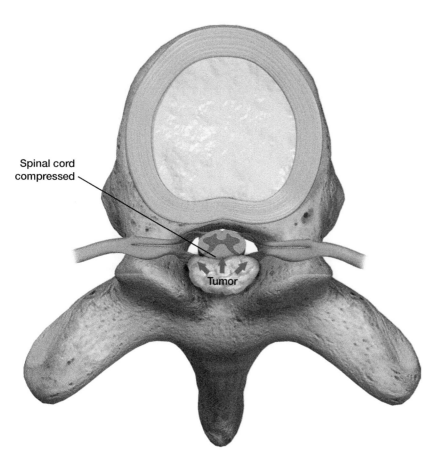

◄ **Figure 18-4** Spinal cord compression.

Spinal cord compressed

Tumor

Radiation therapy can provide pain relief, as well as functional preservation and maintenance of skeletal integrity. Decreasing the tumor burden leads to less stretch of the periosteum and less irritation of the endosteum, thus decreasing bone pain. In a study involving patients who received radiation therapy for painful metastatic bone lesions from prostate or breast cancer at 3 months, after treatment 15% had no pain and were on no narcotics whereas 50% had significantly less pain.[1]

Radiation therapy has another beneficial effect. Metastatic bone lesions weaken the structural matrix of bone by both damaging healthy bone cells and disturbing the normal process of bone turnover. After radiation treatment, a portion of cancer cells die; as a result, healthy bone cells replace the lost tissue, allowing bones to become stronger, less painful, and less likely to break.

Cord Compression Due to Tumor

Patients with cord compression (cancer pressing on the spinal cord) present with acute back pain and neurologic deficits in the lower extremities, which may include sensory changes and/or weakness (Fig. 18-4). They also may present with bowel or bladder incontinence. Bone metastases from breast, prostate, lung, and colon cancers are at particularly high risk for these

changes. Treatment for spinal cord compression includes high-dose corticosteroids and radiation as well as possible surgical decompression. Radiation therapy shrinks the tumor and quickly relieves the pressure on the spinal cord, reducing the pain. Radiation therapy provides definitive treatment in most patients. A wide range of fractional schemes is used in clinical practice with no general consensus: A common scheme is 3 Gy a day for 10 days for a total of 30 Gy.

The key is early recognition of cord compression and addressing the condition as an emergency. Table 18-1 outlines treatment efficacy in relation to point of intervention.

TABLE 18-1 Chance of Remaining Ambulatory with Treatment for Spinal Cord Compression

Point of Intervention	Chance of Remaining Ambulatory
If treatment starts while patient is still able to walk	75%
If treatment starts with partial or incomplete weakness	30–50%
If patient is already paralyzed	10–20%

HOW TO USE

The total dose of radiation is fractionated, which means that it is spread out over time. Fractionizing the total dose produces better results for two reasons. First, cancer cells cannot recover as quickly as normal cells before being exposed to another dose. This favors the targeted death of cancer cells while preserving normal cells. Second, cancer cells that are chronically or acutely hypoxic (therefore more radioresistant because they do not have water that can be ionized into free radicals) may reoxygenate and hydrate between fractions, improving the indirect action of radiation therapy.

More than 40 different radiation therapy fractionation schedules have been reported in the literature, with 30 Gy in 10 fractions being most common in the United States. The specific treatment plan depends on type and extent of the cancer, and is chosen by the radiation oncologist. In some cases, palliative single-fraction radiation therapy is used.

WHEN NOT TO USE AND POTENTIAL SIDE EFFECTS

Radiation treatment itself is painless. This mode of treatment, however, has side effects, which may be categorized as acute or late.

Acute side effects include the following:

● Damage to the epithelial surface where the beam is focused
● Ulceration in the mouth and throat if the head and neck area is treated
● Swelling in the area in which the beam is placed
● Infertility

Late side effects include the following:

● Fibrosis in tissue that has been irradiated.
● Lymphedema in the region treated. This is most common in patients who received treatment for breast cancer, because the axilla is vulnerable.
● Injury to the brachial or lumbosacral plexus, which can occur with direct exposure (Fig. 18-5).

Radiation injury to the brachial plexus may present 1 to 30 years following radiation treatment. Patients commonly describe pain as aching in the shoulder or hand. Other symptoms include paresthesia in the lateral fingers or entire hand. For the lumbosacral region, presenting symptoms include weakness of the legs associated with sensory symptoms, paresthesia, and numbness. Weakness starts distally in the L5 to S1 segments and slowly progresses. Magnetic resonance imaging (MRI) and/or electromyography can help establish the diagnosis. MRI features suggestive of radiation-induced plexopathy

Figure 18-5 Radiation-induced brachial ▶ plexopathy.

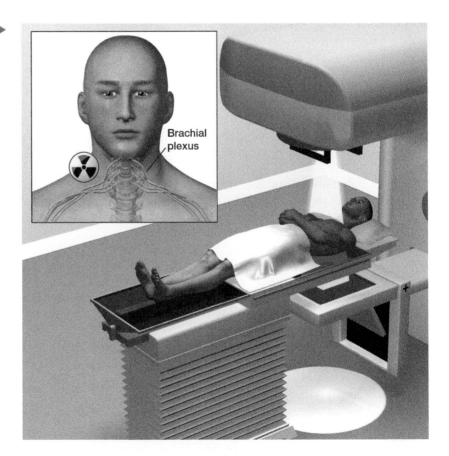

include diffuse, uniform, symmetric swelling, and T2 hyperintensity of the plexus, compared with nonuniform, asymmetric, and focal enlargement, and the presence of a mass with postcontrast enhancement, which is indicative of tumor recurrence. There are no proven methods of reversing this neurologic damage.

Although there is an increased risk for secondary malignancy with radiation exposure, the benefits usually outweigh the risks. When treating an adult with cancer, the chance of causing a new cancer from radiation ranges between 1% and 5% up to 30 years later. Thus, for example, if a 57-year-old patient receiving radiation therapy lives to age 87, that patient will have at most a 1 in 20 chance of developing a radiation-induced cancer.

CASE STUDIES

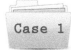

Case 1 A 57-year-old woman with breast cancer diagnosed 2 years ago presents to the emergency department with back pain and some mild weakness in her legs. An MRI performed in the emergency department shows a thoracic metastatic tumor, which is causing compression of the cord at T8. On a visual analog scale, she rates her pain level as 10 out of 10. The woman begins receiving intravenous (IV) Dilaudid 2 mg every 2 hours and IV Solu-Medrol. Four hours later, she rates her pain as 8 out of 10. The patient is admitted to the hospital, where emergent radiation treatment begins. By the end of treatment, the patient is no longer receiving IV narcotics and using a minimal amount of hydrocodone orally for pain as needed.

Case 2 A 78-year-old man with metastatic colon cancer. He is currently taking OxyContin 20 mg every 8 hours and Percocet 7.5/325 every 8 hours as needed for breakthrough pain. The patient states that his back pain is what bothers him the most. On imaging, he has metastatic lesions to L3 and L4. There are no cord abnormalities (remember that the spinal cord usually ends at about L1). You recommend radiation therapy to help with the pain. The patient is worried about making the cancer worse with radiation. You explain that the radiation is targeted directly to where the painful spinal lesions are and that the increased risk of secondary malignancy is very small—if the patient lived to 93, at most he would have a 1 in 10 chance of developing a radiation-induced cancer. After a full discussion, the patient decides to proceed with treatment.

REFERENCE

1. The Bone Metastases and Osteoporosis: Painful Bone Metastases: RTOG Trial 9701 finds that the response rate from 8 Gy single-fraction radiotherapy is as effective as a longer course.

PART III

Interventional Treatments

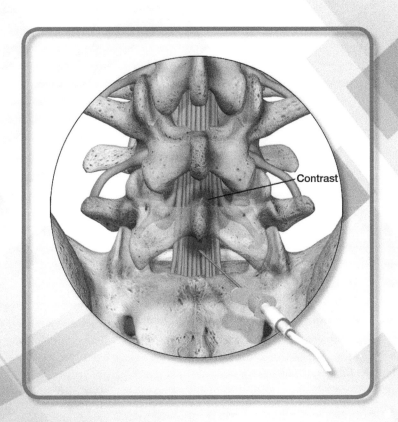

Contrast

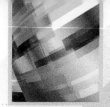

CHAPTER 19

Epidural Steroid Injections

Most people think of an epidural injection as what is administered to a woman for pain control before she delivers her baby. The word *epidural* simply refers to the epidural space. It is the outermost space in the spinal canal, lying outside the dura mater inside the surrounding vertebrae (Fig. 19-1). The superior limit of the epidural space is the foramen magnum, where the spine meets the skull. The inferior limit is the end of the sacrum. The epidural space is important because it is where the nerve roots can be accessed to provide pain relief. There are multiple approaches to this space and different medications that can be injected into it. A catheter may be placed into the epidural space to deliver continuous local anesthetic infusion, which is what the expectant mother receives. After delivery, the infusion is stopped and the catheter is taken out. This chapter addresses epidural steroid injections—injecting steroid into the epidural space to reduce inflammation and decrease pain.

A vertebral disc is built like a jelly doughnut. The inner jelly part is the nucleus pulposus and the outer layer is the anulus fibrosus (Fig. 19-2). The anulus fibrosis can become weak, allowing the nucleus pulposus to herniate into it, and in some cases through it. This herniation of disc material out of its normal position causes compression and irritation of the adjacent nerve root (Fig. 19-3). This is referred to as radicular pain or radiculopathy (irritation of a nerve root). When a nerve root is irritated, it sends an aberrant signal up to the brain, which interprets this as pain along that entire nerve. The brain is tricked into thinking the entire nerve is affected. Furthermore the nucleus pulposus contains inflammatory factors that can leak out through the anulus fibrosus and bathe the

nerve root in an inflammatory matrix. Steroids suppress the autoimmune response triggered by glycoproteins from the nucleus pulposus and exert membrane-stabilizing effects on injured nerve segments, reducing ectopic discharges from the affected nerve roots.[1,3] The combination of both inflammation and physical protrusion of a disc herniation may eventually put pressure on the epidural venous plexus, causing venous obstruction.[1] When the venous side is backed up, it can lead to decreased perfusion of the nerve root from the arterial side. Prolonged irritation and poor blood circulation appear to make these nerve roots hypersensitive,[2] further contributing to prolonged radicular pain.

The disc that lies between the body of the fourth and fifth lumbar vertebral bodies (L4–L5) and the disc that lies between the fifth lumbar vertebral body and the sacrum (L5–S1) are where 90% of disc herniations occur in the lumbar spine. This is a matter of physics. The greatest range of motion in the spine is at the L4–L5 and L5–S1 levels, which makes these discs most vulnerable to herniation. This phenomenon can also occur in the cervical spine. Cervical discs can herniate, causing cervical radiculopathy with paresthesia (a skin sensation of tingling or prickling) radiating down the arm. The location with the greatest range of motion in the cervical spine is at the C5–C6 and C6–C7 levels.

WHEN TO USE

The two most common indications for epidural steroid injections are lumbar and cervical radiculopathy. Another condition that may respond to a series of

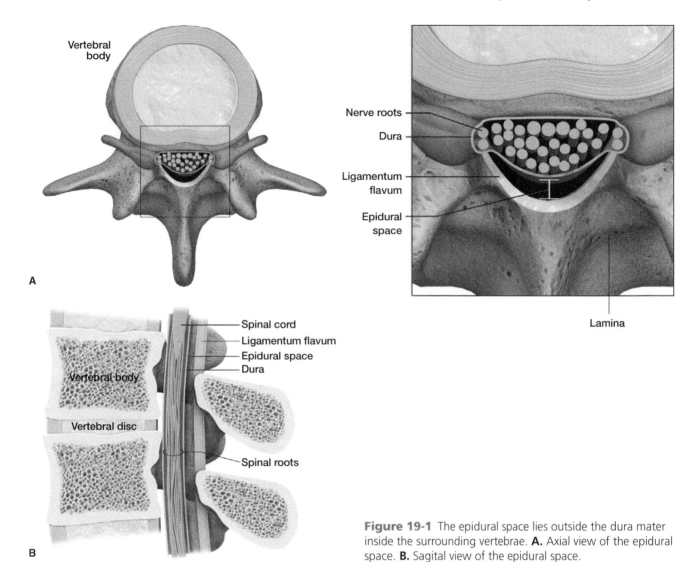

A

B

Vertebral body

Nerve roots
Dura
Ligamentum flavum
Epidural space
Lamina

Spinal cord
Ligamentum flavum
Epidural space
Dura
Vertebral body
Vertebral disc
Spinal roots

Figure 19-1 The epidural space lies outside the dura mater inside the surrounding vertebrae. **A.** Axial view of the epidural space. **B.** Sagital view of the epidural space.

Annulus fibrosus
Nucleus pulposus
Pedicle
Superior articulating facet
Lamina
Spinous process

Superior articulating facet
Transverse process
Inferior articulating facet
Pedicle
Vertebral body

Figure 19-2 Spinal column anatomy.

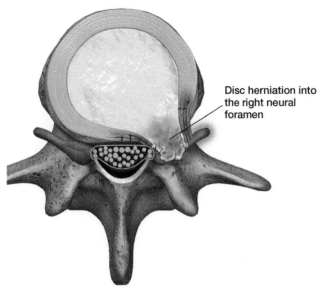

Disc herniation into the right neural foramen

Figure 19-3 Compression and irritation of a nerve root caused by the herniation of disc material.

TABLE 19-1 Equivalent Doses of Other Steroids to Kenalog 40 mg

Trade Name	Generic Name	Equivalent Dose to Kenalog
Depo-Medrol	Methylprednisolone acetate	40 mg
Celestone	Betamethasone acetate	6 mg
Decadron	Dexamethasone acetate	8 mg

epidural steroid injections is spinal canal stenosis. The injections alleviate pressure stemming from the inflamed tissue. Other common indications include postlaminectomy syndrome, vertebral compression fractures, sacral fractures, degenerative disc disease, and postherpetic neuralgia. In postherpetic neuralgia, an epidural steroid injection consisting of a local anesthetic and steroid mixture can help to stabilize an aberrant firing dorsal root ganglion.

Epidural steroid injections remain a conservative traditional alternative to surgery. They can be used in combination with oral medication or as an alternative. Epidural steroid injections deliver a concentrated steroid dose directly to the level of pathology in lower quantities than would be needed via oral or intravenous administration. Theoretically, the epidural steroids are more effective within the first 3 months of radiculopathy, and may help prevent chronic fibrosis and adhesions around the nerve root.

The pain from most disc herniations resolves on its own in around a year. However, with an epidural steroid injection, the patient may not have to spend as much as a year waiting for the symptoms to dissipate. By decreasing pain levels the patient can remain active, avoiding the risk of deteriorating physical condition and missing work. An epidural steroid injection can eliminate the need for pain medications that often have to be taken every day, can have side effects, and may not be effective. For radiculopathy, trying an epidural steroid injection before prescribing narcotic medication is highly appropriate.

In the past physicians performed epidural steroid injections blindly without fluoroscopy (x-ray guidance), and this necessitated injecting a substantial amount of medication. Now that the use of fluoroscopy with epidural steroid injections are routinely used, the doses used have dropped substantially. Patients currently on average can have four injections per year (not three injections in a lifetime, a common misconception) without disrupting the pituitary adrenal axis.

As frequently as these injections are performed, there is no consensus as to what steroid to inject and how much should be injected. I use Kenalog (triamcinolone acetonide) for my injections; reasonable Kenalog doses are provided in the examples to follow. But if you decide to use Depo-Medrol, Celestone, or any other steroid, their proper dose can easily be calculated—for example, 40 mg of Kenalog is equivalent to 6 mg of Celestone (Table 19-1).

The physicians should be sure to tell the patient that steroids take time to work, pain relief may not be noted until 4–7 days post injection, and more than one injection may be necessary to achieve a compounding effect.

HOW TO PERFORM THE PROCEDURE

The two most common forms of the epidural steroid injection are the interlaminar and transforaminal approaches; sometimes it is necessary to use a caudal approach.

Interlaminar Epidural Steroid Injection

It is essential that the procedure be completely explained to the patient, that all questions are answered, and that informed consent obtained.

After the patient is brought to the fluoroscopy suite, he or she should lie on the fluoroscopic table in the prone position (face down). A "time out" is performed

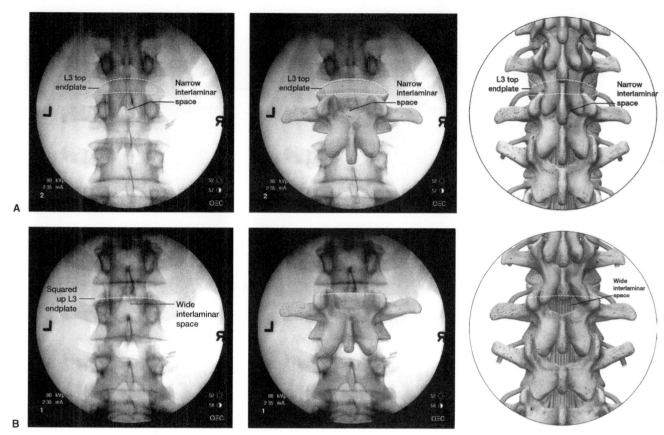

Figure 19-4 The fluoroscope is placed in the anteroposterior (AP) position and tilted, if necessary, in a cephalad to caudad motion to "square up" the endplates of the vertebral bodies. **A.** In the first panel of pictures, the top of the L3 vertebral body is slanted which narrows the entry to the interlaminar space. **B.** In the second panel of pictures the angle of the camera has been adjusted in a cephalad position to "square up" the top of the L3 vertebral body which widens the entry to the intralaminar space making the procedure easier to perform.

prior to the procedure including verbal confirmation of correct patient, procedure & procedural site. Noninvasive hemodynamic monitors and pulse oximetry are placed.

To begin, the skin over the lower back is prepped with Betadine and drapes are placed over the area in standard sterile fashion. The fluoroscope is placed in the anteroposterior (AP) position, tilting it if necessary in a cephalad to caudad motion to "square up" the end plates of the vertebral bodies (Fig. 19-4). Patients with prominent lordosis may require a significant tilt of the fluoroscope. The epidural space of interest is visualized. Using a metal marker and a felt tip marking pen, an "X" is placed on the skin overlying the inferior lamina of the epidural space of interest (Fig. 19-5).

The skin and subcutaneous tissue is anesthetized with 2% lidocaine using a 1.5-in, 25G needle. After the skin is anesthetized, a Tuohy epidural needle

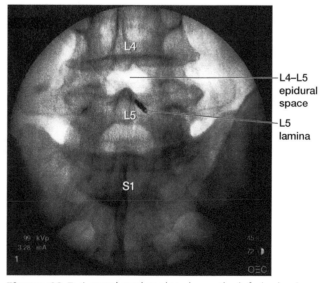

Figure 19-5 A metal marker placed over the inferior lamina of the epidural space of interest.

Figure 19-6 **A.** Tuohy epidural needle. **B.** The slight curve at the end of the needle is a saftey feature. It makes it less likely the dura will be punctured.

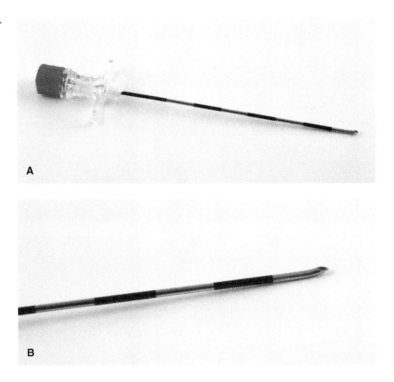

A

B

(Fig. 19-6) is placed through the "X" in a perpendicular fashion to the skin and parallel to the fluoroscope (Fig. 19-7). The Tuohy needle is advanced until the lamina is contacted; the needle is then slightly retracted and advanced superiorly and medially toward the center of the epidural space. The needle then enters the ligamentum flavum, a typically thick ligament that "grabs" the needle as you enter it. At this point, the stylet of the Tuohy needle is removed and a glass syringe is attached to the Tuohy needle. I

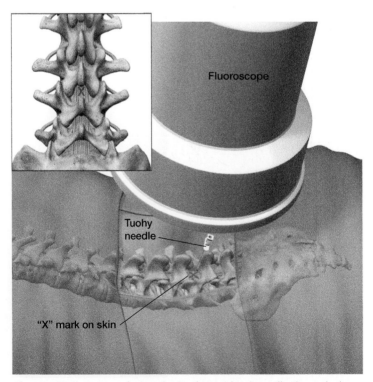

Fluoroscope

Tuohy needle

"X" mark on skin

Figure 19-7 Doctor placing the Tuohy epidural needle through the "X" on the skin in a perpendicular fashion to the skin and parallel to the fluoroscope.

fill the glass syringe with 3 mL of preservative free saline; some doctors use air. When the needle is in the ligamentum flavum, the saline stays in the syringe despite applying light pressure to the plunger. As the needle pushes through the ligamentum flavum the saline is sucked into the epidural space by negative pressure indicating proper position (Fig. 19-8). This is known as the loss-of-resistance technique. Once

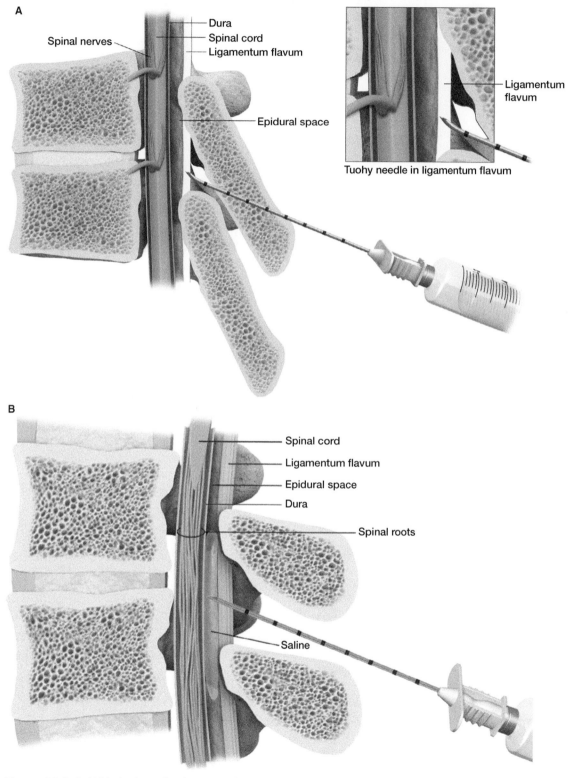

A.

Spinal nerves

Dura
Spinal cord
Ligamentum flavum

Epidural space

Ligamentum flavum

Tuohy needle in ligamentum flavum

B.

Spinal cord
Ligamentum flavum
Epidural space
Dura

Spinal roots

Saline

Figure 19-8 A. With the loss of resistance technique, saline stays in the glass syringe despite light pressure being applied to it as the bevel of the needle is up against the ligamentum flavum. **B.** As the needle pushes through the ligamentum flavum saline is sucked into the epidural space by negative pressure indicating proper position.

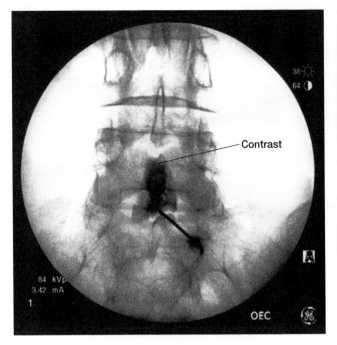
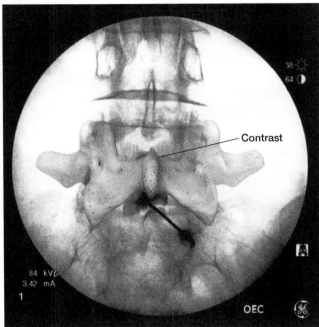
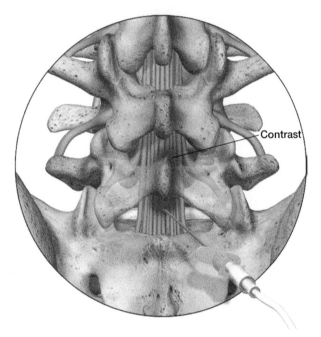

Figure 19-9 Proper contrast spread for a lumbar epidural steroid injection.

this occurs, a 3-mL syringe with tubing containing contrast is connected to the Tuohy needle. Tubing is used so that you can see the contrast being injected under live x-ray without having your hand obscure the image while simultaneously protecting your hand from radiation exposure. Contrast is injected to make sure that there is proper spread into the epidural space (Fig. 19-9). You can also confirm proper contrast spread on a lateral view (Fig. 19-10).

You have now checked proper needle placement under fluoroscopy, using the loss-of-resistance technique and ensuring proper contrast spread. The 3-mL

syringe containing contrast is disconnected from the tubing. A 10-mL syringe with the therapeutic agent, normal saline and a steroid, is connected to the tubing and injected. I use 5 mL of normal saline and 80 mg of Kenalog as my therapeutic agent in the lumbar spine and 3 mL of normal saline and 80 mg of Kenalog as the therapeutic agent in the cervical spine. If the patient has significant central canal stenosis, the volume of medication is decreased. The needle is then removed and a bandage placed.

With the cervical spine unlike the lumbar spine, the injection is typically performed at the C7–T1

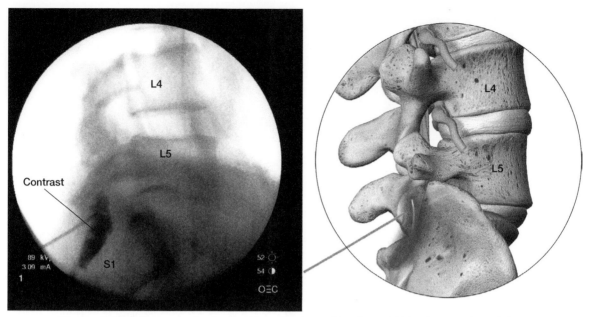

Figure 19-10 Proper contrast spread for a lumbar epidural steroid injection on a lateral view.

level regardless of the level of pathology (Fig. 19-11). This is where the epidural space is the widest. It is the safest level to advance the needle and detect proper loss of resistance. Because the cervical epidural space is much smaller as compared with the lumbar spine, the medication injected can typically flow up to the level of interest—even if the disc herniation is a few levels above the needle entry site. By simply increasing the volume of the therapeutic agent, you can drive the medication to more superior levels. If there is any blockade to the level of interest, a small catheter can be fed through the Tuohy needle into

the epidural space up to the level of interest. The same procedural steps are followed as in the lumbar spine.

Transforaminal Lumbar Epidural Steroid Injection

Nerve roots leave the epidural space on the left and right side of the spine through their respective neural foramen. The vertebral discs lie on the anterior side of the epidural space (toward the stomach) and herniate posteriorly into the neuroforamen. Here the disc contacts the nerve root, for example, the L4 nerve root on

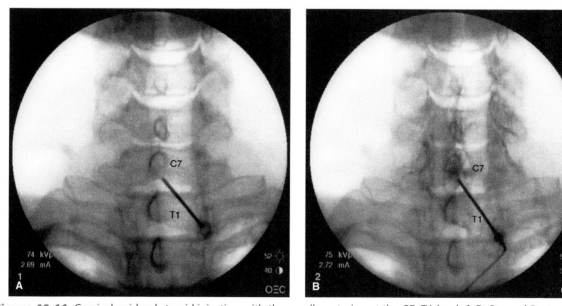

Figure 19-11 Cervical epidural steroid injection with the needle entering at the C7–T1 level. **A,B:** Pre and Post contrast.

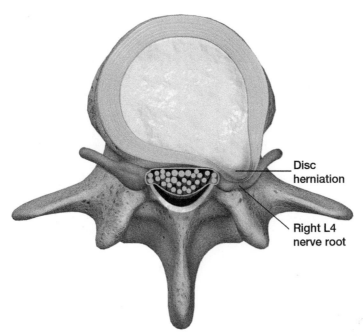

Figure 19-12 Disc herniating into the neural foramen on the right side.

the right (Fig. 19-12). It is possible to advance a needle to the epidural space at a particular neuroforamen. With the foraminal approach, the medication can be delivered directly to the anterior epidural space where the disc is affecting that particular nerve root (Fig. 19-13). As mentioned previously, in the interlaminar approach, medication has to flow from the posterior epidural space to the site of pathology by seeping around the thecal sac and into the ventral epidural space. The transforaminal approach puts medication directly on the area of interest (Fig. 19-14).

It is essential that the procedure be completely explained to the patient, that all questions are answered, and that informed consent obtained.

After the patient is brought to the fluoroscopy suite, he or she should lie on the fluoroscopic table in the prone position (face down). A "time out" is performed prior to the procedure including verbal confirmation of

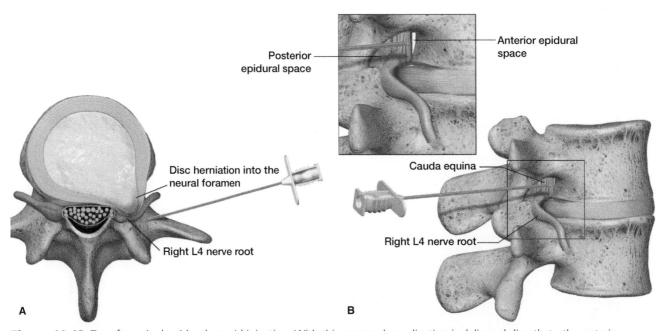

Figure 19-13 Transforaminal epidural steroid injection. With this approach medication is delivered directly to the anterior epidural space where the disc is affecting a particular nerve root.

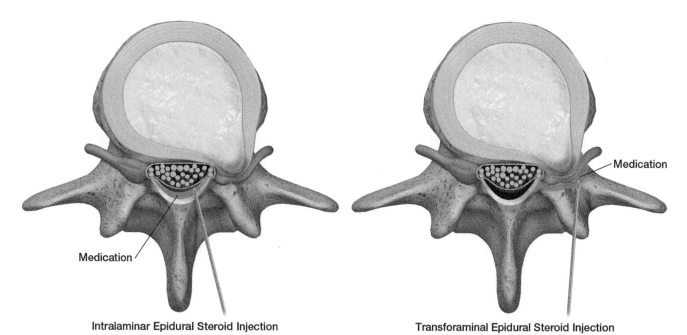

Medication

Medication

Intralaminar Epidural Steroid Injection

Transforaminal Epidural Steroid Injection

Figure 19-14 Intralaminar versus transforaminal epidural steroid injection.

correct patient procedure & procedural site. Noninvasive hemodynamic monitors and pulse oximetry are placed.

To begin, the skin over the lower back is prepped with Betadine and drapes are placed over the area in standard sterile fashion. The fluoroscope is placed in the AP position, tilting it if necessary in a cephalad to caudad motion to "square up" the end plates of the vertebral bodies (Fig. 19-4). Patients with prominent lordosis may require a significant tilt of the fluoroscope.

The epidural space of interest is visualized and the fluoroscope is rotated obliquely toward the side of the pain. The fluoroscope is rotated enough so that the lateral border of the pedicle is 1 to 2 mm from being superimposed on the lateral edge of the vertebral body (Fig. 19-15). This oblique angle is the position that allows best access to the neuroforamen. Using a metal marker and a felt tip marking pen, an "X" is placed on the skin just inferior to the pedicle. This entry point

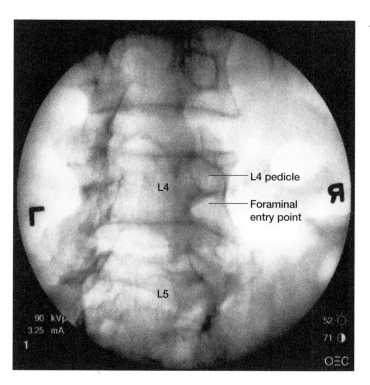

L4

L4 pedicle

Foraminal
entry point

L5

90 kVp
3.25 mA
1

52
71

OΞC

◄ **Figure 19-15** Proper starting oblique view for a transforaminal epidural steroid injection. The camera is in an oblique view, toward the right, the side of pain. The intended target is just below the L4 pedicle for a L4/L5 transforaminal epidural steroid injection on the right.

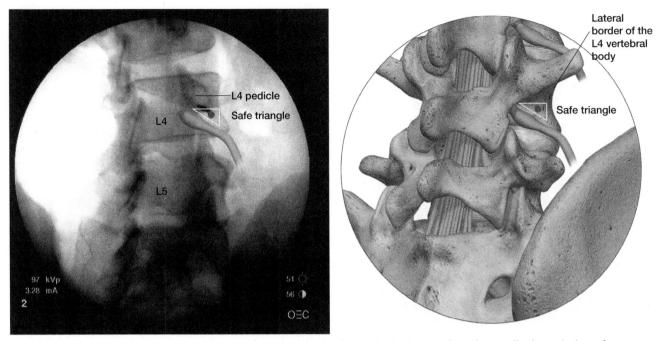

Figure 19-16 Target needle position for a transforaminal epidural steroid injection to place the needle through the safe triangle. The safe triangle is defined by the inferior surface of the transverse process and pedicle, the anticipated course of the emerging nerve root and the lateral border of the vertebral body.

will secure a path through "the safe triangle" (Fig. 19-16). Because the iliac crest can obscure the oblique entrance at the L5/S1 level, this level is the most challenging.

The skin and subcutaneous tissue is anesthetized with 2% lidocaine using a 1.5-in, 25G needle. After the skin is anesthetized, a 5-in, 22G spinal needle (Fig. 19-17) is placed through the "X" in a perpendicular fashion to the skin and parallel to the fluoroscope (Fig. 19-18). The needle is advanced toward the foramen. If your needle is on target, the most you can advance it is to the vertebral body itself. Once insertion is sufficiently deep, the fluoroscope is rotated to the AP position. The AP picture allows the interventionist to know the depth of the needle's entry. The needle should be advanced until its tip is superimposed on the vertebral body, usually to mid-pedicle line (Fig. 19-19). The fluoroscope is then rotated to the lateral position; the needle should be in the epidural space (Fig. 19-20).

If the needle tip is past the epidural space the needle angle was too steep and the needle should be retracted and redirected at a shallower angle conversely if the tip of the needle is posterior to the epidural space or the lateral view the needle should be retracted and redirected at steeper angle. Needle position has now been checked in three different planes of view.

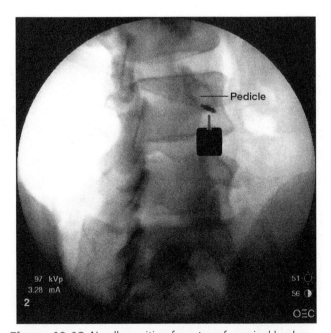

Figure 19-18 Needle position for a transforaminal lumbar epidural steroid injection with the fluoroscopy machine positioned in an oblique view to the right.

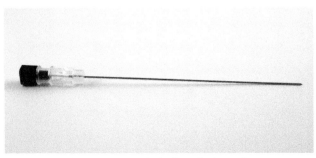

Figure 19-17 Quincke spinal needle.

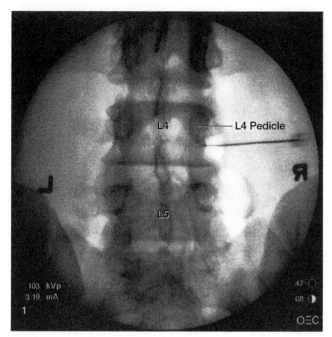

Figure 19-19 AP view with the needle advanced to the mid-pedicle line indicating foraminal position.

Figure 19-20 Needle in the posterior one-third of the epidural space on a lateral view.

The fluoroscope is rotated back to the AP view. The stylet of the 22G, 5-in needle is removed. The stylet is used to prevent tissue from collecting within the needle. A 3-mL syringe with tubing containing contrast is connected to the needle. Tubing is used so that you can see the contrast being injected under live x-ray without having your hand obscuring the image while simultaneously protecting your hand from direct radiation exposure. Contrast is injected to make sure that there is proper spread into the neuroforamen and that there is no contrast taken up by a vessel, indicating that the tip of the needle is in a vessel. Once proper contrast spread is seen (Fig. 19-21), the 3-mL syringe containing contrast is disconnected from the tubing. A 10-mL syringe with the

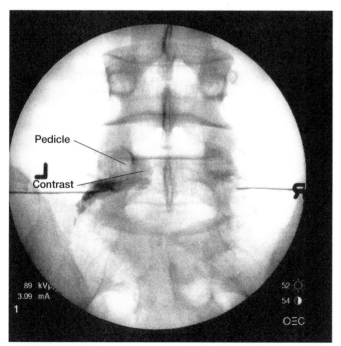

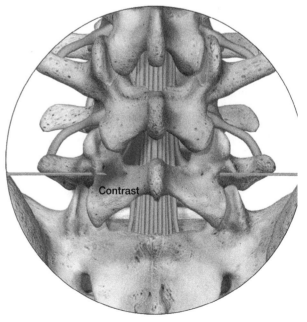

Figure 19-21 Proper spread of contrast for a transforaminal epidural steroid injection at the L5/S1 level. Needles are positioned for a bilateral approach, contrast has only been injected on the left side.

Figure 19-22 Sacral hiatus, a gap at the lower end of the sacrum exposing the vertebral canal. It is closed by the sacrococcygeal ligament and provides access to the sacral epidural space.   ▶

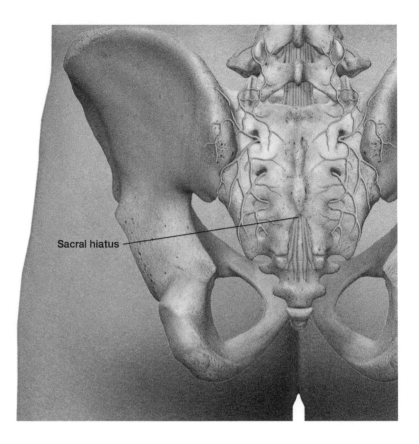

Sacral hiatus

therapeutic agent, a local anesthetic and a steroid, is connected to the tubing and injected. I use a mixture of 2 mL of 1% lidocaine (to aid in postprocedure comfort) and 40 mg of Kenalog as my therapeutic agent for this injection. The needle is then removed and a bandage placed.

More than one level can be treated at a time, for example, the L4/L5 and L5/S1 levels on the left side can be done together. The same steps are performed for each level. For this injection, 40 mg per level would be used for a total of 80 mg of Kenalog. Many practitioners refrain from performing cervical transforaminal epidural steroid injections, as some steroids inadvertently injected into a blood vessel can cause catastrophic results.

Caudal Epidural Steroid Injection

In particular cases it is necessary to use a caudal approach and enter the epidural space through the sacral hiatus (Fig. 19-22). Caudal epidural steroid injections are used to treat the pain from sacral neuropathy, sacral fractures, and coccygodynia. In individuals who have had an extensive posterior fusion the interlaminar approach to the epidural space may be obstructed and therefore a caudal approach is necessary.

The same preprocedural steps are followed as for an interlaminar epidural steroid injection except the fluoroscope is placed in the lateral position rather than the AP position (Fig. 19-23). Using a metal marker and a felt tip marking pen, an "X" is placed on the skin just below the sacral hiatus.

The skin and subcutaneous tissue is anesthetized with 2% lidocaine using a 1.5-in, 25G needle. After the skin is anesthetized, a Tuohy epidural needle is placed through the "X" using a very flat approach. The Tuohy needle is advanced until it enters the sacral hiatus. No

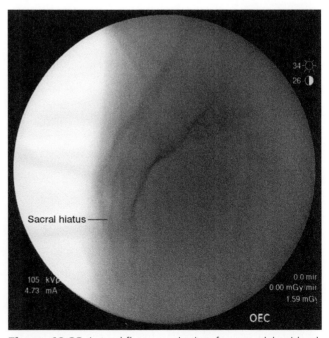

Sacral hiatus

Figure 19-23 Lateral fluoroscopic view for a caudal epidural steroid injection.

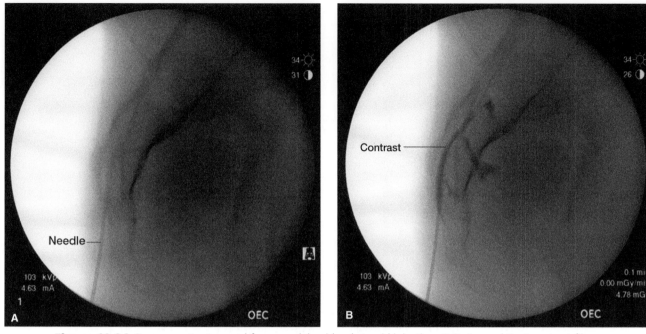

Figure 19-24 Proper contrast spread for a caudal epidural steroid injection. **A,B:** Pre and Post contrast films.

loss of resistance technique is used for a caudal approach. Once the needle is placed, a 3-mL syringe with tubing containing contrast is connected to the Tuohy needle. Tubing is used so that you can see the contrast being injected under live x-ray without having your hand obscure the image while simultaneously protecting your hand from radiation exposure. Contrast is injected to make sure that there is proper spread into the epidural space (Fig. 19-24). Once proper contrast spread is seen, the 3 mL syringe containing contrast is disconnected from the tubing. A 10-mL syringe with the therapeutic agent is connected to the tubing and injected. I use 2 mL of normal saline, 4 mL of 1% lidocaine, and 80 mg of Kenalog as my therapeutic agent for caudal epidural steroid injection. With a caudal approach a greater volume of fluid is needed to drive the medication over a larger area. The needle is then removed and a bandage placed.

Reasons for a Nontherapeutic Response to an Epidural Steroid Injection and Modes of Correction

Blind Injections: Patients who have had epidural steroid injections in the past that were not performed using fluoroscopy require re-evaluation. Identification of the intended level, using surface anatomy, is notoriously unreliable. With blind injections, there is no confirmation that the injected medications reached the epidural space; the medication may have been injected into deep paraspinal muscle or a pad of fat.

Today we are able to confirm needle placement in the epidural space under fluoroscopy. We are able to target the needle not only to the epidural space but directly to the area of pathology within the space. We are able to make sure that adhesions within the epidural space do not block flow of medication to the desired target, and can monitor how the medication spreads.

Use of only an intralaminar approach: The two most common forms of epidural steroid injection are the interlaminar and transforaminal approaches. Studies have shown greater support for the transforaminal approach as compared to the interlaminar approach, and that transforaminal injections decrease the need for operative treatment of lumbar radicular pain.[3] In one study, researchers divided patients with significant lumbar radicular pain who were deemed to be good surgical candidates into two groups. The first group received an interlaminar epidural steroid injection and in that group 25% of patients went on to have surgery. The second group received a transforaminal epidural steroid injection and in that group only 10% went on to have surgery.[4] If a patient did not have a therapeutic response to a interlaminar injection under fluoroscopic guidance it is worth considering a transforaminal epidural steroid injection.

Injections were tried before surgery: Some patients have had an epidural steroid injection in the past that was not helpful and subsequently underwent surgery. If surgery did not help their pain or changed the kind of pain they have, these patients should be re-evaluated for an epidural steroid injection. The patient's anatomy is now different after surgery—the patient's original anatomic structure was not amenable to the injection treatment, whereas altered postoperative anatomy may respond well to the injection.

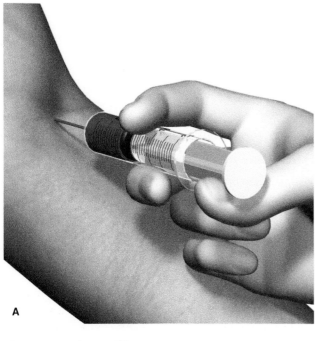

A

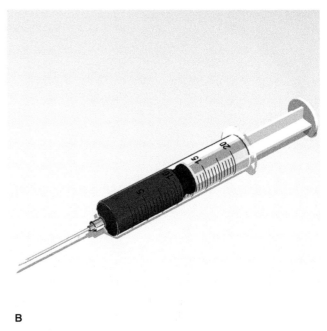

B

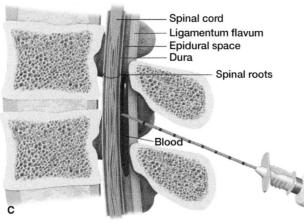

- Spinal cord
- Ligamentum flavum
- Epidural space
- Dura
- Spinal roots
- Blood

C

Figure 19-25 The procedural steps for an epidural blood patch. **A.** A venous puncture is made. **B.** 20 cc of blood is withdrawn. **C.** The blood is slowly injected into the epidural space.

CONTRAINDICATIONS AND POTENTIAL COMPLICATIONS

Contraindications to epidural steroid injections include systemic infection or infection on the site of the skin where the needle is to be inserted. Blood thinners and antiplatelet medications such as Coumadin and Plavix must be withheld. There are no definitive control studies evaluating the need to withhold aspirin (including both the 325- and 81-mg dose). Stopping aspirin, nonsteroidal anti-inflammatory drugs (NSAIDs), and fish oil is at the discretion of the individual practitioner. Pregnancy is a contraindication because of the use of fluoroscopy.

Complications include—but are not limited to—infection, bleeding, and nerve damage. Epidural steroid injection in the hands of a well-trained physician is a safe, well-tolerated procedure. One minor complication to be aware of is the possibility of a lumbar puncture headache. In this situation, the needle is

advanced too deeply passing completely through the epidural space into the intrathecal space. As the needle is removed it has the possibility of leaving a small hole in the dura which cerebral spinal fluid (CSF) can leak out of. This small hole is normally asymptomatic and resolves on its own but in a small percentage of patients a lumbar puncture headache may develop. The decrease in CSF pressure may lead to subsequent stretching of pain-sensitive structures and cerebral vasodilatation. Patients more likely to develop a lumbar puncture headache include those less than 50 years of age. A less stretchable dura mater caused by either atherosclerosis or age-related mechanical changes might explain why the incidence is lower in elderly patients. The key feature of the headache is its positional sense. When the patient lies flat the headache abates but when the patient stands a severe holocephalic headache exists, usually worse in the frontal and occipital region. The onset of headache is usually within 24 to 48 hours after dural puncture. The headache typically subsides with conservative measures such as fluids and caffeine. Presumably the caffeine leads to increased cerebral arterial vasoconstriction. If the headache does not resolve with conservative measures or is severe at onset it may be necessary to perform an epidural blood patch. This procedure uses the same steps as an intralaminar epidural steroid injection but rather the physician injects 20 cc of the patient's own blood into the epidural space instead of a steroid (Fig. 19-25). The blood patches the hole in the dura correcting the cause of the lumbar puncture headache. After the procedure the patient typically lies flat for an hour giving time for the patch to form and time for normal CSF production to raise pressure toward baseline. Lumbar puncture headaches can also be seen in patients who have had an intended lumbar puncture, a myelogram, or an epidural catheter for child birth that inadvertently punctured a hole in the dura.

Success rate of an epidural steroid injection depends on patient selection. As per an article by Abram and Hopewood, factors that predict less favorable results include patients who were unemployed, received compensation, had a long duration of symptoms, and had nonradicular pain complaints.[5]

CASE STUDIES

Case 1 A 48-year-old business executive reports she has had pain for the last 8 weeks in her right buttock that radiates down her right leg. She reports that the symptoms began while on a short business trip, making her way through the airport. The symptoms have gradually increased in intensity. She describes the pain as burning and electric in nature. The pain travels over the lateral-posterior aspect of her right thigh down to her foot. The symptoms are worse with prolonged walking or standing. She has taken over-the-counter Tylenol and Motrin, which have been somewhat helpful. She denies any weakness or change in bladder function. She has no previous history of pain and is on no medications other than acetaminophen and ibuprofen.

On physical examination she is at full strength, her reflexes are normal, and there are no deficits on sensory examination. She has a positive straight leg test on the right. You send her for a magnetic resonance imaging (MRI) of the lumbar spine without contrast. (Contrast is generally reserved for infections, tumor, multiple sclerosis, and if the patient previously had surgery.) She returns to your office with the same pain a week later. The MRI shows a herniated disc at L5/S1, asymmetrical to the right. You explain the risks, benefits, and alternatives to a transforaminal epidural steroid injection. A plastic model of the spine is used to show the patient the level of pathology. The patient has a transforaminal steroid injection at L5–S1 on the right, which is repeated 2 weeks later. The patient has complete relief of her pain, is very happy with the results, and is participating at home in the physical therapy exercises she learned in her training session.

Case 2 An 84-year-old female comes to your office with her daughter. She has pain in her lumbar spine that radiates into both of her legs. It is made worse with prolonged sitting, standing, or walking. She cannot walk more than 5 minutes before she has to sit down. The pain bothers her on a daily basis, for which she takes Tramadol 50 mg every 6 hours. The daughter reports that her mother's quality of life is declining because of pain. A recent MRI shows multilevel spinal canal stenosis, degenerative disc disease, and arthritis. The patient is sent for an intralaminar epidural steroid injection. The patient has about 80% relief for approximately a month after an intralaminar epidural steroid injection, a 50% reduction during the second month, and by the end of the third month the pain has returned to its preinjection level. The patient has an injection scheduled for every 3 months, and with the use of Tramadol her quality of life has increased.

REFERENCES

1. Devor M, Govrin-Lippman R, Raber P. Corticosteroids suppress ectopic neural discharge originating in experimental neuromas. *Pain.* 1985;22:127–137.
2. Riew KD, Yin Y, Gilula L, et al. The effect of nerve-root injections on the need for operative treatment of lumbar radicular pain: A prospective, randomized, controlled, double-blind study. *J Bone Joint Surg Am.* 2000:82a:1589–1593.
3. Marshall LL, Trethewie ER, Curtain CC. Chemical radiculitis: A clinical, physiological and immunological study. *Clin Orthop Relat Res.* 1977;29:61–67.
4. Schaufele M, Hatch L. Interlaminar versus transforaminal epidural injections in the treatment of symptomatic lumbar intervertebral disc herniations. *Arch Phys Med Rehabil.* 2002;83:1661.
5. Abram SE, Hopwood MB. Factors associated with failure of lumbar epidural steroids. *Reg Anesth.* 1993;18:238–243.

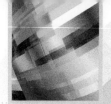

CHAPTER **20**

Facet Joint Procedures: Facet Joint Injections, Medial Branch Blocks, and Radiofrequency Ablation of the Medial Branches of the Spinal Nerve Roots

WHEN TO USE
▶ Diagnostic Injection Versus Diagnostic Therapeutic Injection
▶ Facet Joint Injections Versus Medial Branch Blocks

HOW TO PERFORM THE PROCEDURE
▶ Facet Joint Injections
▶ Medial Branch Blocks

▶ Radiofrequency Ablation of the Medial Branches of the Spinal Nerve Roots

CONTRAINDICATIONS AND POTENTIAL COMPLICATIONS

The facet joint is a synovial-lined joint that links two vertebral bodies posteriorly (Fig. 20-1).

In the lumbar spine, the facet joint is formed by the articulation of the inferior articulating process of one lumbar vertebra with the superior articular process of the next vertebra. Facet joints allow the spine to flex, extend, and rotate. Wear and tear caused by our body movement over time can cause these joints to become arthritic and painful (Fig. 20-2). When our intervertebral discs lose height as part of the normal aging

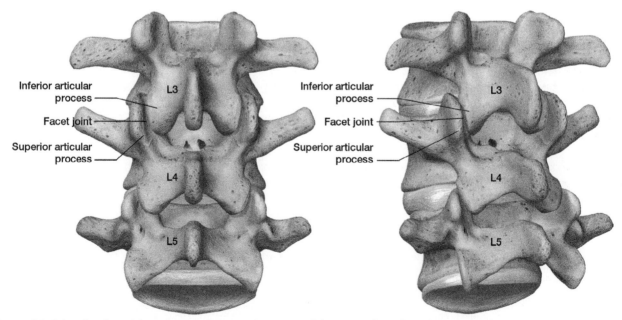

Figure 20-1 Lumbar facet joints connect the posterior aspect of the spine, they allow the spine to flex, extend, and rotate. Facet joints are formed by a inferior and superior articulating processes.

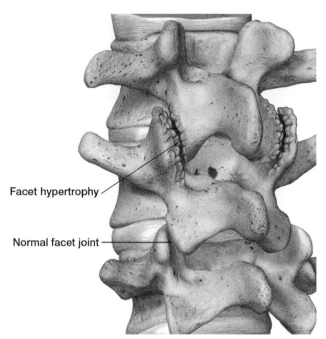

Figure 20-2 Arthritic lumbar facet joints.

Facet hypertrophy

Normal facet joint

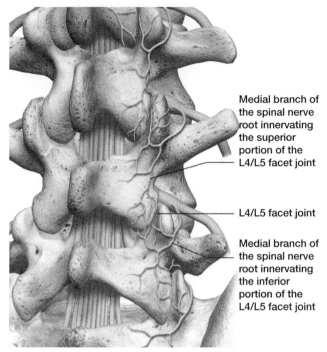

Medial branch of the spinal nerve root innervating the superior portion of the L4/L5 facet joint

L4/L5 facet joint

Medial branch of the spinal nerve root innervating the inferior portion of the L4/L5 facet joint

Figure 20-3 The L4/L5 facet joint innervated by the medial branch of the spinal nerve above and below it. Pain emanating from a facet joint is transmitted to the brain via these medial branches.

process, up to 70% of the compressive force usually applied to the discs may be transferred to the facet joints.[1] The most commonly affected are the lower cervical (C4/C5 and C5/C6) and the lower lumbar (L3/L4, L4/L5, and L5/S1) facet joints. The lumbar facet joints are particularly vulnerable because the distribution of axial weight along the spine is greatest at these levels and because this is where the greatest range of motion in the spine occurs. Pain from a facet joint is transmitted to the brain via the medial branch of the posterior division of the spinal nerve roots. For each facet joint there is a medial branch that innervates the superior aspect of the facet joint and one that innervates the inferior aspect (Fig. 20-3).

Facet joint pain is axial in nature rather than radicular. Radicular pain runs from the lower back to the foot or in the cervical spine from the neck to the hands. Facet pain is often described as deep and achy. The pain is focal over the area of arthropathy. Deep palpation over the facet joint may elicit pain. Some doctors have patients extend the lower back and rotate toward the side of pain as a mechanism to stress the facet joints. From a mechanical point of view, extension and extension rotation stress facet joints but probably stress disc and ligaments more.[2]

The diagnosis of facet joint-mediated pain is obtained by response to a diagnostic block. If based on the history and examination you feel that pain seems to be coming from facet joint arthropathy, it is reasonable to arrange a block for the patient. The facet joints are paired joints—a facet joint on the left and right

sides of the spine links two vertebral bodies. Your patient may have pain over the bottom two facet joints—L4/L5 and L5/S1—on the right only (Fig. 20-4). In this case, you would do a unilateral block of the L4/L5 and L5/S1 facet joints on the right. The diagnosis of

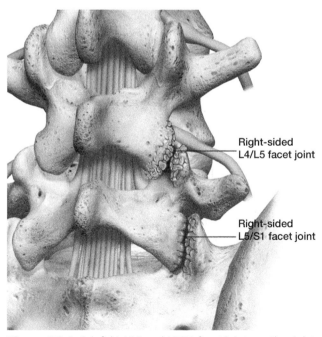

Right-sided L4/L5 facet joint

Right-sided L5/S1 facet joint

Figure 20-4 Painful L4/L5 and L5/S1 facet joints on the right. The left L4/S5 and L5/S1 facet joints are without arthropathy.

facet-mediated pain is clinical and not radiographic. The degree of degeneration identified on radiologic evaluation does not correlate with the severity of facet joint pain. However, if the patient has a normal magnetic resonance imaging (MRI) or computed tomography (CT) scan of their spine it is unlikely their pain is facet joint mediated. There are two ways to perform a diagnostic block: (1) The joint itself is injected with a local anesthetic or (2) anesthetize the medial branches of the spinal nerve roots that innervate a particular facet joint. If the facet joint is the pain generator, both the intra-articular (in the joint) or medial branch diagnostic blocks will temporarily relieve the pain produced from the facet joint. Typically, patients receive a pain diary to fill out before the injection and immediately after the procedure. The diary tracks the visual analog pain score over time. The block is considered positive if it relieves pain in the area from which pain could be expected to be blocked. If the pain is not relieved, a new hypothesis regarding the source of the patient's pain needs to be developed.

It is important to remember that patients may have more than one source of back pain. As wear and tear develops in the spine over the years, there is increased destruction of the facet joints, intervertebral discs, and nerve roots. For example, patients can have facet joint pain and lumbar radiculopathy. A diagnostic injection can help you determine the facet joint generator component of the pain.

If the patient and the patient's pain diary indicate a positive response, the patient undergoes a second diagnostic injection to ensure that the first response was not a false-positive result. Controlled studies have shown that single blocks carry a false-positive rate of 38%.[3] To confirm that the results are repeatable, it is necessary to perform second injection.

If you have targeted which facet joints are the pain generator, and the patient has had two positive responses to diagnostic injections, the next step is to use radiofrequency (RF) ablation for a more permanent block. RF ablation uses a very controlled source of heat to destroy the medial branches that innervate a particular facet joint. The theory is that even though the painful facet joint remains unchanged (unless surgery has been performed), the medial branches of the spinal nerve roots can no longer send painful impulses to the posterior division of the spinal nerve and then up to the brain if it is ablated. This ablation process results in neutralization of the painful facet joints but does not alter the structural integrity of the joint. Pathologic pain is being eliminated—the patient will still have the awareness to properly protect the spine. Typically, the effects last 6 to 18 months because the nerve may regenerate. In a selected group of patients using strict criteria and proper techniques, 87% of patients had a 60% pain reduction at 1 year.[4] If the symptoms return, a repeat procedure is done. There is no cumulative risk to repeating the RF procedure.

There are two common questions regarding facet joint procedures: Diagnostic injection versus diagnostic therapeutic injection and facet joint injections versus medial branch blocks. The following sections discuss these issues.

WHEN TO USE

Diagnostic Injection Versus Diagnostic Therapeutic Injection

The purpose of a diagnostic injection is to identify whether a facet joint or joints are the pain generator. This is accomplished by using a local anesthetic. In academic centers, patients receive two injections. A local anesthetic will be used with the first diagnostic injection and if the patient has pain relief, the second diagnostic injection again using a local anesthetic is performed.

In some academic centers and most private practices, patients often choose to have an injection that can be both diagnostic and therapeutic rather than one that is simply diagnostic—for financial and physiologic reasons. Injection of a steroid–local anesthetic mixture into the facet joint or on the medial branch of the spinal nerve roots is diagnostic, but it may also reduce inflammation, providing a therapeutic effect. Young people with facet pain caused by minor trauma or strain may experience permanent pain relief. Older people with facet pain caused by osteoarthritis may have months of pain relief.

Facet Joint Injections Versus Medial Branch Blocks

In clinical practice, some physicians use intra-articular facet joint injections, whereas others use medial branch blocks. The rationale for using intra-articular injections is that they can be both diagnostic and therapeutic. Injecting steroids into any joint—including painful facet joints—can provide longer-lasting pain relief, thus indicating that the pain originated in the facet joint. The rationale for not using intra-articular facet joint injections as a diagnostic block is that they lack a direct valid subsequent treatment. The next step to a positive diagnostic facet joint block is RF ablation of the medial branches of the respective spinal nerve roots branches not the joint itself. The rationale for not using medial branch blocks as a therapeutic tool rather than strictly a diagnostic injection is if a combination of a steroid and a local anesthetic is used as the therapeutic agent and the steroid is injected near the joint but not into it, the block may not provide long-lasting pain relief.

HOW TO PERFORM THE PROCEDURE

This section discusses the basics of facet joint injections, medial branch blocks, and RF ablation of the medial branches of spinal nerve roots. For all treatments, it is necessary to explain the procedure to the patient completely, answer all questions, and obtain informed consent. On arrival in the fluoroscopy suite the patient lies down on the fluoroscopic table in the prone position (face down). A pillow placed under the abdomen makes the lumbar facet joints more accessible. Facet joint procedures are done under fluoroscopic guidance (live x-ray) for accuracy and safety. A "time out" is performed prior to the procedure including verbal confirmation of correct patient,

procedure and procedural site. Noninvasive hemodynamic monitors and pulse oximetry are placed. Finally, the procedure requires that the skin is prepped with Betadine and drapes are placed over the area in standard sterile fashion.

Facet Joint Injections—Lumbar Spine

The fluoroscope is placed in the anteroposterior (AP) position and tilted if necessary in a cephalad to caudad motion to "square up" the endplates of the vertebral bodies (Fig. 20-5). Patients with prominent lordosis may require a significant tilt of the fluoroscope. The fluoroscope is then put in the oblique position, at an approximate 25- to 30-degree angle, toward the left or right side depending on which side is painful. Using a metal marker and a felt-tip marking pen, an "X" is placed on the skin overlying the inferior aspect of each facet joint that is to be blocked

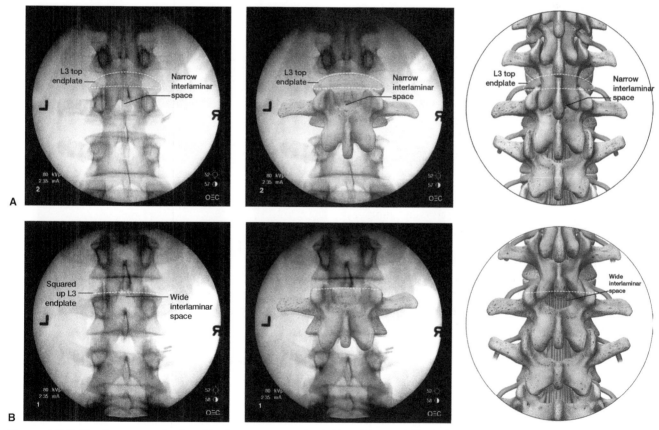

Figure 20-5 The fluoroscope is placed in the anteroposterior (AP) position and tilted, if necessary, in a cephalad to caudad motion to "square up" the endplates of the vertebral bodies. **A.** In the first panel of pictures the top of the L3 vertebral body is slanted which will make it more challenging to obtain a clear image of the facet joints. **B.** In the second panel of pictures the angle of the camera has been adjusted in a cephalad position to "square up" the top of the L3 vertebral body which will make it easier to obtain a crisp image of the facet joints.

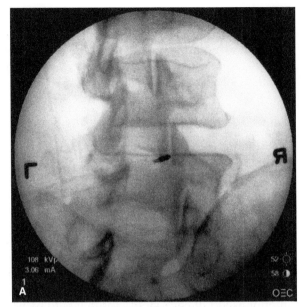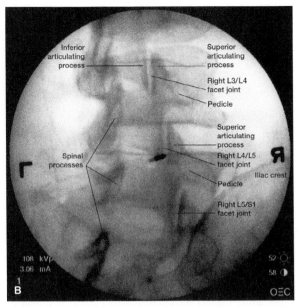

Figure 20-6 The intended target for a lumbar facet joint injection is the inferior aspect of the facet joint. In this case the L4/L5 facet joint on the right.

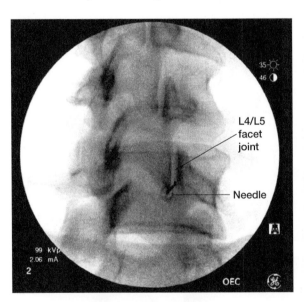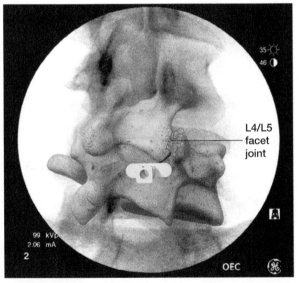

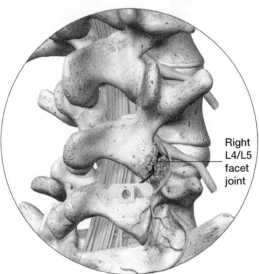

Figure 20-7 Needle inserted into the L4/L5 facet joint on the right, with fluoroscopic guidance.

(Fig. 20-6). The skin and subcutaneous tissue are anesthetized with 2% lidocaine using a 1.5-in, 25-gauge needle. After the skin is anesthetized, a 3.5-in (5 in for larger patients), 22-gauge spinal needle is placed through the "X" in a perpendicular fashion to the skin and parallel to the fluoroscope. A small bend at the tip of the needle can be made to help with steering. The needle is advanced until it enters the facet joint. This is confirmed under fluoroscopic guidance when bone contact is made (Fig. 20-7). The stylet of the needle is then removed. This step is repeated for all the facet joints that are to be blocked. A 10-mL syringe is filled with a mixture of a local anesthetic and steroid and then is injected. I use 1.5 mL of 0.5% bupivacaine and 20 mg of Kenalog (triamcinolone acetonide) per facet joint: For example, if three facet joints are injected—the L3/L4, L4/L5, and L5/S1 facet joints on the right—I will draw up 60 mg of Kenalog and 4.5 mL of 0.5% bupivacaine into the same syringe, dividing the medication equally over the three facet joints. The needles are then removed and a bandage placed. If the L3/L4, L4/L5, and L5/S1 facet joints are going to be blocked bilaterally (six total facet joints), I will draw up 120 mg of Kenalog and 9 mL of 0.5% bupivacaine into the same syringe, dividing the medication equally over the six facet joints. In the recovery room, the preoperative pain scores are compared with the postoperative score to see if the facet joints are indeed the pain generator.

Intra-articular facet joint injections are reserved for the lumbar spine and are usually not performed for the cervical spine—the cervical facet joints are so small that a proper amount of medication cannot be delivered effectively into the joint space.

Medial Branch Blocks

Lumbar Spine: Each facet joint is innervated by the medial branch of two consecutive spinal nerve roots, one medial branch from the superior aspect of the joint and one from the inferior aspect of the joint. Each medial branch runs from the facet joint and hugs around the superior articulating process, where it is covered by the mamillo-accessory ligament, tracking to the intervertebral foramen where it enters the dorsal rami of its respective spinal nerve root on its way up to the brain (Fig. 20-8).

To perform the procedure, place the fluoroscope in the AP position, tilted if necessary in a cephalad to caudad motion to "square up" the endplates of the vertebral bodies (Fig. 20-5). Patients with prominent lordosis may require a significant tilt of the fluoroscope. Then put the fluoroscope in the oblique position, at an approximate 25- to 30-degree angle toward the left or right side depending on which side is painful. Using a metal marker and a felt-tip marking pen, an "X" is placed on the skin where the superior articulating process and transverse process meet at the

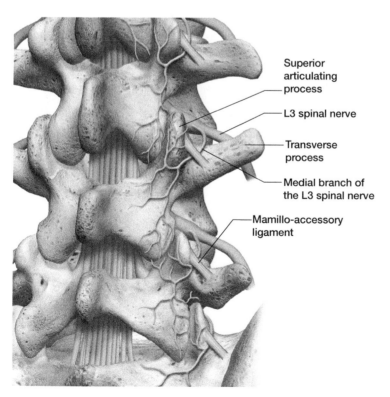

Superior articulating process

L3 spinal nerve

Transverse process

Medial branch of the L3 spinal nerve

Mamillo-accessory ligament

◀ **Figure 20-8** Medial branch of each lumbar dorsal ramus spinal nerve transversing the area where the superior articulating process and transverse process meet. The nerve is held in place by the mamillo-accessory ligament.

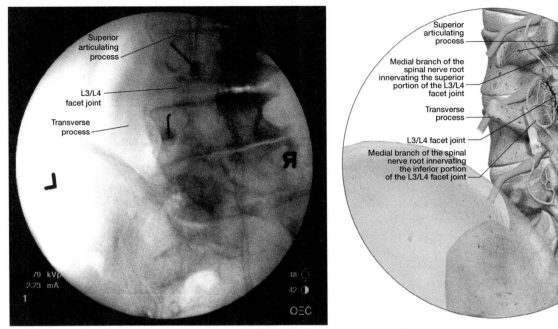

Figure 20-9 Medial branch block of the L3/L4 facet joint on the left. The bony target is where the transverse process and inferior articulating process meet which is along the patch of the medial branch of the lumbar spinal nerve.

level above and below the facet joint to be blocked (Fig. 20-9). If the pedicle was a clock face the intended target would be 10 O'clock for the left side and 2 O'clock for the right side. This is often described as the "eye of the Scotty Dog"; this is the path of the medial branch nerve.

The medial branch that innervates the S1 articulating process takes a slightly different route, crossing the ala of the sacrum (Fig. 20-10). The golden rule is that you need to block one more medial branch than the number of facet joints you are blocking—for example, if a procedure involves blocking the medial branches that

Figure 20-10 The medial branch nerve that innervates the S1 portion of the L5/S1 facet joint crossing the ala of the sacrum.

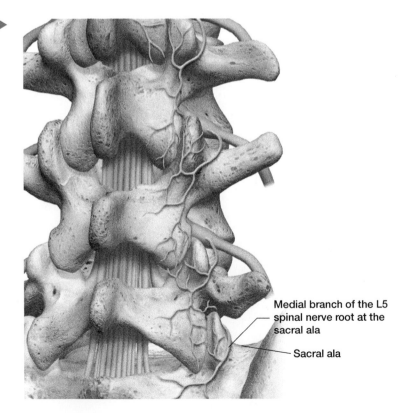

innervate the L3/L4 facet joint, it is necessary to block two medial branches for this one facet joint. Another example, if you are blocking three facet joints you need to block four medial branches. Contiguous facet joints are blocked in clinical practice—let us say that the L3/L4, L4/L5, and L5/S1 facet joints on the right are to be blocked. In this case you need to block the following nerves.

- The medial branch that innervates the L3 portion of the L3/L4 joint.
- The medial branch that innervates both the L4 portion of the L3/L4 facet joint and L4 portion of the L4/L5 facet joint.
- The medial branch that innervates both the L5 portion of the L4/L5 facet joint and L5 portion of the L5/S1 facet joint.
- The medial branch that innervates the S1 portion of the L5/S1 facet joint (Fig. 20-11).

At the sites, an "X" is marked on the skin and subcutaneous tissue is anesthetized with 2% lidocaine using a 1.5-in, 25-gauge needle. After the skin and subcutaneous tissue are anesthetized, a 3.5-in (5 in for larger patients), 22-gauge spinal needle is placed through the "X" in a perpendicular fashion to the skin and parallel to the fluoroscope. The needle is advanced until it touches bone in the path of the intendes medial branches.

Cervical Spine: For the cervical spine the anatomy is different: The medial branches curve around "the waist" of the articular pillar. This is where access is possible (Fig. 20-12). The cervical medial branches are bound by fasciae, which hold them against the articular pillar. The cervi-

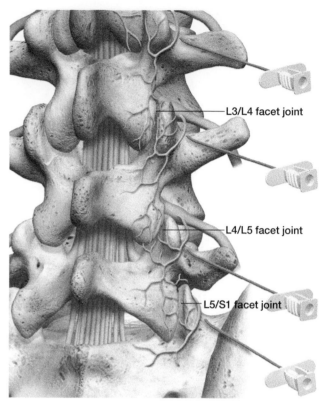

Figure 20-11 A right side L3/L4, L4/L5, L5/S1 medial branch block.

cal facet joints extend from C2/C3 to C7/T1. The same preparatory steps are performed as for a lumbar medial branch nerve block. Rather than obliquing the camera, the medial branch nerves are accessed using an AP view. The needle is advanced until bone contact is made at the

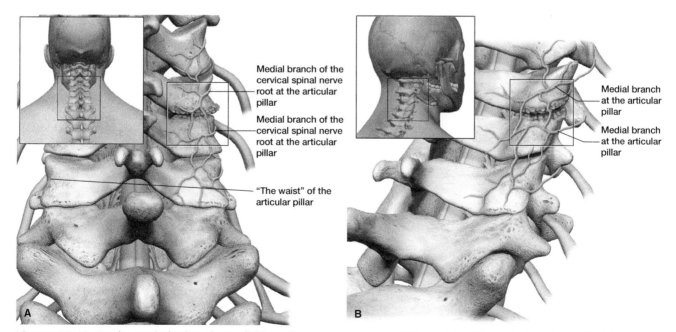

Figure 20-12 For the cervical spine, the medial branch nerve curves around "the waist" of the articular pillar and this is where they should be blocked.

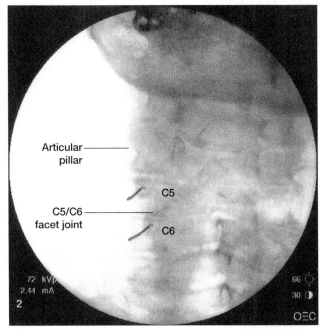

Figure 20-13 Cervical medial branch block at C5/C6 on the left. The needles are placed at the "the waist" of the articular pillar.

articular pillar then redirected so that it sits on the lateral margin of the pillar (Fig. 20-13).

This step is repeated for the predetermined medial branches. The camera is then rotated to a lateral view to confirm proper needle placement (Fig. 20-14). The local anesthetic is drawn up in a single syringe. I use 1.5 mL of

0.5% bupivacaine per medial branch: For example, if three facet joints are to be blocked (four medial branches), 6 mL of 0.5% bupivacaine is drawn up into a single syringe and divided equally over the four medial branches. The needles are then removed and a bandage placed. In the recovery room, the preoperative pain score is compared with the postoperative score to see if the cervical facet joints blocked are indeed the pain generator.

Radiofrequency Ablation of the Medial Branches of the Spinal Nerve Roots

The science behind RF is an electric field is established around the needle tip. This field oscillates with alternating RF current causing movement of ions. This movement of ions creates friction in the tissue surrounding the catheter tip producing heat. Which causes ablation of the medial branch of the spinal nerve root. Cells become damaged at 45°C. At temperatures 60°C to 100°C, there is induction of protein coagulation leading to cell death. Standard ablation settings are 80°C for 60 seconds.

RF machines can be programmed with the physicians preferred settings for sensory testing, motor testing, and ablation temperature and duration.

Lumbar Spine: In the lumbar spine, the same fluoroscopic landmarks as a diagnostic medial branch block are used for RF ablation. At the sites marked with an "X," anesthetize the skin and subcutaneous tissue with 2% lidocaine using a 1.5-in, 25-gauge needle. Upon

Figure 20-14 Lateral view of proper needle ▶ position for a cervical medial branch block.

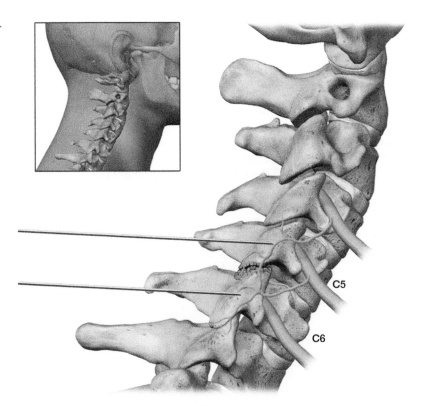

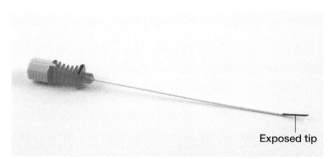

Figure 20-15 3.5-in, 22-gauge, Teflon-coated radiofrequency needle with a 10-mm exposed tip.

anesthetization, a 3.5-in, 22-gauge, Teflon-coated RF needle with a 10-mm exposed tip (Fig. 20-15; the RF needle comes in a straight- or curved-tip form—the curved tip is often easier to guide) is placed through the "X" in a perpendicular fashion to the skin and parallel to the fluoroscope. A 5-in needle may be required in larger patients. The needle is advanced until it touches bone in the path of the medial branch of the spinal nerve root. Repeat this step for the predetermined medial branches.

Once all RF needles are in position, check their location using both sensory and motor stimulations. Electrical stimulation at 50 hz should produce sensory stimulation of the intended medial branches if the tips of the needles are properly placed. To perform sensory testing the stylet of the RF needle is removed and the RF probe is placed into the needle (Fig. 20-16). The jack from the RF cable is connected to the RF machine. The RF machine is able to send a small amount of electrical stimulation to the tip of the needle. The machine is set to sensory testing and the operator slowly increase the sensory impulse up to 50 hz. If the needle is placed correctly the patient will feel a small tapping or buzzing sensation at the targeted facet joint as the medial branch is stimulated. If the needle sits to close to the spinal nerve root, the patient will feel a shooting sensation down the leg. After proper sensory stimulation is confirmed, motor stimulation is next checked. Motor stimulation confirms a safe distance from the unintended motor fibers of the spinal nerve root. The RF machine is set to motor testing and the operator slowly increase the

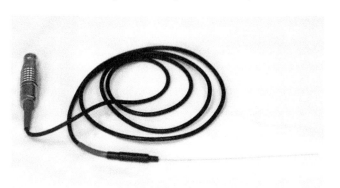

Figure 20-16 Radiofrequency probe.

motor impulse up to 2 hz. Motor stimulation at 2 hz should evoke contraction of the ipsilateral paraspinal muscles with out limb contraction. Small lumbar multifidus muscles which are paraspinal in location receive motor innervation from the medial branches. With proper motor stimulation contraction of the lumbar paraspinal muscles are seen. This is normal indicating proper needle placement. However, if the needle tip is too close to the spinal nerve root leg contraction is seen. In this case reposition the needle until proper motor stimulation is achieved. Destruction of the medial branch nerve does not cause clinically consequential lumbar weakness. Once needle placement is properly confirmed via both fluoroscopy and electrical stimulation, remove the RF probes and anesthetize the medial branch nerves using a local anesthetic. The local anesthetic is drawn up in a single syringe. I use 1.5 mL of 0.5% bupivacaine per medial branch nerve. For example, for blocking the facet joints (four medial branch nerves), 6 mL of 0.5% bupivacaine are drawn up into a single syringe and divided equally over the four medial branches. The area is anesthetized so that this is painless for the patient.

The RF probes are reinserted the RF machine set to ablation and the ablation process begins (Fig. 20-17). The needle is then removed and a bandage placed.

Cervical Spine: For the cervical spine, the medial branches of the cervical spinal nerves curve around "the waist" of the articular pillar; this is where they are accessed. The cervical medial branches are bound by fasciae that hold them against the articular pillar. A

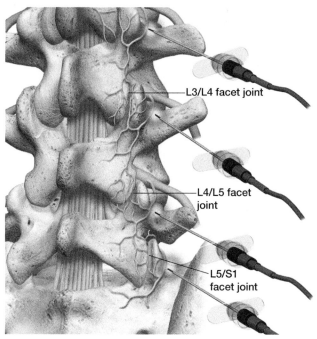

Figure 20-17 Radiofrequency ablation of the medial branch nerves innervating the L3/L4, L4/L5, and L5/S1 facet joint on the right.

Teflon-coated RF needle with a 5-mm exposed tip is used rather than the 10-mm exposed tip in the lumbar spine. The same safety checkpoints and ablation protocol used for the lumbar spine are applicable for the cervical spine.

CONTRAINDICATIONS AND POTENTIAL COMPLICATIONS

Contraindications for facet joint procedures include systemic infection and infection of the skin where the needle is inserted as well as pregnancy. Blood thinners must be withheld for the procedure. For diagnostic blocks, the patient must understand the details of the procedure and have the ability to tolerate the block; otherwise the block should not take place. For the RF procedure, the possibility of motor weakness and sensory loss is possible but in well-trained hands the procedure is safe.

CASE STUDIES

Case 1

A 47-year-old male presents with low back pain that does not radiate down his leg. The patient states that the pain is deep and that he has a dull ache along the lower part of his spine. The pain has been gradually increasing over the last year and a half, and is somewhat helped with ibuprofen. The pain is aggravated with prolonged standing and walking. Of note, the patient has the least discomfort when he lies flat on his back. Any Valsalva maneuver such as coughing, sneezing, or straining does not affect the pain, nor is it affected by leaning forward.

The patient has a history of hypothyroidism but is otherwise healthy.

On examination the patient has pain on palpation of the L4/L5 and L5/S1 facet joint on the right. Reflexes are normal and strength is good. Imaging shows facet degenerative changes along the lumbar spine with the right side clearly worse. The patient undergoes a diagnostic therapeutic intra-articular block of the L4/L5 and L5/S1 facet joints on the right. A month later the patient comes back to your office and he states that his pain is about 75% less. A repeat injection eliminates the pain.

Case 2

The patient from the first case is so happy with your care that he brings in his 77-year-old father to see you. His father has very similar symptoms, with axial low back pain. He has had this pain for at least 5 years. Imaging shows facet degenerative changes along the lumbar spine with no particular joint clearly worse. The patient has a diagnostic therapeutic intra-articular block of the L4/L5 and L5/S1 facet joints bilaterally. A month later, the patient comes back to your office and states that his pain was gone for the first few weeks after the procedure but over the month the pain has increased. At this point, his back is hurting at the same level as before he had the procedure. The injection is repeated with a very similar response. Having now had pain relief with facet joint injections on two separate occasions you and the patient decide to proceed with RF denervation. This leads to a significant reduction in the patient's axial low back pain and increase in daily function for about 8 months, at which time the pain begins to return.

REFERENCES

1. Lynch MC, Taylor JF. Facet joint injection for low back pain: A clinical study. *J Bone Joint Surg Br.* 1986;68:138–141.
2. Revel M, Poiraudeau S, Auleley GR, et al. Capacity of the clinical picture to characterize low back pain relieved by facet joint anesthesia: Proposed criteria to identify patients with painful facet joints. *Spine.* 1998;23:1972–1977.
3. Schwarzer AC, Aprill CN, Derby R, et al. The false-positive rate of uncontrolled diagnostic blocks of the lumbar zygapophysial joints. *Pain.* 1994;58:195–200.
4. Dreyfuss P, Halbrook B, Pauza K, et al. Efficacy and validity of radiofrequency neurotomy for chronic lumbar zygapophysial joint pain. *Spine (Phila Pa 1976).* 2000;25(10):1270–1277.

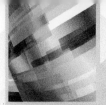

CHAPTER 21

Sacroiliac Joint Injections

The sacroiliac (SI) joint is the weight-bearing joint between the sacrum at the base of the spine and its connection to the ileum of the pelvis (Fig. 21-1). The location of the SI joints is visible at the gluteal dimples (Fig. 21-2). There is both a left and right SI joint. The SI joints are located where the spine connects to the pelvis, and they are subject to a good amount of stress by virtue of their function. The SI joints are a common origin of pain, being the source in 13% to 19% of patients with chronic low back pain.[1,2] SI joint degeneration develops more often in patients who have had lumbosacral fusion regardless of the number of fusion segments. On history, patients describe SI joint pain as achy and sharp. Sometimes they report that climbing stairs makes it worse. The pain may radiate into the thigh or groin, mimicking facet or hip joint pain. On physical examination, when the hips are pushed together SI pain might be elicited. However, physical examination is notoriously unreliable for teasing out SI pain. The pain may affect one SI joint (unilateral) or both SI joints (bilateral).

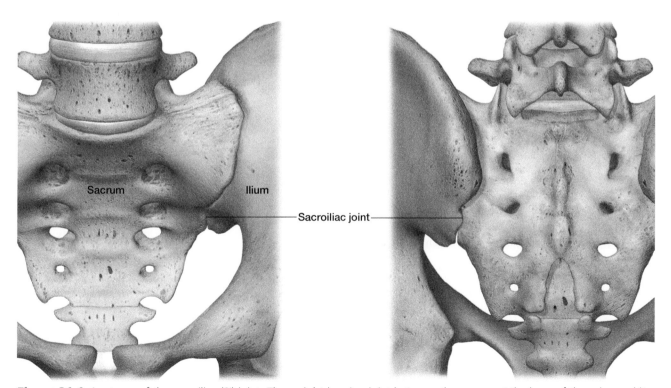

Figure 21-1 Anatomy of the sacroiliac (SI) joint. The weight-bearing joint between the sacrum at the base of the spine and its connection to the ileum of the pelvis.

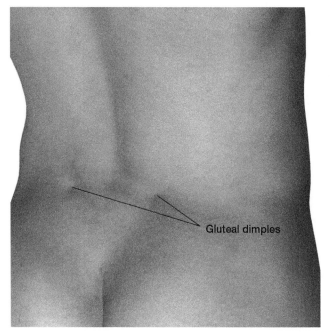

Figure 21-2 The SI joints are located at the gluteal dimples.

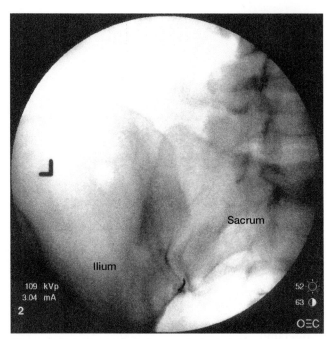

Figure 21-3 The intended target is the inferior aspect of the SI joint.

WHEN TO USE

SI joint injections can be both diagnostic and therapeutic. As previously mentioned, it is difficult relying on history and examination to clearly identify if the SI joint or joints are the source of pain. A diagnostic block is a reliable way to determine definitively whether the SI joint or joints in question are the source of pain: If anesthetic relieves the pain, this confirms the diagnosis. Diagnostic blocks help protect the patient from undergoing needless pursuit of competing diagnoses and from undergoing presumptive treatment that is not appropriate for SI joint pain. If the SI joint is indeed the source of pain, the patient should feel relief in this area after the procedure. The patient may not be relieved of 100% of their pain, as there may be several other pain generators.[3] However, the percentage of the patient's back pain that stems from the SI joint can be determined by this method.

Before the procedure, it is predetermined whether to block a single SI joint or both SI joints based on the patient's pain. If the pain is confirmed to be coming from the SI joint or joints with a diagnostic block, there are interventional therapeutic options. Patients may receive therapeutic injections of cortisone directly into the joint. Another therapeutic option is radiofrequency (RF) ablation of the nerves that transmit painful impulses from the painful SI Joint.

HOW TO PERFORM THE PROCEDURE

Diagnostic Sacroiliac Joint Injections

It is necessary to explain the procedure to the patient completely, answer all questions, and obtain informed consent. For accuracy and safety, SI joint injections are performed under fluoroscopic guidance (live x-ray).

After arrival at the fluoroscopy suite the patient lies on the fluoroscopic table in the prone position (face down). A "time out" is performed prior to the procedure including verbal confirmation of correct patient, procedure and procedural site. Noninvasive hemodynamic monitors and pulse oximetry are placed. The fluoroscope is placed in the anteroposterior (AP) position. Radiographically the SI joint does not have a single silhouette of its articular cavity. To help isolate the posterior margin of the joint the C-arm of the fluoroscope should be rotated usually to the contralateral side until the medial inferior aspect of the joint is maximally crisp. Usually 5–20 degrees of contralateral rotation is necessary to properly improve the picture. The target is, approximately 1–2 cm cephalad of the most inferior aspect of the joint. The skin is prepped with betadine and drapes are placed over the area in standard sterile fashion. Using a metal marker and a felt-tip marking pen, an "X" is placed on the skin overlying the intended target, the inferior aspect of the SI joint (Fig. 21-3). The skin is anesthetized with lidocaine using a 1.5-in, 25-gauge needle. After the skin is anesthetized a 3.5-in, 22-gauge spinal needle with a curve at the end—the physician typically bends the needle to create a curve (Fig. 21-4)—is placed through the "X" in a perpendicular fashion to the skin and parallel to the fluoroscope (Fig. 21-5). The needle is advanced until it enters the SI joint and bone is touched. The stylet of the needle is then removed. A 3-mL syringe with tubing containing contrast is connected to the needle. Tubing

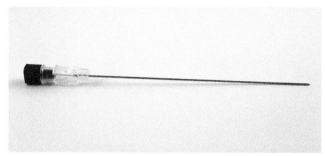

Figure 21-4 3.5-in, 22-gauge quincke spinal needle.

is used so that you can see the contrast being injected under live x-ray without having your hand obscure the image and to protect your hand from radiation exposure. A small amount (1 mL) of contrast is injected to make sure that it spreads in the intra-articular joint space. Once proper contrast spread is seen (Fig. 21-6), the 3-mL syringe is disconnected from the tubing. A local anesthetic is then injected via a 10-mL syringe connected to the tubing. I use 1.5 mL of 0.5% bupivacaine as my diagnostic agent. The needle is removed and a bandage placed. In the recovery room, the preoperative pain score is compared with the postoperative score to see if the SI joint or SI joints are the pain generator.

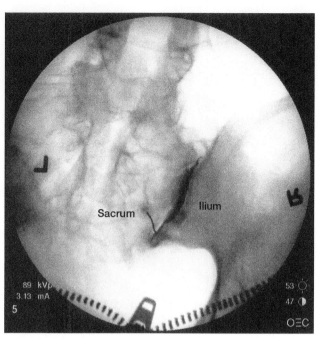

Figure 21-6 Proper contrast spread for an SI joint injection.

Nonfluoroscopic-guided injections, known as "blind injections," rarely place medication into the intra-articular portion of the joint.[4] The results of these injections should be interpreted with great caution.

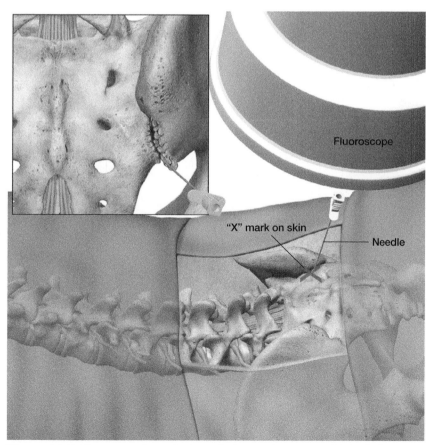

Figure 21-5 Placement of needle through the "X" in a perpendicular fashion to the skin and parallel to the fluoroscope toward the inferior aspect of the SI joint.

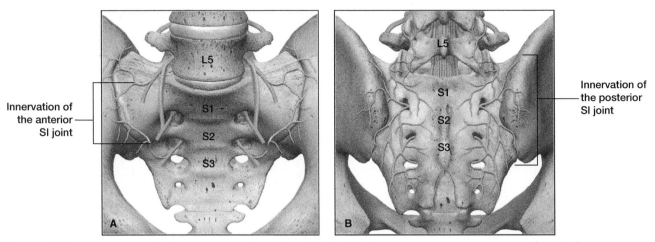

Figure 21-7 A. Anterior and **B.** Posterior innervation of the SI joint. Only the posterior nerves are engaged for radiofrequency ablation (RFA).

Therapeutic Sacroiliac Joint Injection

The same exact steps for the diagnostic SI joint injection are performed for a therapeutic injection except that a steroid is administered, typically 40 mg of Kenalog or 40 mg of Depo-Medrol (methylprednisolone acetate) per SI joint. Many doctors, myself included, perform a simultaneous diagnostic–therapeutic injection in one sitting by combining a local anesthetic and a steroid. I use 40 mg of Kenalog in 1.5 mL of 0.5 bupivacaine as my therapeutic agent per SI joint. For financial and psychological reasons, patients usually choose to have the injection that is diagnostic and therapeutic rather than one that is simply diagnostic.

Sacroiliac Joint Radiofrequency

The science behind RF is an electric field is established around the needle tip. This field oscillates with alternating RF current causing movement of ions in the tissue. This friction in the tissue surrounding the needle tip produces heat. Cells become damaged at 45°C. At temperatures 60°C to 100°C there is induction of protein coagulation leading to cell death.

There are various techniques of performing RF for the SI joint. No single technique has been shown to be the gold standard. One approach is intra-articular; it involves placement of an RF needle in the joint and ablation of the nerves lying in the posterior joint surface. Another

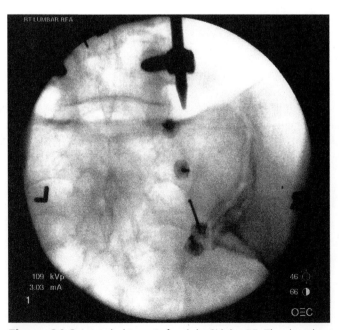

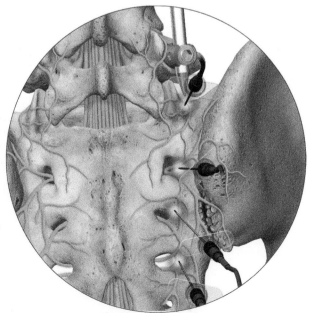

Figure 21-8 Intended targets for right SI joint RF: The dorsal ramus of the L5 medial branch nerve and lateral branches of the S1, S2, and S3 spinal nerves, for a total of four lesions. In this illustration the patient has had a previous fusion.

technique is extra-articular; it involves ablating the nerves that carry pain impulses from the SI joint. RF ablation for SI joint pain can be challenging for two reasons.

- The nerves are inconsistent in their anatomic location, varying from patient to patient, side to side, and level to level.
- The nerves that transmit pain from the SI joint run their anatomic course at different depths, with some embedded in soft tissue and some lying on the bone.

It is possible to safely engage the nerves that lie on the posterior aspect of the joint with RF. However, this is not true for the nerves on the anterior surface; the operator would have to go anteriorly through the pelvis. Because of this, RF can help with only a portion of the inervation of the SI joint, at best (Fig. 21-7).

The following discussion presents a common procedural protocol for RF lesioning of the medial branch nerves innervating an SI joint. The practitioner performs the same preprocedural steps as described for an SI joint injection. The fluoroscope is placed in the AP position and the L5 vertebral body and sacrum are brought into focus. Using a metal marker and a felt-tip marking pen, an "X" is placed on the skin at the four points that correspond to the medial branch of the dorsal ramus of the L5 spinal nerve and lateral branches of the S1, S2, and S3 spinal nerves (Fig. 21-8). At the sites where you have placed an "X," the skin and subcutaneous tissue are anesthetized with 2% lidocaine using a 1.5-in, 25-gauge needle. After the skin and subcutaneous tissue are anesthetized, a 3.5-in, 22-gauge, Teflon-coated RF needle with a 10-mm exposed tip is placed through the "X" in a perpendicular fashion to the skin and parallel to the fluoroscope. The needle comes in straight or curved-tip versions, the curved tip is often easier to guide. The needle is advanced until it touches bone in the path of the medial branch of the L5 spinal nerve and lateral branches of the S1, S2, and S3 spinal nerves.

Once all RF needles are in position under fluoroscopic guidance, the position of the needle over the medial branch of the L5 spinal nerve is checked using both sensory and motor stimulations. To do this the stylet on the needle corresponding to the medial branch of the L5 spinal nerve is removed and the RF probe is placed into the needle. The jack from the RF needle is connected to the RF machine. Sensory testing is done

first; a small amount of electrical stimulation is driven to the tip of the needle. Typical settings are 50 Hz for sensory testing. If the needle is properly placed, the patient will feel a small tapping or buzzing sensation at the targeted area as the medial branch nerve is stimulated. If the needle sits too close to the nerve root, the patient will feel a shooting sensation down the leg. Motor stimulation is tested next. If the needle sits too close to the nerve root, it will cause motor contraction of the leg muscles. The needle may stimulate the lumbar multifidus muscle, which is a paraspinal muscle that receives its motor enervation from the medial branch nerve. This contraction of the lumbar paraspinal muscles is normal and indicates proper needle placement. Motor stimulation at 2 Hz should evoke contraction of the ipsilateral paraspinal muscles without limb contraction if the needle is properly placed. Destruction of the medial branch nerve while denervating this small muscle does not cause clinically consequential lumbar weakness. The remaining three lateral branches overlying the sacrum are not typically tested using motor and sensory stimulations as the area is devoid of large motor nerve roots. The RF probes are removed and the nerves are anesthetized using a local anesthetic.

I use 1.5 mL of 0.5% bupivacaine per nerve: As four nerves are going to be anesthetized, 6 mL of 0.5% bupivacaine are drawn up into a single syringe and divided equally over the four nerves. The RF probes are placed back into the RF needles and the ablation process now begins. The area has been anesthetized so that this is painless for the patient. Standard ablation settings are 80° C for 60 seconds. The needles are then removed and a bandage placed.

CONTRAINDICATIONS AND POTENTIAL COMPLICATIONS

Contraindications include systemic infection and infection on the skin where the needle is inserted. The procedure is contraindicated if the patient is or may be pregnant. Some doctors perform non fluoroscopic-guides injections, known as "blind injections", which rarely place medication into the intra-articular portion of the joint.[4] The results of these injections should be interpreted with great caution. For the RF procedure, the possibility of motor weakness and sensory loss exists but in well-trained hands the procedure is safe.

CASE STUDY

Case

Twin sisters—61-year-old women—come to see you with isolated low back pain. The pain is on the right side of the lower back, and they describe it as deep, constant, and achy. The pain does not radiate into the right leg. The women have had the pain for the past 8 months. Magnetic resonance imaging studies are identical in both patients, revealing no disc herniation and facet arthropathy at L5/S1 with the right side being affected greater than left.

Both patients have a pain level that ranges between 6 and 8 on a 10-point visual analog scale. Their physical examinations are normal except that they both have pain on palpation of the lumbar paraspinal region on the right side. Based on examinations and histories, it is unclear if the pain is from the L5/S1 facet joint on the right or the SI joint on the right.

To clearly identify the source of pain, both patients undergo a diagnostic–therapeutic right SI joint injection with 1.5 mL of 0.5% bupivacaine and 40 mg of Kenalog under fluoroscopic guidance. In the recovery room, their reports of pain differ. The first twin states that her pain level is the same after the injection. The second twin states that her pain level went down from a 7 out of 10 to 0 out of 10, indicating that the SI joint is the source of her pain. The first twin, who had no pain relief, most likely has pain from the facet joint, which is confirmed by a medial branch block of the L5/S1 facet joint during her next visit.

REFERENCES

1. Schwarzer AC, Aprill CN, Bogduk N. The sacroiliac joint in chronic low back pain. *Spine (Phila Pa 1976)*. 1995;20:31–37.
2. Maigne JY, Aivaliklis A, Pfefer F. Results of sacroiliac joint double block and value of sacroiliac pain provocation tests in 54 patients with low back pain. *Spine (Phila Pa 1976)*. 1996;21:1889–1892.
3. Slipman CW, Lipetz JS, Plastaras CT, et al. Fluoroscopically guided therapeutic sacroiliac joint injections for sacroiliac joint syndrome. *Am J Phys Med Rehabil*. 2001;80:425–432.
4. Rosenberg JM, Quint TJ, de Rosayro AM. Computerized tomographic localization of clinically-guided sacroiliac joint injections. *Clin J Pain*. 2000;16:18–21.

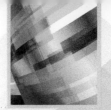

CHAPTER **22**

Trigger Point Injections for Myofascial Pain

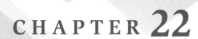

> **WHEN TO USE**
>
> **HOW TO PERFORM THE PROCEDURE**
>
> **CONTRAINDICATIONS AND POTENTIAL COMPLICATIONS**

In order for a muscle to contract, actin and myosin strands slide over each other. These filaments then release, sliding back to their starting position. A taught muscle band is a part of the muscle where the contraction cannot release. A trigger point is a painful taut muscle band (Fig. 22-1). According to experts, an abnormal neuromuscular junction may lead to the development of this. The neuromuscular junction, where the nerve transmits signals to the muscle, is a highly excitable region, where each strand of muscle tissue obtains information on when to contract. If this charged, hyperexcitable region becomes overexcited, those muscle filaments remain contracted. Evidently, this contracted muscle state causes an increased metabolic demand and region of local ischemia. It may help

to think of static cling in pants as an analogy for over-contraction. Too much electric charge causes pants to bunch up in some areas instead of lying flat.

Trigger points often cause regional persistent pain that can result in decreased range of motion. They commonly develop along the weight-bearing axial skeleton used to maintain body posture such as the neck, shoulder, or back. Skeletal muscle is subject to wear and tear just like the bones, joints, and bursa, which predisposes it to pathologic changes. Palpation of the trigger point elicits pain at the affected area and/or causes radiation of pain toward a zone of reference.[1] Trigger points are a clinical diagnosis—there is no specific laboratory test, imaging study, or interventional modality such as EMG or muscle biopsy useful in establishing a diagnosis.[2] By palpating the region of pain with your finger pad, specific trigger points can often be identified by verbal confirmation from the patient. A patient may have one or a multitude of trigger points.

Trigger point injections are thought to diffuse the abnormal electrical charge at the neuromuscular junction; this leads to restoration of normal muscle contraction sequelae. A variety of fluids have been injected into trigger points over the years including saline, local anesthetic, corticosteroids, Vitamin B solution, ketorolac (a nonsteroidal anti-inflammatory drug [NSAID]), and botulinum toxin. Usually a local anesthetic such as 2% lidocaine or 0.5% bupivacaine, or a combination of both, is used.

Currently, there is no consensus on the benefit of injecting any of these solutions over dry needling. Dry needling is the practice of breaking up the taut muscle band and diffusing the abnormal neuromuscular junction without injecting solution. In the United States, a local anesthetic is typically used because it may provide benefit by reducing pain and irritation caused by the needling itself.[3] In one study, patients who underwent

Trigger points in muscle fibers

Figure 22-1 Trigger points within skeletal muscle.

trigger point injections with lidocaine and participated in physical therapy had less pain at 4-week follow-up as compared with the control group that underwent trigger point injections with dry needling and also participated in physical therapy.[4] Using botulinum toxin type A in varying strengths showed no advantage over using a local anesthetic.[4] In clinical practice some doctors also include a steroid to cure any local inflamation contributing to the trigger point.

WHEN TO USE

Trigger point injection is a relatively safe procedure that can be used to control the symptoms of myofascial pain. As long as trigger points can clearly be identified, trigger point injections may be effective. Trigger point injections discharge the aberrant neuromuscular junction, mechanically disrupt abnormally functioning contractile elements, and wash out any nerve-sensitizing substances. They also inactivate any pathologic neural feedback mechanism. It is best to use injections in combination with physical therapy for myofascial pain.

HOW TO PERFORM THE PROCEDURE

Start by asking the patient to identify the painful areas by having the patient push on the painful areas. Then palpate the region of pain with the pad of your index and trigger fingers and ask the patient to identify when you have pushed on a trigger point, a point that elicits pain. When you push on an identified a trigger points, make an "X" on that area with a marking pen. Then start the examination from the beginning, ignoring the just-marked "X's." Once again, place an "X" over the patient-identified trigger points. Places that have two "X" marked are your high-yield, repetitive trigger points.

The area is vigorously prepped with alcohol. A 1.5-in, 25-gauge needle is attached to a 10-mL syringe containing a local anesthetic. The needle is inserted through the "X" on the skin as you hold the muscle in place. After negative aspiration, the local anesthetic is injected at the trigger point. The needle is then withdrawn and redirected superiorly, inferiorly, laterally, and medially to disrupt the muscle band (Fig. 22-2). You can often feel resistance as you break through the

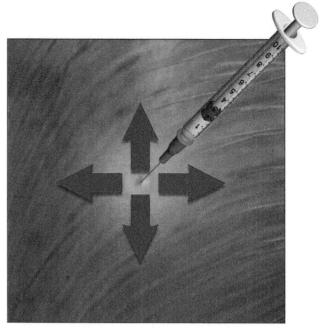

Figure 22-2 When injecting at a trigger point the needle should be inserted and then redirected superiorly, inferiorly, laterally, and medially.

trigger point. The needle is used to break up the taut band thoroughly. The needle is then removed from the skin and the procedure performed at all predetermined marked spots. The medication in the syringe should be distributed equally among the sites. Once the procedure is completed, a bandage is placed over the area as needed. I use an equal part mixture of 0.5% bupivacaine and 2% lidocaine, injecting 3 mL of solution per trigger point.

CONTRAINDICATIONS AND POTENTIAL COMPLICATIONS

Trigger point injections are a safe procedure that does not require fluoroscopic guidance. Contraindications include systemic infection, infection on the skin where the needle is passed, bleeding disorders, and acute muscle trauma. Special care is necessary when the procedure is performed in the cervical region or lung fields. In the cervical region intrathecal and arterial injections have been reported. The needle should remain in the muscle.

CASE STUDY

Case

A 38-year-old man comes to your office complaining of pain at the back of his neck. The pain is between the shoulder blades and in both trapezius muscles. The pain, which was mild at first, has occurred for the past 4 months. The man states that the pain does not radiate down his arms but is rather axial in nature and worse as the day goes on. He has tried over-the-counter acetaminophen (Tylenol) and ibuprofen with mild benefit. The patient describes his muscles as feeling tight and tense. He has tried stretching out the region on his own. On examination, he has full range of motion of the cervical spine, full strength in his upper extremities, and normal reflexes. He notes pain when you mildly palpate the cervical paraspinal muscles and trapezius muscles. He has had cervical x-rays, which are normal.

You ask the patient to press on the areas that are painful. You palpate those areas and the patient identifies four trigger points; you mark each one with an "X" using a marking pen. You repeat the examination and he indicates pain in three of the four previously marked spots. After explaining the procedure and obtaining informed consent, you clean the back with alcohol. You take a 10-mL syringe filled with 5 mL of 2% lidocaine and 5 mL of 0.5% bupivacaine. You enter all three points with the needle as the medication should be administered equally into all trigger points. The needle passes back and forth into every aspect of the trigger point. After the procedure, you place a bandage on the area. You prescribe physical therapy for a complete approach to the patient's pain and have the patient schedule a follow-up appointment for 1 month.

REFERENCES

1. Fricton JR, Kroening R, Haley D, et al. Myofascial pain syndrome of the head and neck: A review of clinical characteristics of 164 patients. *Oral Surg Oral Med Oral Pathol.* 1985;60(6):615–623.
2. Kamanli A, Kaya A, Ardicoglu O, et al. Comparison of lidocaine injection, botulinum toxin injection, and dry needling to trigger points in myofascial pain syndrome. *Rheumatol Int.* 2005;25(8):604–611.
3. Scott NA, Guo B, Barton PM, et al. Trigger point injections for chronic non-malignant musculoskeletal pain: A systematic review. *Pain Med.* 2009;10(1):54–69.
4. Alvarez DJ, Rockwell PG. Trigger points: Diagnosis and management. *Am Fam Physician.* 2002;65(4):653–660.

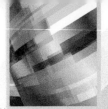

CHAPTER **23**

Joint and Associated Bursa Injections: Shoulders, Elbows, Hips, and Knees

Joints and their associated bursas can be injected with a corticosteroid and local anesthetic to reduce both pain and inflammation. These injections also help increase the range of motion of painful joints. Injections may be into the joint (intra-articular) in cases of arthritis or next to the joint (para-articular) in cases of bursitis. Bursitis is the painful inflammation of the bursa, a pad-like sac found in the areas subject to friction. Conditions often treated with these injections include osteoarthritis, bursitis, tendinitis, and frozen shoulder.

A number of different local anesthetics and steroids are used in combination for joint and bursa injections.

One syringe holds both the local anesthetic and the corticosteroid solution. The local anesthetic is useful because it provides immediate pain relief and confirms proper needle location. It also enables dispersion of steroid in a large joint space or bursa. The corticosteroid is useful because it decreases inflammation in three ways. One, it reduces excess synovial blood flow, which is increased because of vasodilation. Two, it lowers the local leukocyte and inflammatory modulatory response.[1-3] Three, it alters collagen synthesis and may, in moderate doses, retard bone and cartilage destruction (Fig. 23-1). In addition, the corticosteroid provides long-lasting pain relief.

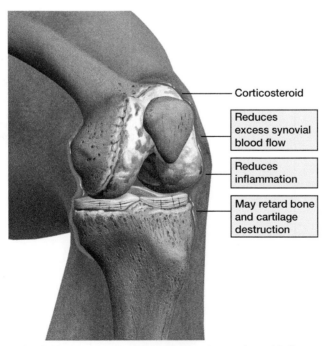

Corticosteroid

Reduces excess synovial blood flow

Reduces inflammation

May retard bone and cartilage destruction

Figure 23-1 How corticosteroids work to reduce pain and inflammation.

TABLE 23-1 Primary Corticosteroids Currently Available and Their Equivalent Doses

Trade Name	Generic Name	Equivalent Dose (mg)
Kenalog	Triamcinolone acetonide	40
Depo-Medrol	Methylprednisolone acetate	40
Celestone	Betamethasone acetate	6
Decadron	Dexamethasone acetate	8

TABLE 23-2 Comparison of Action of Lidocaine and Bupivacaine

Local Anesthetic	Onset of Action	Duration of Action (h)
Lidocaine	45–90 s	1–2
Bupivacaine	1–5 min	2–6

The primary corticosteroids on the market are listed in Table 23-1. There is no particular steroid that is more appropriate over another. I use Kenalog (triamcinolone acetonide) for my injections; standard Kenalog doses are presented in the examples to follow. If you decide to use any other steroid, its proper dose can easily be calculated: For example, 40 mg of Kenalog is equivalent to 6 mg of Celestone (Table 23-1).

Two types of local anesthetics are primarily used for joint and bursa injections: Lidocaine and bupivacaine, which both work by blocking fast voltage-gated sodium channels (Fig. 23-2). This prevents neuronal depolarization, blocking the painful nerve impulses that are sent to the brain. Doses of 1% lidocaine and 0.25% bupivacaine are equivalent to each other; however, they differ in their time of onset and length of duration (Table 23-2). I prefer bupivacaine because of its duration of action, but either local anesthetic is fine.

The following guidelines should be followed for joint and associated bursa injections. The total volume injected into medium-size joints such as the elbow, can be 2 mL. The total volume injected into larger-size joints such as the shoulders, hips, or knees can be 5 mL. The most common ratio of local anesthetic to corticosteroid is 2:1 or 3:1.

Repeated steroid injections for osteoarthritis are safe and do not accelerate disease progression.[4] Studies suggest that cartilage damage over time in patients with osteoarthritis is likely caused by the underlying disease rather than any deleterious effect of steroids. The recommended interval between intra-articular injections is 3 months.[5]

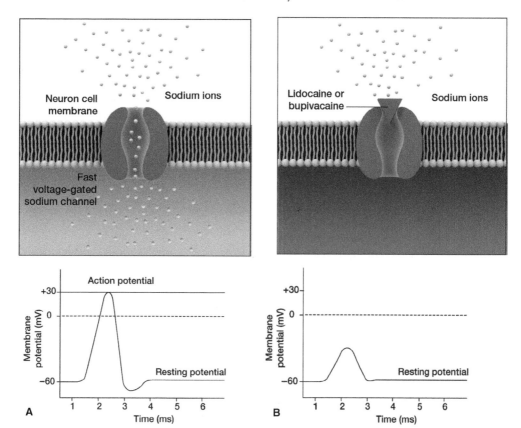

Figure 23-2 Lidocaine and bupivacaine block fast voltage-gated sodium channels, preventing neuronal depolarization. This blocks the transmission of pain. **A.** Sodium channel triggered action potential. **B.** Sodium channel action potential being inhibited by a local anesthetic.

WHEN TO USE

There are three primary reasons for joint and bursa injections.

The first reason is curative, in cases such as greater trochanteric bursitis (hips). After a single injection for greater trochanteric bursitis, patients often report a prolonged improvement in pain and disability.[6] A 2005 paper reported that in a 5-year follow-up there was a 2.7-fold increase in the number of patients who were pain free after a single corticosteroid injection compared with those who did not receive an injection.[7] In cases such as lateral epicondylitis (tennis elbow), corticosteroid injections are superior to nonsteroidal drug therapy and physical therapy before 6 weeks.[8,9]

The second reason is provision of a pain-free window. Often this gives the patient an ability to participate fully in physical therapy. Complete participation in rehabilitative exercises may lead to the resolution of forms of tendinopathy or bursitis.

The third reason is diagnostic, to help determine if pain is coming from the primary site or is referred: For example, identifying the hip as a main pain generator rather than being referred from the lumbar spine via a diagnostic block. If the patient has pain relief with a local anesthetic in the hip joint, it is most likely the pain generator and not referred from the back. This helps protect the patient from undergoing the needless pursuit of competing diagnoses, and from undergoing presumptive treatment that is not appropriate.

HOW TO PERFORM THE PROCEDURE

Shoulder Region

The shoulder is a ball and socket joint. The ball is the top, rounded part of the humerus; the socket is the outer edge of the scapula (the glenoid, Fig. 23-3). The joint is held together by muscles, ligaments, and tendons. This joint is flawed by design. The ball is too big for the relatively flat socket. This allows for the joints significant range of motion. The glenohumeral joint is a common pain generator. Patients also have pain at the superior aspect of the shoulder, where the clavicle and the acromion (part of the scapula) join. This area, commonly referred to as the acromioclavicular (AC) joint, is subject to friction, and consequently arthritis. Bursitis of the shoulder occurs at the subacromial bursa, which separates the supraspinatus tendon (one of the four tendons of the rotator cuff) from the coracoid process ligament (Fig. 23-4). When the arm is resting at the side, the subacromial bursa lies laterally below the acromion. When the arm is abducted, it moves medially beneath the bone where it can be impinged. To better understand which type of shoulder injection is appropriate for your patient, see the shoulder pain section of Chapter 1, Musculoskeletal Pain.

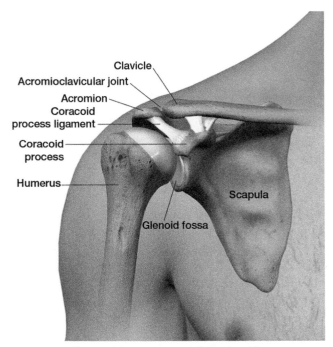

Figure 23-3 Anatomy of the shoulder.

Shoulder (Glenohumeral) Joint Injection: The patient is seated. The major landmark for this joint is the coracoid process (Fig. 23-5). Standing in front and just lateral to the painful shoulder, this knob of bone can be palpated. The injection point is 2 cm lateral to the inferior edge of the coracoid. Mark an "X" on this point using a felt-tip marking pen. The skin is prepped with betadine. A 5-mL syringe should be filled with a mixture of local anesthetic and steroid; an 18-gauge needle is used to draw up the medication. The needle is then removed once the medications have been drawn up and a 1.5-in, 25-gauge needle is employed next. A longer

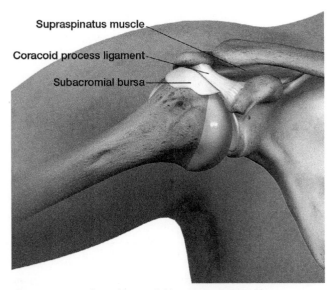

Figure 23-4 The subacromial bursa separating the supraspinatus tendon and coracoid process ligament.

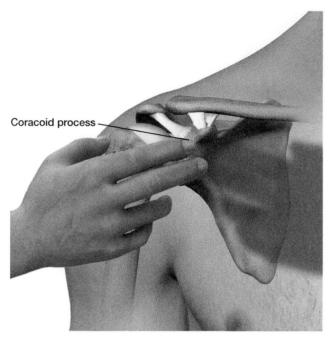

Figure 23-5 Physician palpating the coracoid process.

needle may be needed on larger patients. I use a mixture of 3 mL of 0.25% bupivacaine and 40 mg of Kenalog as my therapeutic agent. The needle is placed through the "X" that was marked on the skin (Fig. 23-6). The needle is advanced toward the humeral head until the needle tip touches bone. The needle is retracted 1 to 2 mm and the therapeutic agent is injected. The needle is then withdrawn, the betadine wiped away, and a bandage is placed. The patient is asked to move the shoulder through a full range of motion, which helps to distribute the therapeutic solution.

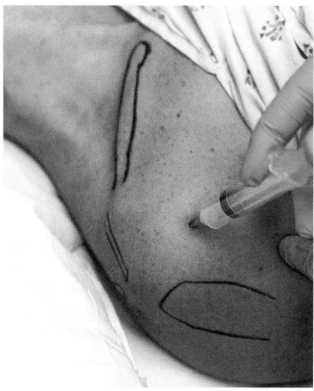

Figure 23-6 Skin entry point for a shoulder (glenohumeral) joint injection.

Shoulder (Acromioclavicular) Joint Injection: The patient is seated. Standing in front and just lateral to the painful shoulder, the clavicle is palpated in a medial to lateral direction. There is a small depression at the lateral aspect of the clavicle that can be tender. This is the AC joint (Fig. 23-7). Mark an "X" on this

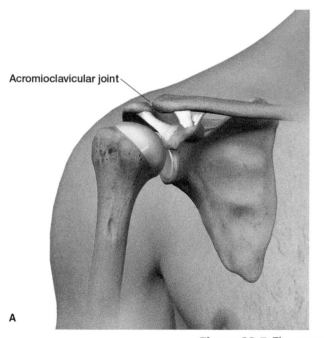

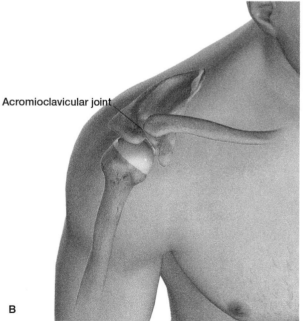

A

B

Figure 23-7 The acromioclavicular (AC) joint.

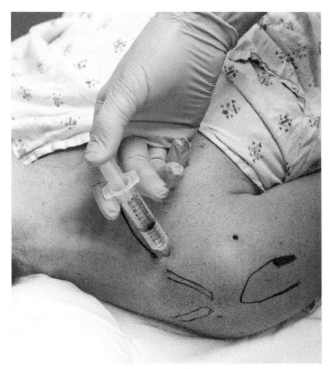

Figure 23-8 Skin entry point for an AC joint injection.

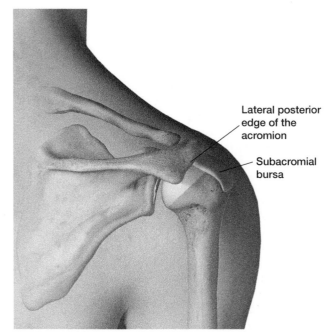

Lateral posterior
edge of the
acromion

Subacromial
bursa

Figure 23-9 Lateral posterior edge of the acromion can be palpated to help locate the subacromial bursa.

point using a felt tip marking pen (Fig. 23-8). The skin is prepped with betadine. A 5-mL syringe should be filled with a mixture of local anesthetic and steroid; an 18-gauge needle is used to draw up the medication. The needle is removed once the medications have been drawn up and a 1.5-in, 25-gauge needle is employed next. I use a mixture of 1 mL of 0.25% bupivacaine and 20 mg of Kenalog as my therapeutic agent. The needle is placed through the "X" that was marked on the skin and advanced toward the target until the needle tip touches bone and then withdrawn 1 to 2 mm. This is very superficial. The therapeutic agent is then injected. The needle is withdrawn, the betadine wiped away, and a bandage is placed.

Shoulder (Subacromial Bursa) Injection: The patient is seated. Standing in back and just lateral to the painful shoulder, the lateral posterior edge of the acromion is palpated (Fig. 23-9). Mark an "X" 2 cm below this point using a felt-tip marking pen (Fig. 23-10). The skin is prepped with betadine. A 5-mL syringe should be filled with a mixture of local anesthetic and steroid; an 18-gauge needle is used to draw up the medication. The needle is removed once the medications have been drawn up and a 1.5-in, 25-gauge needle is employed next. I use a mixture of 2 mL of 0.25% bupivacaine and 40 mg of Kenalog as my therapeutic agent. The needle is placed through the "X" that was marked on the skin, with the needle tip pointed cephalad toward the acromion. The needle is advanced toward the target until the

tip touches bone, the undersurface of the acromion. The needle is withdrawn 1 to 2 mm. The therapeutic agent is then injected. The needle is withdrawn, the betadine wiped away, and a bandage is placed. The patient is asked to move the shoulder through a full range of motion, which helps to distribute the therapeutic agent.

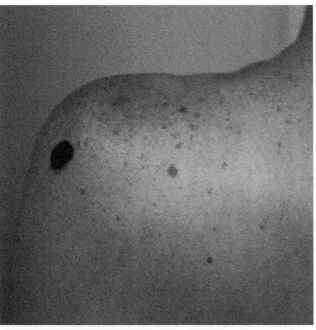

Figure 23-10 Skin entry point for a subacromial bursa injection.

Elbow Region

The elbow joint is formed by three bones. The humerus of the upper arm, the bones of the forearm, the radius laterally and the ulna medially. It is a hinge joint moving in one direction permitting only flexion and extension.

Lateral Epicondylitis (Tennis Elbow) Injection:

Tennis elbow is an overuse injury. The lateral epicondyle is the origin of the wrist extensor and supinators (Fig. 23-11). It is an idiopathic condition of middle-aged people characterized by the outer part of the elbow becoming painful and tender. Gripping and wrist extension movement are painful.

The patient is seated, and rests the arm on a table with the affected elbow slightly flexed. The wrist is in a neutral position. The elbow is supported with a towel. Standing in front and just lateral to the painful elbow, the lateral epicondyle is palpated for the maximum tender spot. Mark an "X" on this point using a felt-tip marking pen (Fig. 23-12). The skin is prepped with betadine. A 5-mL syringe should be filled with a mixture of local anesthetic and steroid; an 18-gauge needle is used to draw up the medication. The needle is removed once the medications have been drawn up and 1.5-in, 25-gauge needle is employed next. I use a mixture of 2 mL of 0.25% bupivacaine and 20 mg of Kenalog as my therapeutic agent. The needle is placed through the "X" that was marked on the skin and is advanced toward the target until the needle tip touches bone. This is very superficial. The needle is withdrawn 1 to 2 mm. The therapeutic agent is then injected. The needle is withdrawn, the betadine wiped away, and a bandage is placed. The patient is asked to move both the wrist and elbow through a full range of motion, which helps to distribute the therapeutic solution. Lateral epicondylitis is more common than medial epicondylitis, to be discussed next.

Medial Epicondylitis (Golfer's Elbow) Injection:

Golfer's elbow is an overuse injury. This syndrome is analogous to lateral epicondylitis and involves the wrist

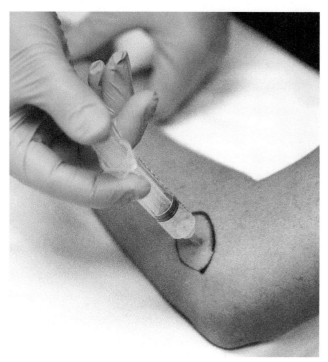

Figure 23-12 Skin entry point for a, lateral epicondyl, tennis elbow injection.

flexors on the medial side of the elbow (Fig. 23-13). Pain is exacerbated by resisted wrist flexion. Of note, golfers are more likely to get tennis elbow as tennis elbow is so prevelant. The ulnar nerve runs just posterior and inferior to the medial epicondyle. The local anesthetic, when injected, can spread and may involve the ulnar nerve. Before the injection, the patient should be informed that there may be transient numbness in the lateral aspect of the hand as well as the fourth and fifth digits, which are innervated by the ulnar nerve.

The patient is in the supine position on the examination bed. The arm rests by the patient's side, with the affected elbow slightly flexed. The wrist is in a neutral position. The elbow is supported with a towel. Standing in front and just lateral to the painful elbow, the medial epicondyle is palpated for the maximum tender spot. Mark an "X" on this point using a felt-tip

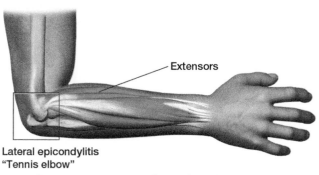

Lateral epicondylitis
"Tennis elbow"

Figure 23-11 Tennis elbow—lateral epicondylitis.

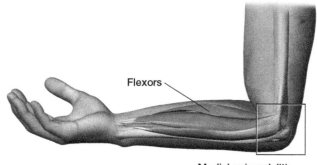

Medial epicondylitis
"Golfer's elbow"

Figure 23-13 Golfer's elbow—medial epicondylitis.

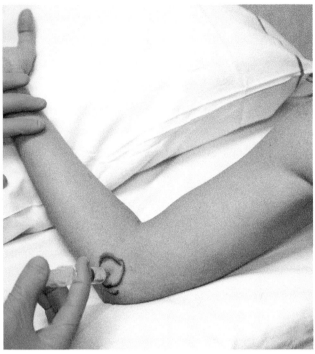

Figure 23-14 Skin entry point for a, medial epicondyle, golfer's elbow injection.

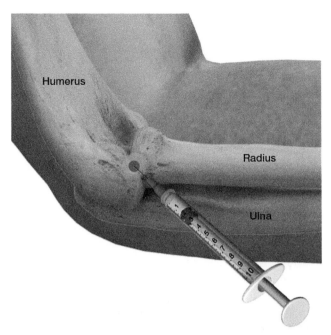

Figure 23-15 Landmark for elbow joint injection: Medial groove between the head of the radius and the humerus.

marking pen (Fig. 23-14). The skin is prepped with betadine. A 5-mL syringe should be filled with a mixture of local anesthetic and steroid; an 18-gauge needle is used to draw up the medication. The needle is removed once the medications have been drawn up and a 1.5-in, 25-gauge needle is employed next. I use 2 mL of 0.25% bupivacaine and 20 mg of Kenalog as my therapeutic agent. The needle is placed through the "X" that was marked on the skin and is advanced until the tip touches bone. This is very superficial. The needle is withdrawn 1 to 2 mm. The therapeutic agent is then injected. The needle is withdrawn, the betadine wiped away, and a bandage is placed. The patient is asked to flex and extend both the wrist and elbow through, which helps to distribute the therapeutic solution.

Elbow Joint Injection: The elbow joint is formed by three articulating surfaces: Where the humerus meets the radius, where it meets the ulna, and where the radius and ulna meet. To perform the procedure, have the patient place the painful elbow on the examining table with the arm bent at 45 degrees and the hand palm down on the table. Your landmark is the groove between the head of the radius (lateral aspect of the elbow) and the humerus (Fig. 23-15). Mark an "X" on this point using a felt-tip marking pen (Fig. 23-16). The skin is prepped with betadine. A 5-mL syringe should be filled with a mixture of local anesthetic and steroid; an 18-gauge needle is used to draw up the medication. The needle is removed once

the medications have been drawn up and a 1.5-in, 25-gauge needle is employed next. I use a mixture of 2 mL of 0.25% bupivacaine and 20 mg of Kenalog as my therapeutic agent. The needle is placed through the "X" that was marked on the skin and is advanced toward the target until the needle tip touches bone.

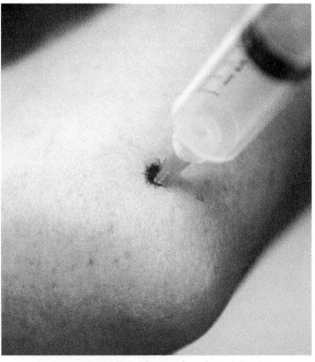

Figure 23-16 Site of entry for elbow injection.

This is very superficial. The needle is withdrawn 1 to 2 mm. The therapeutic agent is then injected. The needle is withdrawn, the betadine wiped away, and a bandage is placed.

Olecranon Bursa Injection: The olecranon bursa is the fluid-filled sac over the extensor aspect of the ulna (Fig. 23-17). In olecranon bursitis often a fluid collection develops at the elbow. The injection consists of two parts, aspiration and injection. The same patient positioning is used as an elbow joint injection. The area of maximum tenderness over the olecranon bursa is palpated, which is your target. The skin is prepped with betadine. The area of maximum tenderness is anesthetized using lidocaine with a 1.5-in, 25-gauge needle. After the skin is anesthetized an 18-gauge needle attached to a 10-cc syringe is entered at the area of maximum tenderness and advanced into the center of the area. The area is then aspirated. Prior to the procedure a 5-mL syringe should be filled with a mixture of local anesthetic and steroid; a separate 18-gauge needle is used to draw up the medication. I use a mixture of 2 mL of 0.25% bupivacaine and 40 mg of Kenalog as my therapeutic agent. Detach the 10-cc syringe from the 18-gauge needle after aspiration, grasp the hub of the needle, and attach your 5-cc syringe carrying the therapeutic agent. The therapeutic agent is then injected. The needle is withdrawn, the betadine wiped away, and a bandage is placed.

Hip Region

The hip joint is a ball and socket joint between the femoral head and the acetabulum cup (Fig. 23-18). Because

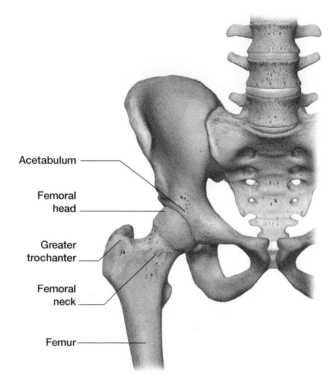

Figure 23-18 Anatomy of the hip joint.

of the lack of palpable structures, especially in larger individuals, fluoroscopy or ultrasound is needed for proper needle placement. The fluoroscopic approach will be described.

Intra-articular Hip Injection: The patient is brought to the fluoroscopy suite and placed on the fluoroscopic table in the supine position (face up). The painful hip is placed in a frog-leg position to open up the joint (Fig. 23-19). The fluoroscope is placed in the anteroposterior (AP) position. The skin is prepped with betadine and drapes are placed over the area in standard sterile fashion. Using a metal marker and a felt-tip marking pen, an "X" is placed on the skin overlying the

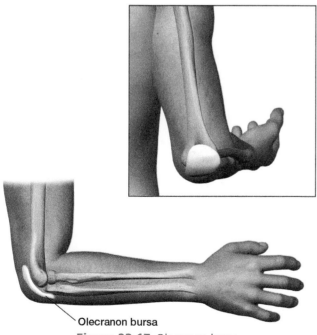

Figure 23-17 Olecranon bursa.

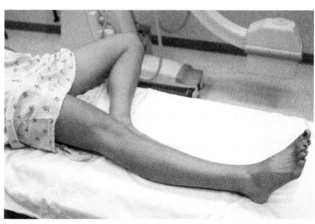

Figure 23-19 Left hip in frog-leg position.

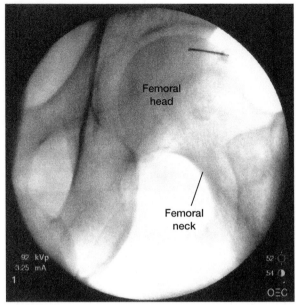

Figure 23-20 Target for a hip injection, the middle to lateral femoral head (*fluoroscopic view*).

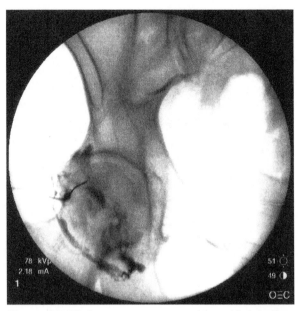

Figure 23-22 Proper contrast spread for a hip injection.

target, the middle to lateral femoral head (Fig. 23-20). The skin is anesthetized with 3 to 4 mL of lidocaine using a 1.5-in, 25-gauge needle. After the skin is anesthetized, a 3.5-in, 22-gauge spinal needle (Fig. 23-21) is placed through the "X" in a perpendicular fashion to the skin and parallel to the fluoroscope, advanced until it touches the femoral head, then retracted 1 to 2 mm. The stylet of the needle is removed. A 3-mL syringe with tubing containing contrast is connected to the needle. Tubing is used so that you can see the contrast being injected under live x-ray without your hand obscuring the image and to protect your hand from radiation exposure. Contrast is slowly injected to make sure it spreads properly over the femoral head. Once proper contrast spread is seen (Fig. 23-22), the 3-mL syringe containing the contrast is disconnected from the tubing. A 10-mL syringe with the therapeutic agent is then connected to the tubing and injected. I use a mixture of 4 mL of 0.25% bupivacaine and 40 mg of Kenalog as my therapeutic agent. The needle is then removed, the betadine wiped away, and a bandage is placed.

Nonfluoroscopic-guided injections (known as "blind injections") rarely place medication into the intra-articular portion of the joint. The results of these injections should be interpreted with great caution because of their imprecision in delivering medication to the desired location.

Greater Trochanteric Bursa Injection: The greater trochanteric bursa can become inflamed by repeated rubbing of the insertion of the gluteus maximus over the bursa, which causes friction against the femur (Fig. 23-23). In slender patients, the injection can be

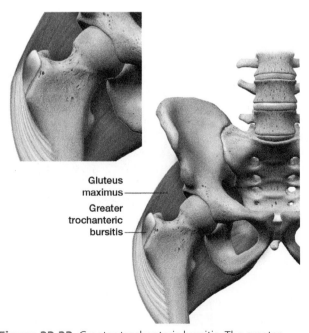

Figure 23-23 Greater trochanteric bursitis. The greater trochanteric bursa being irritated by friction of the gluteus maximus over the femur.

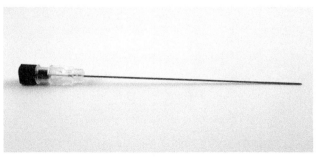

Figure 23-21 A 3.5-in, 22-gauge spinal needle.

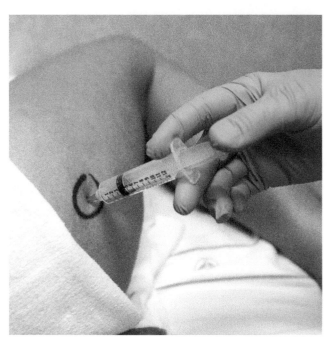

Figure 23-24 Skin entry point for a greater trochanteric bursa injection when not using fluoroscopy.

mal tenderness. Mark an "X" over the area of maximal tenderness using a felt-tip marking pen (Fig. 23-24). The skin is prepped with betadine. A 5-mL syringe should be filled with a mixture of local anesthetic and steroid; an 18-gauge needle is used to draw up the medication. The needle is removed once the medications have been drawn up and a 2.5-in, 25-gauge needle is employed next. I use a mixture of 4 mL of 0.25% bupivacaine and 40 mg of Kenalog as my therapeutic agent. The needle is placed through the "X" that was marked on the skin and advanced toward the target until the tip touches bone. A longer needle may be needed on bigger patients. The needle is then retracted 1 to 2 mm and the therapeutic agent is injected. Fan this injection to deliver the therapeutic agent over a wider area. The needle is withdrawn, the betadine wiped away, and a bandage is placed.

Trochanteric bursa injection under fluoroscopic guidance. The patient is brought to the fluoroscopy suite and placed on the fluoroscopic table in the prone position (face down). The fluoroscope is placed in the AP position. The skin of the buttock and lateral hip is prepped with betadine and drapes are placed over the area in standard sterile fashion. Using a metal marker and a felt-tip marking pen, an "X" is placed on the skin overlying the target, the greater trochanter (Fig. 23-25). The skin is anesthetized with 3 to 5 mL of lidocaine using a 1.5-in, 25-gauge needle. A 5-in, 22-gauge spinal needle is placed through the "X" in a perpendicular fashion to the skin and parallel to the fluoroscope in the AP view. The needle is advanced until it touches the lateral aspect of the greater trochanter, retracted

performed in the examination room. In most patients, fluoroscopy should be used.[10] Both the "blind" and fluoroscopic approaches will be described.

Trochanteric bursa injection in the examination room. The patient is placed in the lateral decubitus position, painful side up with the hip bent to 40 degrees. Stand behind the patient. The lateral aspect of the trochanter of the hip is palpated to find the site of maxi-

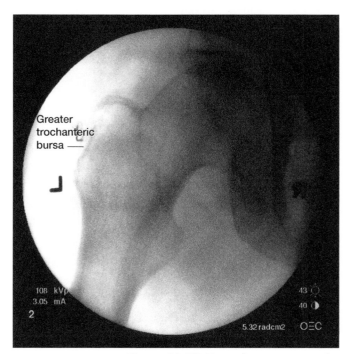

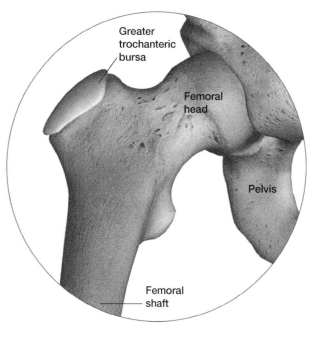

Figure 23-25 Target for a greater trochanteric bursa injection (*fluoroscopic view*).

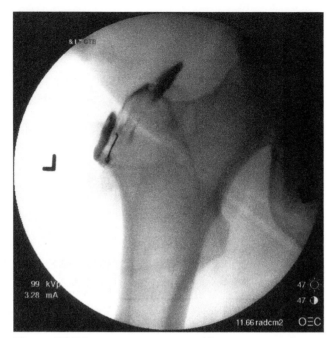

Figure 23-26 Proper contrast spread for a greater trochanteric bursa injection under fluoroscopic guidance.

1 to 2 mm, then the stylet of the needle is removed. A 3-mL syringe with tubing containing contrast is connected to the needle. Tubing is used so that you can see the contrast being injected under live x-ray without your hand obscuring the image and to protect your hand from radiation exposure. Contrast is injected to make sure it spreads properly over the greater trochanter (Fig. 23-26). Once proper contrast spread is seen, the 3-mL syringe containing contrast is disconnected from the tubing. A 5-mL syringe with the therapeutic agent is connected to the tubing and injected. I use 4 mL of 0.25% bupivacaine and 40 mg of Kenalog as my therapeutic agent. The needle is then removed, the betadine wiped away, and a bandage is placed.

Knee Region

Entry to the knee joint is possible from four different quadrants: Above or below the patella, or from the medial or lateral aspect of the joint. All points work well when entered properly. The intra-articular injection below describes the inferior lateral approach, because it is the easiest entry point for most practitioners. The same technique applies for the injection of a mixture of local anesthetic and steroid as well as for the injection of a hyaluronic acid viscosupplement. The only difference is that injection of the viscosupplement requires a bigger needle—22-gauge rather than 25-gauge—because of the viscosity of the viscosupplement.

Corticosteroid injections for osteoarthritis of the knee have a long-standing clinical beneficial track record for treating both pain and function. These injections, along

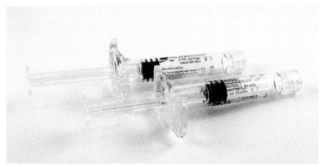

Figure 23-27 Hyaluronic acid viscosupplementation. Its method of action most likely involves acting as a physical cushion for a joint, anti-inflammatory properties, and stimulation of endogenous hyaluronan.

with physical therapy and NSAID use, remain a cornerstone of treatment.

For osteoarthritis of the knee only, the FDA has approved hyaluronic acid viscosupplementation injections (Fig. 23-27). These injections are good for patients who have derived no pain relief from corticosteroid injections and those with poorly controlled diabetes. The exact mechanism of action of hyaluronic acid viscosupplementation is unknown but most likely involves physical cushioning of the knee joint, anti-inflammatory properties, and stimulation of endogenous hyaluronan. Hyaluronan is a major component of the synovial fluid and was found to increase the viscosity of the fluid, providing joint lubrication and shock absorbency. In osteoarthritic joints, the concentration of hyaluronan is decreased by 32%, limiting its role in maintaining normal joint function.[11] It is also an important component of articular cartilage. Injectable hyaluronan (viscosupplementation) is commercially available in various forms (Table 23-3). They are all derived from the comb of a rooster with the exception of Euflexxa. If the patient has an allergy to egg products Euflexxa should be used, being the sole viscosupplement not derived from rooster combs. Injection schedules for the different forms of injectable hyaluronan are presented in Table 23-3.

Intra-articular Knee Injection: The patient is seated. The leg is allowed to hang naturally. Standing

TABLE 23-3 Viscosupplementation Guidelines

Injectable Hyaluronan Products	Instructions
Synvisc	Once a week for 3 wk
Orthovisc	Once a week for 3 wk
Hyalgan	Once a week for 5 wk
Supartz	Once a week for 5 wk
Euflexxa	Once a week for 3 wk

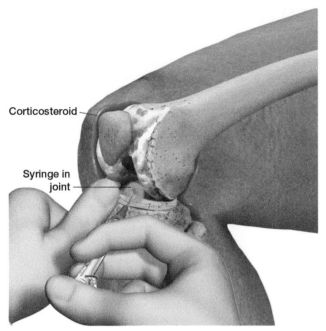

Figure 23-28 Anatomical window for a knee injection.

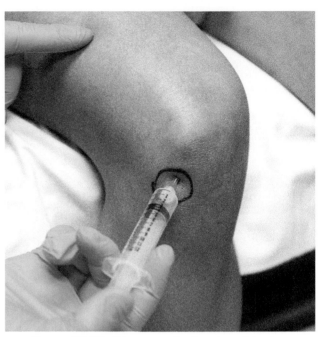

Figure 23-29 Skin entry point for a knee injection.

in front and just lateral to the painful knee, the groove between the fibula and tibia is palpated (Fig. 23-28). Using a felt-tip marking pen, mark an "X" at a point just superior and slightly medial to the groove (Fig. 23-29). The skin is prepped with betadine. A 5-mL syringe should be filled with a mixture of local anesthetic and steroid; an 18-gauge needle is used to draw up the medication. The 18-gauge needle is removed once the medications have been drawn up and a 1.5-in, 25-gauge needle is employed next. I use 3 mL of 0.25% bupivacaine and 40 mg of Kenalog as my therapeutic agent. The needle is placed through the "X," aiming at the center of the knee, medial and superior from the entry position, and advanced toward the target until the hub touches the skin. If the needle touches bone it should be redirected, usually more medial and superior. The therapeutic agent is then injected. The needle is withdrawn, the betadine wiped away, and a bandage is placed. The patient is asked to move the knee through a full range of motion, which helps to distribute the therapeutic agent.

For a hyaluronic acid viscosupplement injection, the prepackaged sterile syringe is attached to a 22-gauge needle and implemented following the same steps as described previously. Because the needle is larger for a viscosupplement injection, the skin should be numbed with 2 to 3 mL of lidocaine using a 1.5-in, 25-gauge needle before using the 22-gauge needle.

CONTRAINDICATIONS AND POTENTIAL COMPLICATIONS

Contraindications include systemic infection, infection on the skin where the needle is inserted, and especially infection in the joint itself. The presence of an osteochondral/intra-articular fracture or severe joint destruction contraindicates injection. Blood thinners should be withheld for hip injection. Blood thinners are not typically withheld for shoulder, elbow and knee injections.

The most common complication of intra-articular injections is postinjection flair of pain in 2% to 10% of patients. It is advised that patients wait at least 3 to 4 weeks between intra-articular injections. The effect of corticosteroids on tendon/ligament properties is poorly understood. There seems to be a transient biochemical weakness that returns to control levels. Used at standard joint injection doses, corticosteroids do not have any effect on the strength of bone and do not lead to bone destruction.

Injecting corticosteroids in the subcutaneous tissue can result in skin atrophy and hypopigmentation. To prevent this, it is best to avoid injection until the needle has passed through the subcutaneous tissue.

CASE STUDIES

Case 1

A 65-year-old woman reports pain in the right knee that is worse with prolonged standing or walking. She describes the pain as deep, achy, and dull. It has increased in severity over the past year and a half. She has been taking over-the-counter ibuprofen to control the pain. Examination shows that the woman has full strength in her lower extremities, with no signs of instability. X-rays of the right knee show osteoarthritis.

After discussing treatment options, you and the patient decide to proceed with a local anesthetic/corticosteroid injection of the right knee. You perform the injection with 40 mg of Kenalog and 3 mL of 0.25% bupivacaine. You also prescribe physical therapy. For the next 5 years, the patient does well with an injection every 6 months. At year 5, the patient reports that the injections are not relieving the pain for the full 6 months. At this point, you initiate a series of hyaluronic acid viscosupplementation injections. You choose Euflexxa, because the patient has an egg allergy. The patient has one injection a week of Euflexxa for 3 weeks. This helps with the pain such that she is once again able to have the local anesthetic and cortisone injection intervals of 6 months and even longer.

Case 2

A 53-year-old woman comes to the office complaining of right hip pain. It had become so bad that she went to the emergency department (ED) the day before. While in the ED, she had an x-ray, which was normal. After receiving a shot of morphine, she was released for follow-up with you the next day. The woman reports that the pain started about 3 weeks ago and has increased in intensity quickly. She cannot understand how her x-ray is normal when the pain is so bad. The pain is at the posterior lateral aspect of her hip, with no radiation into the groin or down the leg. The patient denies any trauma.

On examination, the patient has full range of motion of the hip and exquisite tenderness over the right greater trochanteric bursa. You explain that she has bursitis, which does not show up on an x-ray. You perform a right greater trochanteric bursa injection, and the patient has a significant reduction in pain.

REFERENCES

1. Caldwell JR. Intra-articular corticosteroids. Guide to selection and indications for use. *Drugs.* 1996;52(4):507–514.
2. Lavelle W, Lavelle ED, Lavelle L. Intraarticular injections. *Med Clin North Am.* 2007;91(2):241–250.
3. Wei AS, Callaci JJ, Juknelis D, et al. The effect of corticosteroid on collagen expression in injured rotator cuff tendon. *J Bone Joint Surg Am.* 2006;88(6):1331–1338.
4. Bellamy N, Campbell J, Robinson V, et al. Intraarticular corticosteroid for treatment of osteoarthritis of the knee. *Cochrane Database Syst Rev.* 2006;(2):CD005328.
5. Raynauld JP, Buckland-Wright C, Ward R, et al. Safety and efficacy of long-term intraarticular steroid injections in osteoarthritis of the knee: A randomized, double-blind, placebo-controlled trial. *Arthritis Rheum.* 2003;48(2):370–377.
6. Shbeeb MI, O'Duffy JD, Michet CJ Jr, et al. Evaluation of glucocorticosteroid injection for the treatment of trochanteric bursitis. *J Rheumatol.* 1996;23(12):2104–2106.
7. Lievense A, Bierma-Zeinstra S, Schouten B, et al. Prognosis of trochanteric pain in primary care. *Br J Gen Pract.* 2005;55(512):199–204.
8. Smidt N, van der Windt DA, Assendelft WJ, et al. Corticosteroid injections, physiotherapy, or a wait-and-see policy for lateral epicondylitis: A randomised controlled trial. *Lancet.* 2002;359(9307):657–662.
9. Bisset L, Beller E, Jull G, et al. Mobilisation with movement and exercise, corticosteroid injection, or wait and see for tennis elbow: Randomised trial. *BMJ.* 2006;333(7575):939.
10. Cohen SP, Narvaez JC, Lebovits AH, et al. Corticosteroid injections for trochanteric bursitis: Is fluoroscopy necessary? A pilot study. *Br J Anaesth.* 2005;94(1):100–106.
11. Watterson JR, Esdaile JM. Viscosupplementation: Therapeutic mechanisms and clinical potential in osteoarthritis of the knee. *J Am Acad Orthop Surg.* 2000;8(5):277–284.

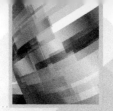

CHAPTER 24

Sympathetic Blocks: Stellate, Celiac, Lumbar, Superior Hypogastric, and Ganglion Impar

WHEN TO USE

HOW TO PERFORM THE PROCEDURE
▷ Stellate Ganglion Block
▷ Celiac Plexus Block
▷ Neurolytic Celiac Plexus Block for Cancer Pain
▷ Lumbar Sympathetic Ganglion Block (Paravertebral block)

▷ Superior Hypogastric Plexus Block
▷ Neurolytic Superior Hypogastric Block for Cancer Pain
▷ Ganglion Impar (Ganglion of Walther) Block
▷ Neurolytic Ganglion Impar Block for Cancer Pain

CONTRAINDICATIONS AND POTENTIAL COMPLICATIONS

The sympathetic chain is a bundle of nerves that runs from the base of the skull to the tip of the spine. The sympathetic chain runs along the vertebral bodies in a paravertebral fashion (Fig. 24-1). At points the nerves bundle together into ganglia. Ganglia are groups of nerve cells forming a nerve center located outside the brain. Each ganglion is responsible for providing neural transmission to and from different parts of the body. These ganglia make up the sympathetic chain.

The sympathetic chain is part of the autonomic nervous system, which controls functions that occur automatically and unconsciously (dilation of a blood vessel, changes in heart rate, or contraction of a sphincter) compared with the somatic nervous system, which controls motor and sensory function (skeletal muscle control, e.g., flexing a bicep, and sensation, such as feeling sandpaper). Table 24-1 gives the name, location, and corresponding body part for each sympathetic ganglion.

WHEN TO USE

Sympathetic blocks have three main indications.

First they are indicated for the treatment of sympathetically maintained pain. It has been shown that by blocking the sympathetic ganglion, pain relief can be achieved in the corresponding body part that lasts longer than the expected duration of a local anesthetic injected. Therefore, aberrant actions of the sympathetic nervous system may generate pain in peripheral tissues. The classic example of this is complex regional pain syndrome (CRPS, formerly known as reflex sympathetic

dystrophy [RSD]). The presence of regional edema in the skin and accompanying irregularities in blood flow/temperature and pseudomotor regulation suggests an autonomic component to the disease. A stellate ganglion block is used for the treatment of upper extremity CRPS whereas a lumbar sympathetic block is used for the treatment of lower extremity CRPS.

Second indication is for pancreatic, pelvic, or peritoneal pain. The classical example of this is a celiac plexus block for pancreatic pain. Fibers that conduct painful impulses from the pancreas are transmitted to the brain along the celiac plexus. By blocking these fibers, it is possible to control pathologic painful impulses. For noncancerous pain, such as pancreatitis, a sympathetic block with a local anesthetic can help break the pain cycle. For cancer pain, a diagnostic block using a local anesthetic is necessary—if positive, a neurolytic block consisting of using pure alcohol or phenol. Phenol causes nerve destruction by inducing protein precipitation, leading to a separation of the myelin sheath from the axon and axonal edema. Six percent phenol produces nerve necrosis within 24 hours. Alcohol causes nerve destruction by extracting phospholipids, cholesterol, and cerebroside from neural tissues. Although 50% to 100% alcohol is used as a neurolytic agent, the minimum concentration required for neurolysis has not been established. Neurolytic sympathetic blocks are reserved for cancer pain because they can lead to deafferentation pain. Deafferentation pain is a complex pain syndrome characterized by burning pain and marked sensitivity to touch in the distribution of a chemically lysed ganglion. In oncology

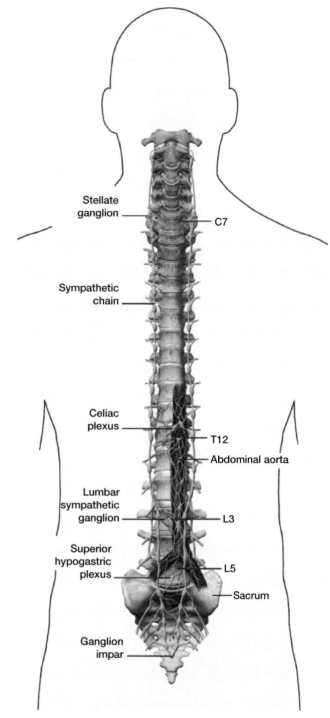

Figure 24-1 Anatomy of the sympathetic chain.

Labels in figure: Stellate ganglion, C7, Sympathetic chain, Celiac plexus, T12, Abdominal aorta, Lumbar sympathetic ganglion, L3, Superior hypogastric plexus, L5, Sacrum, Ganglion impar

TABLE 24-1 Spinal Location of Sympathetic Chain in the Body and Body Part they are Associated With

Ganglion or Plexus	Spinal Level	Body Part
Stellate ganglion	C6–T1	Upper extremity, neck, head
Celiac plexus	T12	Pancreas
Lumbar sympathetic ganglion	L2–L3	Lower extremities
Superior hypogastric plexus	L5–S1	Pelvis
Ganglion impar (ganglion of Walther)	Sacrococcygeal junction	Perineum

crossover of innervation with the ganglion impar which is used classically for cancer pain from rectal, vulva, or distal third of the vagina.

Third they are indicated for ischemic syndrome of a limb. This includes peripheral vascular disease, gangrene, arterial embolism, and frostbite. In a patient with peripheral vascular disease, a sympathetic block can relieve the tonic baseline level of arterial vasoconstriction, allowing for increased circulation as well as decreased pain.

HOW TO PERFORM THE PROCEDURE

Each of these procedures described involve the same initial steps. Fully explain the procedure to the patient, answer all questions, and obtain informed consent. Ensure that intravenous (IV) access has been placed, because all sympathetic blocks can cause hypotension. IV access should be available in the rare instances that it is necessary to give fluids to provide pressure support after a block. The patient lies on the fluoroscopic table. For accuracy and safety, all procedures are performed under fluoroscopic guidance (live x-ray). A "time out" is performed prior to the procedure including verbal confirmation of correct patient, procedure and procedural site. Noninvasive hemodynamic monitors and pulse oximetry are placed.

Stellate Ganglion Block

The stellate ganglion is formed by the fusion of the inferior cervical ganglion and the first thoracic ganglion. It is typically located at the level of C7 (seventh cervical vertebrae), anterior to the transverse process of C7 (Fig. 24-2). Anatomical variation does exist and the ganglion may be anterior to the transverse process of C6.

patients deafferentation pain is not usually of concern, because by the time it develops the patients will most likely have succumbed to the disease. A superior hypogastric block is used primarily to control pelvic cancer pain from the bladder, urethra, uterus, vagina, vulva, perineum, prostate, penis, testes, or rectum. There is a

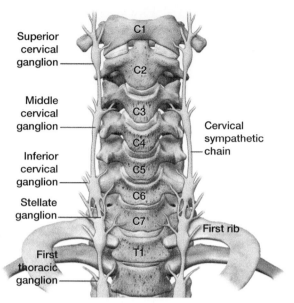

Figure 24-2 The stellate ganglion.

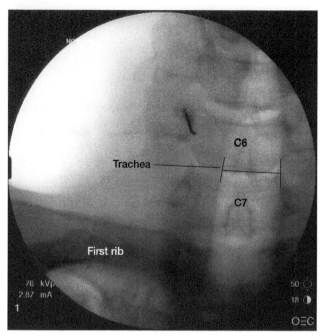

Figure 24-3 The intended target for a stellate ganglion block.

One expected result of a stellate ganglion block is an ipsilateral Horner syndrome (ptosis, miosis, and anhydrosis) because of the sympathetic blockade. Horner syndrome dissipates as the local anesthetic wears off. The patient should be informed of the expected after-block facial changes before the procedure.

The patient should be in the supine position (face up) on the fluoroscopic table. The fluoroscopy machine is placed in the anteroposterior (AP) position. The skin between the chin and the nipple on the side of pain is prepped with betadine and drapes are placed over the area in standard sterile fashion. The tubercle of the C6 vertebral body, Chassaignac tubercle, on the side of pain is brought into focus. Needle placement at C6, rather than C7, provides sufficient clearance from the top of the lung fields yet is still anatomically close enough for proper medication diffusion over the area. Using a metal marker and a felt-tip marking pen, an "X" is placed on the skin overlying the intended target (Fig. 24-3). The skin is anesthetized with lidocaine using a 1.5-in, 25-gauge needle (Fig. 24-4). After the skin is anesthetized, a 2.5-in, 22-gauge spinal needle is placed through the "X" in a perpendicular fashion to the skin and parallel to the fluoroscope. The needle is advanced until it comes in contact with the bone of the C6 tubercle. The needle should remain lateral to the trachea. It may be necessary to manually maneuver the trachea gently to clear a path for the needle. After bony contact, the needle is withdrawn 2 mm to bring the needle tip out of the body of the longus colli muscle. The stylet of the needle is then removed. A 3-mL syringe filled with contrast is connected to tubing (the tubing primed) and is connected to the needle. Tubing is used so that you can see the contrast being injected under live x-ray without having your hand obscure the image and to protect your hand from radiation exposure. Aspirate with the 3-mL syringe to check for blood or cerebrospinal fluid (CSF) return. After negative aspiration, the contrast is injected to make sure that it spreads over the area of the stellate ganglion and that no contrast is taken up by a vessel, indicating that the

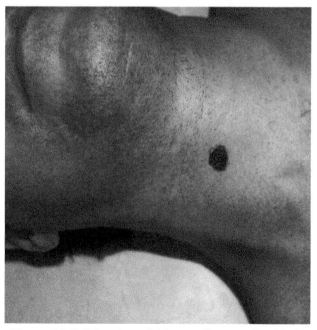

Figure 24-4 Skin entry point for a stellate ganglion block.

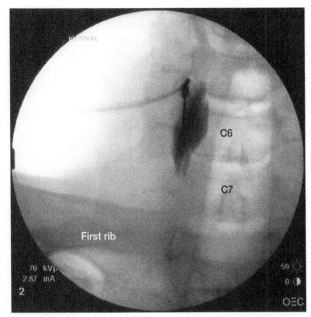

Figure 24-5 Proper contrast spread for a stellate ganglion block.

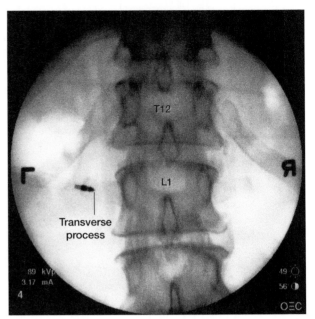

Figure 24-6 Initial entry point target, the lateral aspect of the transverse process of the L1 vertebral body, for a celiac plexus block.

tip of the needle is in a vessel. Once proper contrast spread is seen (Fig. 24-5), the 3-mL syringe containing contrast is disconnected from the tubing. A 10-mL syringe with the therapeutic agent, a local anesthetic, is connected to tubing and injected in 2.5-mL aliquots. I use a mixture of 4 mL of 2% lidocaine and 4 mL of 0.5% bupivacaine in a 10-mL syringe as my therapeutic agent. The needle is then removed and a bandage placed.

Celiac Plexus Block

There are many effective approaches to blocking the celiac plexus. Following discussion describes the standard splanchnic approach.

The patient is placed on the fluoroscopic table in the prone position (face down) with a pillow under the abdomen to flex the thoracolumbar spine. The fluoroscopy machine is placed in the AP position. The back is prepped with betadine and drapes are placed over the area in standard sterile fashion. The L1 vertebral body is brought into focus. Using a metal marker and a felt-tip marking pen, an "X" is placed on the skin overlying the lateral aspect of transverse process of the L1 vertebral body (Fig. 24-6). The skin is anesthetized with lidocaine using a 1.5-in, 25-gauge needle. After the skin is anesthetized, a 5-in spinal needle with at least a 30 degree curve at the end—the physician typically bends the needle to create a curve (Fig. 24-7)—is placed through the "X" in a perpendicular fashion to the skin and a parallel fashion to the camera. The curve at the tip of the needle is key in helping steer the needle medially in the latter part of the procedure. A 7-in needle may be needed for heavier patients. The needle is advanced until it comes in contact with the bone of the

lateral aspect of the L1 transverse process. After contacting the transverse process, the needle is then slightly withdrawn and redirected toward the lateral aspect of the T12 vertebral body (toward the head) and further advanced (Fig. 24-8). This nondirect approach to the anterior border of the T12 vertebral body is used to avoid the lung fields. At this point, the camera is switched to a lateral view. When the needle touches the lateral aspect of the T12 vertebral body, the curved point is rotated away from the vertebral body so that it can be advanced further anteriorly. The needle is then rotated back medially to continue medially toward the celiac plexus, which lies near the anterior border of the T12 vertebral body (Fig. 24-9). Once the needle is brought into final position, just anterior to the T12 vertebral body, the stylet of the needle is removed. A 5-mL syringe is tightened on the spinal needle and aspirated to check for blood or CSF. If blood is withdrawn the needle tip is located too anterior and should be repositioned. After negative aspiration, the 5-mL syringe is

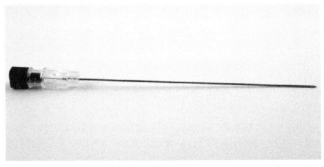

Figure 24-7 Five-inch spinal needle with a curve at the end.

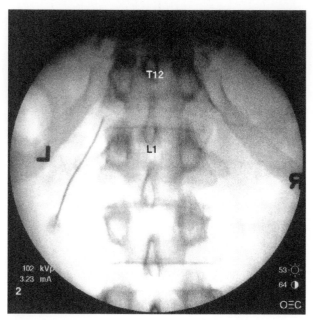

Figure 24-8 Redirection of the needle toward the T12 vertebral body, superior and medially.

disengaged and a 3-mL syringe with tubing containing contrast is connected to the needle. Tubing is used so that you can see the contrast being injected under live x-ray without having your hand obscure the image and to protect your hand from radiation exposure. The contrast is injected to make sure that it spreads over the area of the celiac plexus and that no contrast is taken up by a vessel, indicating that the tip of the needle is in a vessel. If the needle is advanced too far anteriorly,

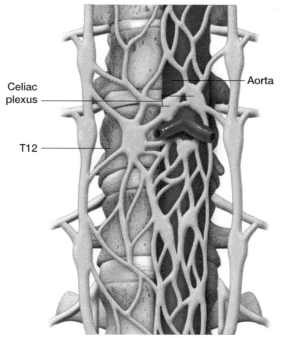

Figure 24-9 Celiac plexus at the anterior aspect of the T12 vertebral body.

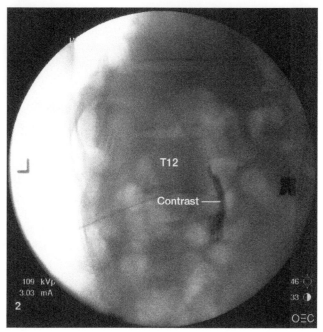

Figure 24-10 Proper contrast spread for a celiac plexus block.

you will see blood on aspiration or the contrast being whisked away under fluoroscopy. At this point, guide the needle posteriorly, toward you, until the needle is in proper position. Once proper contrast spread is seen (Fig. 24-10), the 3-mL syringe containing contrast is disconnected from the tubing. The spinal needle is now properly placed.

Due to the celiac plexus medial location a bilateral approach is usually required. The same steps are followed to place a needle on the contralateral side of the needle already placed. Once this is done, a 20-mL syringe with the therapeutic agent, a local anesthetic, is connected to tubing and injected in 2.5-mL aliquots, 7.5 mL into each needle. I use 7.5 mL of 2% lidocaine and 7.5 mL of 0.25% bupivacaine mixed in the 20-mL syringe as my therapeutic agent. Some physicians will add a steroid, 80 mg of kenalog when treating pancreatitis to curb any irritation of the celiac plexus. The needles are then removed and a bandage placed.

Neurolytic Celiac Plexus Block for Cancer Pain

The same steps are performed as described in the celiac plexus block. After the contrast is injected, showing proper spread, a long-acting local anesthetic (8 mL of 0.25% bupivacaine) is divided equally and injected into both syringes. This is done to ensure comfort during the injection of the neurolytic agent. An injection of 10 mL of the neurolytic agent, 6% phenol, is administered; 5 mL of phenol is injected into each needle. Rather than phenol 10 mL of 100% alcohol can also be used. If done properly, the celiac ganglion block facilitates increased bowel motility by about 50%. This is because of uncontested parasympathetic control of the intestines. However, most pancreatic cancer patients are on a narcotic, which decreases their bowel motility, thus increased motility is not usually a problem and often welcomed.

Lumbar Sympathetic Ganglion Block (Paravertebral block)

The lumbar sympathetic chain is situated in the retroperitoneal connective tissue in a paravertebral plane alongside the L2, L3, or L4 vertebral body. It is most often present opposite the anterior one third of the body of the third lumbar vertebra and at the disks above and below (Fig. 24-11). Lumbar sympathetic blocks are often performed for the treatment of CRPS.

The patient should be informed that the temperature of the leg on the ipsilateral side of the block is going to increase after the procedure. Blood vessels dilate because of uncontested parasympathetic activity. I often tell my patients that blood is going to rush into the areas of pain where it was not able to travel before, which is why the leg is going to heat up.

The patient is placed on the fluoroscopic table in the prone position (face down). The fluoroscopy machine is placed in the AP position. The back is prepped with betadine and drapes are placed over the area in standard sterile fashion. The L3 vertebral body is brought into focus. The camera is then obliqued toward the side of pain until the tip of the transverse process lies at the lateral edge of the vertebral body in the picture. As the camera is rotated at an oblique angle you will see the transverse process radiographically disappear. Using a metal marker and a felt-tip marking pen, an "X" is

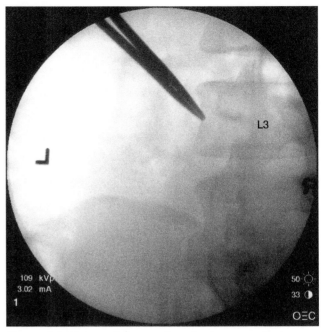

Figure 24-12 Intended target for a lumbar sympathetic block. The fluoroscope has an oblique to the left in this picture.

placed on the skin overlying the lateral aspect of the L3 vertebral body, the intended target (Fig. 24-12). The skin is anesthetized with lidocaine using a 1.5-in, 25-gauge needle. After the skin is anesthetized, a 5-in spinal needle with a curve at the end—the physician typically bends the needle to create a curve (Fig. 24-6)—is placed through the "X" in a perpendicular fashion to the skin and parallel fashion to the camera (Fig. 24-13).

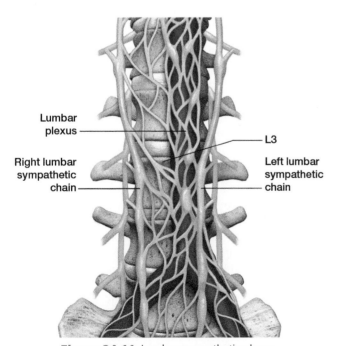

Figure 24-11 Lumbar sympathetic plexus.

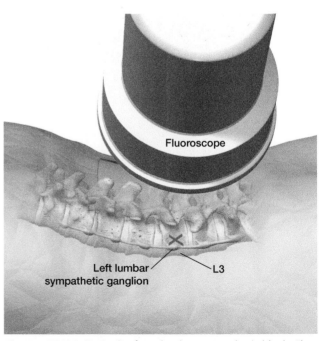

Figure 24-13 Entry site for a lumbar sympathetic block. Fluoroscope machine oblique with "X" on the lateral aspect of the L3 vertebral body.

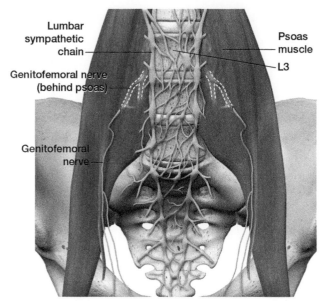

Figure 24-14 The lumbar sympathetic chain and its relation to the genitofemoral nerve. The lumbar sympathetic chain lies medial to the psoas muscle. The genitofemoral nerve lies laterally on the psoas muscle.

A 7-in needle may be needed for heavier patients. The needle is advanced until it comes in contact with the L3 vertebral body. The camera is then rotated to a lateral view. The needle is rotated with the curved end away from the vertebral body to come off the bone, so that it can be advanced further anteriorly, then is rotated back to keep the needle medially. This process may need to be repeated more than once. After the needle is guided into proper place, the anterior aspect of the L3 vertebral body, the stylet of the needle is removed. The lumbar sympathetic chain lies medial to the psoas muscle. The genitofemoral nerve lies laterally on the psoas muscle (Fig. 24-14). If the patient notes groin pain during the procedure, the needle is near the genitofemoral nerve and needs to be readjusted medially. A 5-mL syringe is tightened on the spinal needle, which is aspirated to check for blood or CSF. After negative aspiration, the 5-mL syringe is disengaged and a 3-mL syringe with tubing containing contrast is connected to the spinal needle. Tubing is used so that you can see the contrast being injected under live x-ray without having your hand obscuring the image and to protect your hand from radiation exposure. Contrast is injected to make sure contrast spreads over the area of the lumbar sympathetic ganglion and that no contrast is taken up by a vessel, indicating that the tip of the needle is in a vessel. Once good contrast spread is seen (Fig. 24-15), the 3-mL syringe containing contrast is disconnected from the tubing. A 10-mL syringe with the therapeutic agent, a local anesthetic, is connected to the tubing and injected in 2.5-mL aliquots. I use a mixture of 5 mL of 2% lidocaine and 5 mL of 0.5% bupivacaine mixed together in a 10-mL syringe as my therapeutic agent. Some physicians will add a steroid, 40 mg of kenalog. The needle is then removed and a bandage placed.

Superior Hypogastric Plexus Block

The superior hypogastric plexus is situated in the retroperitoneum, bilaterally extending from the lower third

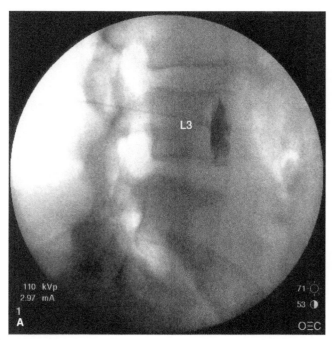

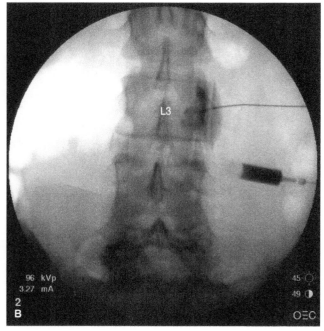

Figure 24-15 Proper contrast spread for a lumbar sympathetic block. **A.** Lateral view with contrast seen over the anterior one third of the L3 vertebral body. **B.** AP view with contrast seen behind the L3 vertebral body.

Figure 24-16 Superior hypogastric plexus and ▶
ganglion impar.

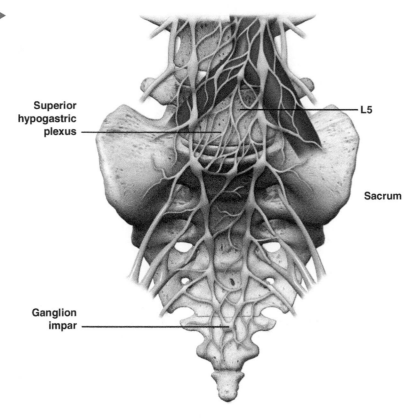

of the fifth lumbar vertebral body to the upper third of the first sacral vertebral body (Fig. 24-16). Superior hypogastric blocks are often performed for the treatment of pelvic pain.

The patient is placed on the fluoroscopic table in the prone position (face down). The fluoroscopy machine is placed in the AP position. The low back is prepped with betadine and drapes are placed over the area in standard sterile fashion. The L5 vertebral body is brought into focus. The camera is then obliqued toward one side. Obscuration from the iliac crest may limit the degree to which the picture can be "obliqued." Using a metal marker and a felt-tip marking pen, an "X" is placed on the skin overlying the lateral aspect of the L5 vertebral body, the intended target (Fig. 24-17). The skin is anesthetized with lidocaine using a 1.5-in, 25-gauge needle.

Figure 24-17 Initial fluoroscopic view for a superior ▶
hypogastric block when entering on the left side. The right-sided needle in this picture is already placed and contrast has been injected on the right side.

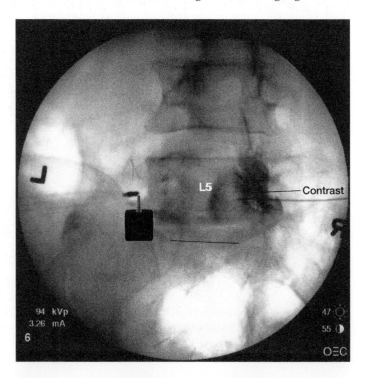

After the skin is anesthetized, a 5-in spinal needle with a curve at the end—the physician typically bends the needle to create a curve (Fig. 24-6)—is placed through the "X" in a perpendicular fashion to the skin and parallel fashion to the camera. The curve at the tip on the needle is key in helping steer the needle medially in the latter part of the procedure. A 7-in needle may be needed for heavier patients. The needle is advanced until it comes in contact with the L5 vertebral body. Care should be taken to avoid the L5 nerve root. The camera is then rotated to a lateral view. The tip of the needle is rotated with the curved end away from the vertebral body to come off the bone, so that it can be advanced anteriorly and then rotated back toward the medial aspect of the L5 vertebral body (this process may need to be repeated). After the needle is placed at the medial anterior aspect of the L5 vertebral body, the stylet of the needle is removed. A 5-mL syringe is tightened to the needle, which is aspirated to check for blood or CSF. If blood is returned often the needle tip is too lateral and should be repositioned more medially after negative aspiration, the 5-mL syringe is disengaged and a 3-mL syringe with tubing containing contrast is connected to the needle. Tubing is used so that you can see the contrast being injected under live x-ray without having your hand obscure the image and to protect your hand from radiation exposure. Contrast is injected to make sure that contrast spreads over the area of the superior hypogastric sympathetic ganglion and that no contrast is taken up by a vessel, indicating that the tip of the needle is in a vessel. Once good contrast spread is seen (Fig. 24-18), the 3-mL syringe containing contrast is disconnected. The needle is now properly placed.

Because the superior hypogastric plexus is a paired ganglion with half located on the right side of the vertebral body and the other half on the left, a bilateral approach is needed. The same steps are followed to place a needle on the contralateral side of the needle already placed. A 20-mL syringe with the therapeutic agent, a local anesthetic, is connected to tubing and injected in 2.5-mL aliquots; 7.5 mL is injected into each needle. I use 7.5 mL of 2% lidocaine and 7.5 mL of 0.5% bupivacaine mixed together in a 20-mL syringe as my therapeutic agent. Some physicians will add a steroid, 80 mg of kenalog, when performing a superior hypogastric block to curb any local inflammatory effect. The needles are then removed and a bandage placed.

Neurolytic Superior Hypogastric Block for Cancer Pain

To perform this block, complete the same steps described for the superior hypogastric plexus block. After injecting the contrast, add a long-acting local anesthetic (3 mL of 0.25% bupivacaine) to each needle to ensure comfort during the injection of the neurolytic agent. Follow this with insertion of 3 mL of the neurolytic agent 6% phenol into each needle for a total injection of 6 mL. Also, 100% alcohol is an appropriate neurolytic agent.

Ganglion Impar (Ganglion of Walther) Block

The ganglion impar is the most inferior, unpaired ganglion of the sympathetic trunk located anterior to the coccyx (Fig. 24-15). Ganglion impar blocks are often performed for the treatment of pelvic perineal pain.

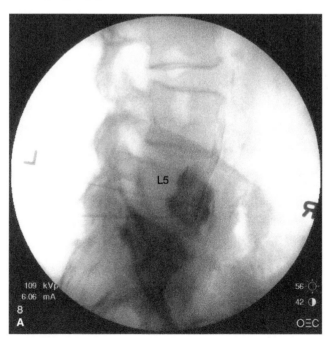
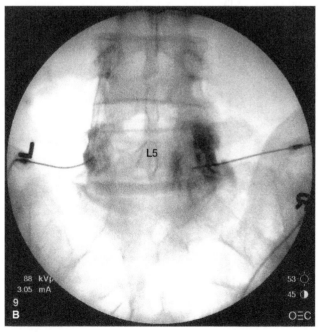

Figure 24-18 Proper contrast spread for a superior hypogastric block. **A.** Lateral view showing proper contrast spread over the anterior one third of the L5 vertebral body. **B.** AP view showing contrast behind the L5 vertebral body on the right. The left needle is in place but no contrast has been injected on that side yet.

The patient lies on the fluoroscopic table in the prone position (face down). The fluoroscopy machine is placed in the lateral position (rather than AP or oblique position, as with the other sympathetic blocks). The low back and buttock are prepped with betadine and drapes are placed over the area in standard sterile fashion. The coccyx is then brought into focus. Anatomical midline is established by palpating the coccyx. Using a metal marker and a felt-tip marking pen, an "X" is placed on the skin overlying the sacrococcygeal ligament, the intended target (Fig. 24-19). The skin is anesthetized with lidocaine using a 1.5-in, 25-gauge needle. After the skin is anesthetized, a 2-in, 22-gauge spinal needle is placed through the "X" in a perpendicular fashion to the skin and parallel to the fluoroscope. The needle is advanced until it comes in contact with the sacrococcygeal ligament. The needle is then advanced to and through the sacrococcygeal ligament to its anterior border. The stylet of the needle is then removed. A 5-mL syringe is tightened on the needle, which is aspirated to check for blood or CSF. After negative aspiration, the 5-mL syringe is disengaged and a 3-mL syringe with tubing containing contrast is connected to the needle. Tubing is used so that you can see the contrast being injected under live x-ray without having your hand obscure the image and to protect your hand from radiation exposure. Contrast is injected to make sure that it spreads over the area of the ganglion impar and that no contrast is taken up by a vessel, indicating that the tip of the needle is in a vessel. Once good contrast spread is seen (Fig. 24-20), the 3-mL syringe containing contrast is disconnected from the tubing. The ganglion impar is a single ganglion (rather than paired); only one needle is needed as compared to the celiac and superior hypogastric approaches,

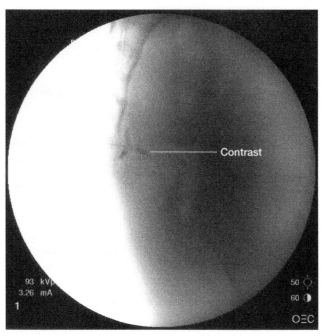

Figure 24-20 Proper contrast spread for a ganglion impar block.

which are bilateral. A 10-mL syringe with the therapeutic agent, a local anesthetic, is connected to tubing and injected. I use a mixture of 1.5 mL of 2% lidocaine and 1.5 mL of 0.5% bupivacaine in a 5-mL syringe as my therapeutic agent. The needle is removed and a bandage placed. Some physicians will add a steroid, 40 mg of kenalog, when performing a superior hypogastric block to curb any local inflammatory effect.

Neurolytic Ganglion Impar Block for Cancer Pain

Perform the same steps described for the ganglion impar block. After injecting the contrast, inject a long-acting local anesthetic (3 mL of 0.25% bupivacaine) to ensure comfort during the injection of the neurolytic agent. Then inject 3 mL of the neurolytic agent, 6% phenol. Also, 3 mL of 100% alcohol is appropriate.

CONTRAINDICATIONS AND POTENTIAL COMPLICATIONS

Contraindications include systemic infection, infection of the skin where the needle is inserted, and pregnancy. Blood thinners must be withheld for the procedure. All of these sympathetic blocks can produce hypotension, because the tonic sympathetic contraction of blood vessels is blocked. In rare cases, IV fluids may be necessary to give pressure support; therefore, it is recommended that IV access be obtained before the procedure. In addition, because the ganglia lie intimately next to the dural sac and blood vessels, it is essential to confirm needle position at all times to avoid improper injection. If medication is improperly injected into a blood vessel, it can cause a seizure.

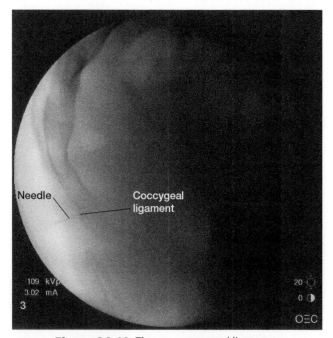

Figure 24-19 The sacrococcygeal ligament.

With stellate ganglion blocks, if the needle is not properly placed, a pneumothorax can result by puncturing the top of the lung fields. Therefore, it is important that bilateral stellate ganglion blocks not be performed. In the rare cases in which bilateral blocks are necessary, the physician performs the block on one side, and the patient returns later for the block on the other side. Bilateral stellate ganglion blocks may be problematic for another reason. Temporary vocal cord paralysis can develop on one side, and a contralateral stellate ganglion block has the potential to block the only working vocal cord, causing airway obstruction. If medication leaks onto the cervical plexus during a stellate ganglion block, the patient will experience weakness in the upper extremity until the local anesthetic wears off. Attention should also be given during stellate ganglion blocks to avoid the trachea which appears as a radiolucent shadow or the fluoroscopy film.

CASE STUDIES

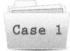

Case 1 A 55-year-old man has been diagnosed with pancreatic cancer and is currently on Percocet 10/325, which he takes four times a day to combat his pain. His current pain intensity is a 7 out of 10. Pain treatment options are reviewed with the patient, including escalation of his narcotics, and he elects to proceed with a celiac plexus block. A diagnostic injection is performed using a mixture of lidocaine and bupivacaine. The patient reports that his pain level went from a 7 out of 10 to no pain after the procedure. Based on these results, it is determined that the patient should respond to a neurolytic phenol block. The patient is brought back to the fluoroscopy suite 3 days later and the injection is repeated, using phenol. The patient's need for opioids diminishes dramatically and his sensorium is clear. He succumbs to the disease 8 months later.

Case 2 A 33-year-old female patient has a painful distal right upper extremity 2 months after right-elbow surgery. Both the surgery and the immediate postoperative period were unremarkable. The patient needed very little postoperative pain medication for the first 3 weeks but has since noted increasing pain. Pain can be elicited by simply touching the skin. There are no noticeable hair, or nail bed changes. The patient does note at times during the day her skin will change color for a few minutes, then revert back to its normal hue. The patient has good peripheral pulses and an ultrasound was normal. Postoperative x-rays are appropriate. The pain does not follow the distribution of a single nerve.

You diagnose this as CRPS. You have the patient schedule a right stellate ganglion block, once a week for 5 weeks. After each stellate ganglion block, the patient has clear signs of sympathetic blockade such as ptosis and miosis. After the third block, the patient reports very little pain relief. At this point, you reevaluate the diagnosis. Based on history and clinical examination, the primary diagnosis is still CRPS. You know all cases of CRPS do not have sympathetically maintained pain. This was the catalyst for the name change of the disease from RSD to CRPS. Based on the patient's continued pain, you book the patient for a spinal cord stimulator trial.

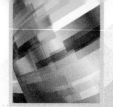

CHAPTER 25

Vertebroplasty and Kyphoplasty

WHEN TO USE

HOW TO PERFORM THE PROCEDURES

CONTRAINDICATIONS AND POTENTIAL COMPLICATIONS

Vertebral compression fractures (VCFs) are a significant problem. In the United States, more than 700,000 age-related osteoporotic compression fractures occur per year. One in two women and one in four men aged 50 years and older will have an osteoporosis-related fracture in their remaining lifetime.[1] The lifetime risk of VCFs is 16% in women and 5% in men.[2] VCFs are of significant importance; they can lead to chronic pain and kyphotic deformity, which can decrease pulmonary function and impair mobility.[3]

VCFs occur for a number of reasons, the most common being osteoporosis. The second most common cause of VCFs is tumors, both benign and metastatic. Cancers that tend to metastasize to the bone originate in the breast, lung, thyroid, kidney, and prostate. The bones in the axial skeleton, ribs, pelvis, and spine are normally the first involved. In breast cancer, pathologic fractures are common because of the lytic nature of the lesions. In lung cancer, they are uncommon because of patient's short lifespan, and in prostate cancer, they are rare, because the lesions tend to be osteoblastic rather than lytic. The third most common cause of VCFs is trauma.

Patients with VCFs present with deep focal pain at the level of the fracture. Activity exacerbates the pain, and lying down relieves it. Any palpation over the area elicits pain. New onset of back pain in a patient with known history of cancer warrants evaluation for compression fracture from metastatic disease. Plain x-rays can confirm a fracture.

Vertebroplasty and kyphoplasty are two minimally invasive procedures used to treat pain from VCFs (Fig. 25-1). Both procedures also prevent further pain and functional decline because of instability stemming from the fractured vertebral body. Vertebroplasty, which was initially developed for the treatment of aggressive spinal hemangiomas, was first performed in France in

1984 and was introduced in the United States in 1993. Kyphoplasty was later introduced in 1998. Both procedures involve injecting a cement-like substance, polymethyl methacrylate, into a fractured vertebral body via a large bore needle under fluoroscopy (x-ray guidance). They significantly reduce pain and improve mobility in patients with VCFs.[4] Kyphoplasty, which is slightly more invasive than vertebroplasty, involves inflation of a balloon, creating a cavity prior to the injection of bone cement. Kyphoplasty also poses a lower risk of bone cement leakage. Both procedures

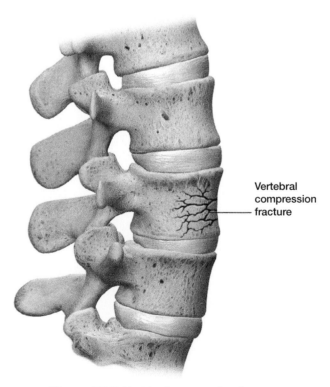

Vertebral compression fracture

Figure 25-1 Vertebral compression fracture.

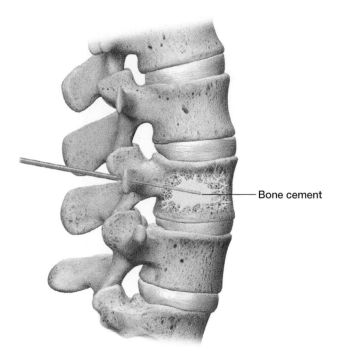

Figure 25-2 Vertebroplasty (cement working through trabecular bone).

are performed on an outpatient basis (Figs. 25-2 and 25-3).

WHEN TO USE

Vertebroplasty and kyphoplasty are used for stability, pain relief, and to improve mobility in patients with VCFs because of a variety of reasons such as osteoporosis, benign tumors, multiple myeloma, metastatic tumors, and trauma.[5] Patients who are likely to bene-

fit are those with a well-localized, deep, intense pain associated with imaging of a new or progressive compression fracture.[6] It has been reported that 95% of people treated with these two procedures immediately experienced partial or complete relief from their pain.[7] In 91% of patients receiving these treatments, required significantly less daily oral analgesic.[8] However, recent studies have challenged the merits of these two procedures.

Magnetic resonance imaging (MRI) is the gold standard for imaging VCFs. An MRI allows for the evaluation of the central spinal canal and neuroforamen, and makes possible identification of other potential sources of pain. When ordering an MRI to investigate a VCF, sagittal short tau inversion recovery (STIR) images should be requested. STIR distinguishes new or unhealed fractures from healed fractures. New or unhealed fractures show hyperintense signals within the bone marrow.

Treatment of VCFs varies. Initial noninterventional conservative treatment includes a nonsteroidal antiinflammatory drug, a waiting period, and a back brace as needed. Even with medical management, 33% patients with VCFs have persistent pain. Bed rest is often useful for pain reduction but can result in increased bone loss caused by inactivity, further increasing the risk of vertebral fracture.[9] In addition, medical management does not prevent the development of kyphotic deformity. Although surgery is an option, many people who develop VCFs are elderly and not ideal surgical candidates. The poor bone quality of osteoporotic fractured vertebrae, when fixated with screws, is a primary reason that surgical fixation often fails.[10] Patients with cancer who have metastatic VCFs may also be poor surgical candidates. Those who are

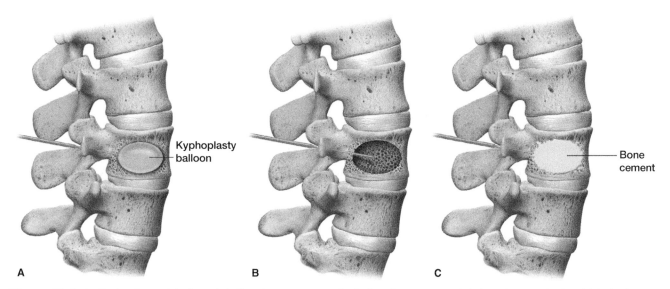

Figure 25-3 A. Kyphoplasty: A balloon is inflated to create a cavity before bone cement is injected. **B.** Cavity in which the bone cement is to be injected. **C.** Bone cement placed into the cavity for pain relief and stabilization of the VCF.

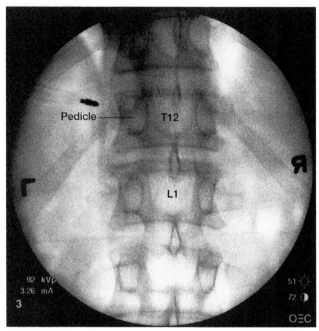

Figure 25-4 The skin entry position is just superior and lateral to the upper outer quadrant of the pedicle of the fractured vertebra. In this case T12 is the fractured vertebra.

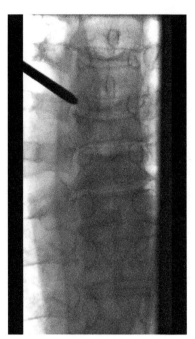

Figure 25-6 Trocar needle advanced under fluoroscopy to come in contact with the pedicle.

suitable surgical candidates may not want to go through the postsurgical recovery process.

HOW TO PERFORM THE PROCEDURES

After completely explaining the procedure to the patient and answering all questions, it is essential to obtain informed consent. Anesthesia may be either general or local. Limited data supporting or opposing the use of preoperative antibiotics are available.

The patient is positioned on the fluoroscopic table in a prone position (face down). The back is prepped in standard sterile fashion. The vertebra of pathology is magnified under fluoroscopic view. The fluoroscope is rotated 15 degrees toward the side being entered. Typically, the side facing the fluoroscopy machine is entered

first, which gives the operator the most room to work. Using a metal marker and a felt-tip marking pen, an "X" is placed on the skin overlying the skin entry point, just superior and lateral to the upper outer quadrant of the pedicle of the fractured vertebra (Fig. 25-4). Using 2% lidocaine, the skin and subcutaneous tissue are anesthetized.

A small (2-mm) incision is made through the anesthetized skin to allow for passage of the trocar needle (Fig. 25-5). The trocar is placed through the skin and advanced under fluoroscopy until it comes in contact with the pedicle (Fig. 25-6). The trocar is inserted through the cortex of the bone at the pedicle by controlled malleting. Caution is taken to avoid the medial border of the pedicle until the posterior vertebral body wall has been entered through the pedicle. The trocar is

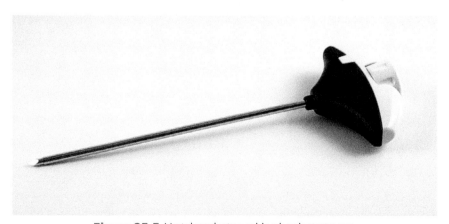

Figure 25-5 Vertebroplasty and kyphoplasty trocar.

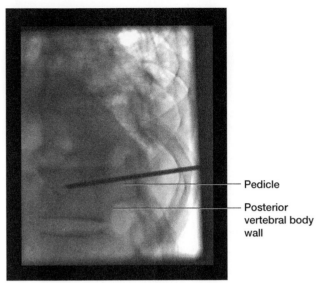

Figure 25-7 Lateral view with trocar advanced into the vertebral body.

then advanced approximately 1 cm past the posterior vertebral body wall. Access to a biplanar fluoroscopy machine, which facilitates simultaneous anteroposterior (AP) and lateral views, is ideal. If a biplanar machine is not available, the fluoroscopy machine needs to be rotated between AP and lateral views. After the trocar is past the spinal canal, it is redirected further medially and advanced to the middle third of the vertebral body in the lateral view (Fig. 25-7). The trocar is removed and the working cannula is left in place. Through the working cannula, a hand drill is placed into the vertebral body (Fig. 25-8). Under fluoroscopic guidance the hand drill is rotated and advanced, creating a channel from the tip of the working cannula toward the anterior cortex. Drilling into the anterior cortex should be avoided. After the channel is made, the hand drill is removed. The same steps are repeated on the contralateral side to place a working cannula, a bipedicular approach (Fig. 25-9). The placement of two cannulas into a single vertebral body decreases the risk of cement leakage.[11] For thoracic spinal fractures, if the vertebral body is small and the needle is placed in the middle, a unilateral approach is all that is needed.

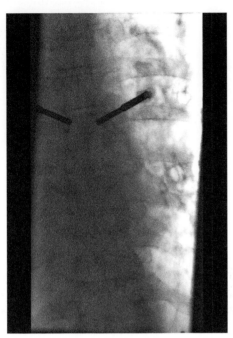

Figure 25-9 Bipedicular approach.

These initial steps are the same for both vertebroplasty and kyphoplasty. An additional step is performed for kyphoplasty: An inflatable balloon catheter is inserted through each of the working cannulae and advanced under fluoroscopic guidance into the channels previously created. There are radiopaque marker bands on the deflated balloon that can be identified with fluoroscopy. The deflated balloon needs to sit fully outside the working cannula so that it can be properly inflated. If the channel is not long enough, the handheld drill needs to be reinserted to create a deeper channel. If there is still not enough room, the working cannula should be gently retracted to create room. A hand pump containing contrast is connected to the balloon catheter (Fig. 25-10). On the

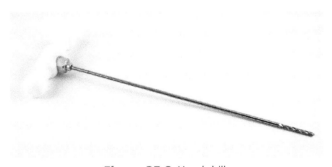

Figure 25-8 Hand drill.

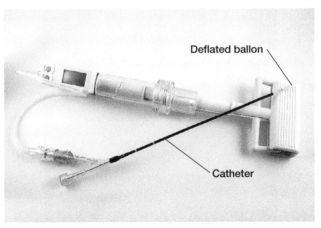

Figure 25-10 The hand pump containing contrast is connected to the balloon catheter.

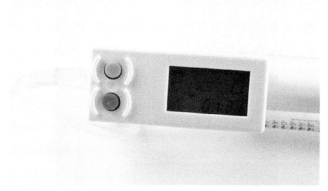

Figure 25-11 Hand pump, indicating milliliters and psi.

pump is a digital readout indicating milliliters injected and pressure (Fig. 25-11). The balloon is slowly inflated sequentially in increments of 0.25 mL of contrast, with careful attention being paid to inflation pressure and balloon position until it reaches 300 psi (Fig. 25-12). At 300 psi, the balloon is deflated by pulling back on the release lever on the hand pump. The balloon catheters are removed. When there is a fracture at more than one level, the identical procedure can be performed at the other levels.

During the balloon inflation step of the procedure, the polymethyl methacrylate bone cement is mixed to toothpaste consistency (usually done by the scrub nurse). For the vertebroplasty technique, bone cement mixing can begin when you are in the latter part of placing your second working cannula. The bone cement is loaded into a medium-sized hollow cannula that can be placed into your larger working

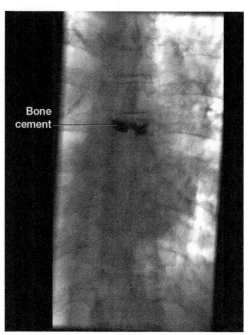

Figure 25-13 Postoperative kyphoplasty films.

cannula. Under fluoroscopic imaging, the bone cement is slowly injected. The cement is made with barium sulfate so that it can be visualized fluoroscopically and its movement can be tracked at all times (Fig. 25-13). The fluoroscope is in the lateral position, which is required when injecting bone cement to ensure that the cement does not violate the posterior one-third of the vertebral body, which contains the spinal cord and central neurostructures. The fluoroscopy monitors are closely watched for any signs of extravasation of bone cement. Bone cement is slowly injected until the core of the vertebral body is filled to roughly 50% to 70% of the residual volume of the compressed vertebra. This is usually 4 to 8 mL for a lumbar vertebra and 2 to 4 mL for a thoracic vertebra. If any bone cement extravagates, the procedure should be discontinued immediately. Once the vertebral body is filled with bone cement, a bone tamp is inserted to clear any cement that may be left in the working cannula or around its edges. The working cannulae are then slowly removed under x-ray guidance. The practitioner watches the monitors to ensure that no cement is dragged out of the vertebral body onto critical structures. If a cement "tail" is seen, the bone tamp should be reinserted to properly clear the working cannula. Once the working cannulae have been removed, the skin is closed typically with Dermabond.

The patient is kept in the prone position for approximately 10 minutes post cement injection then taken to recovery. The patient is monitored in recovery, lying flat for 3 hours. The cement is 90% fixed at 1 hour.

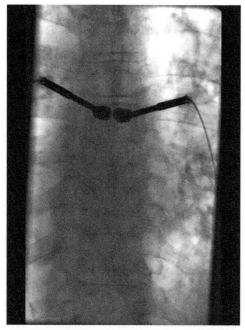

Figure 25-12 Bilateral inflated kyphoplasty balloons.

CONTRAINDICATIONS AND POTENTIAL COMPLICATIONS

Contraindications to vertebroplasty and kyphoplasty are infection, bleeding disorders, or allergies to any of the medications used in the procedures. An additional contraindication is retropulsed fragments into the spinal canal or neuroforamen; injecting cement may push these fragments further toward the spinal cord or nerve roots. Relative contraindications include vertebral collapse to less than one-third the original height and lesion above the fourth thoracic vertebra.

Major complications occur in less than 1% of patients treated for compression fractures secondary to osteoporosis and in less than 5% of treated patients with neoplastic involvement.[2] Rib fractures or pedicle fractures can occur during needle placement. Potential complications include pulmonary venous migration of cement because of the vascularity of the vertebral body.[12] Injection or migration of the cement to any place other than the vertebral body can cause devastating effects, including paraplegia.

In kyphoplasty, a cavity is created within the vertebral body by the inflation of the balloon, allowing for low-pressure cement filling of the cavity. In contrast, in vertebroplasty, the cement is directly injected into the trabecular bone, requiring a higher-pressure injection. A thicker cement is used with kyphoplasty because of the cavity formation. Both the lower pressure and thicker cement combined lead to lower rates of bone cement leakage with kyphoplasty.

CASE STUDY

Case

A 71-year-old woman presents with focal pain in her lower back. The pain, which started while she was lifting a pot out of the oven, began 8 weeks ago. She describes the pain as a constant and deep pain, which has progressively become more intense. It does not radiate into the legs, and she does not have any weakness or bowel/bladder problems. The patient has tried bed rest and both acetaminophen and ibuprofen. Lying flat helps, and activity makes the pain worse. The woman reports never having pain like this before. Her visual analog pain score is an 8 out of 10.

On taking her medical history, you learn that the patient has hypertension and osteoporosis. She denies any weight loss. On examination, the patient has pain over a discrete focal area in her lower thoracic spine. X-ray shows that the patient has a compression fracture of the eighth thoracic vertebra without any retropulsion. Once the compression fracture is confirmed, you decide to obtain an MRI (with STIR images) to better visualize the area. The MRI confirms an osteoporotic compression fracture with 30% loss of height at the eighth thoracic vertebra. There are no retropulsed fragments into the spinal canal or neuroforamen.

After discussing treatment options, you and the patient decide to treat the pain and stabilize the fracture with kyphoplasty. After the procedure, the patient is pain free. A medical regimen is put into place to treat the patient's osteoporosis to help prevent future fractures.

REFERENCES

1. Brunton S, Carmichael B, Gold D, et al. Vertebral compression fractures in primary care: Recommendations from a consensus panel. *J Fam Pract.* 2005;54(9):781–788.
2. McGraw JK, Cardella J, Barr JD, et al. Society of Interventional Radiology quality improvement guidelines for percutaneous vertebroplasty. *J Vasc Interv Radiol.* 2003;14(7):827–831.
3. Garfin SR, Yuan HA, Reiley MA. New technologies in spine: Kyphoplasty and vertebroplasty for the treatment of painful osteoporotic compression fractures. *Spine (Phila Pa 1976).* 2001;26(14):1511–1515.
4. Taylor RS, Taylor RJ, Fritzell P. Balloon kyphoplasty and vertebroplasty for vertebral compression fractures: A comparative systematic review of efficacy and safety. *Spine (Phila Pa 1976).* 2006;31(23):2747–2755.
5. Cotton A, Boutry N, Cortet B, et al. Percutaneous vertebroplasty: State of the art. *Radiographics.* 1998;18:311–320.
6. Gilbert HA, Kagam AR, Nussbaum H, et al. Evaluation of radiation therapy for bone metastases: Pain relief and quality of life. *AJR Am J Roentgenol.* 1977;129:1095–1096.
7. Hiwatashi A, Westesson PL. Vertebroplasty for osteoporotic fractures with spinal canal compromise. *AJNR Am J Neuroradiol.* 2007;28(4):690–692.
8. McGraw JK, Lippert JA, Minkus KD, et al. Prospective evaluation of pain relief in 100 patients undergoing percutaneous vertebroplasty: Results and follow-up. *J Vasc Interv Radiol.* 2002;13(9 Pt 1):883–886.
9. Coumans JV, Reinhardt MK, Lieberman IH. Kyphoplasty for vertebral compression fractures: 1-year clinical outcomes from prospective study. *J Neurosurg.* 2003;99(suppl 1):44–50.
10. Hulme PA, Krebs J, Ferguson SJ, et al. Vertebroplasty and kyphoplasty: A systematic review of 69 clinical studies. *Spine (Phila Pa 1976).* 2006;31(17):1983–2001.
11. Mathis JM, Wong W. Percutaneous vertebroplasty: Technical considerations. *J Vasc Interv Radiol.* 2003;14(8):953–960.
12. Krane SM, Holick MF. Metabolic bone disease. In: Fauci AS, Braunwald E, Isselbacher KJ, eds. *Harrison's Principles of Internal Medicine.* 14th ed. New York, NY: McGraw-Hill; 1998:2247–2259.

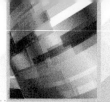

CHAPTER 26

Injections for Headache (Occipital Nerve Blocks and Botulinum Toxin Injections)

WHEN TO USE
▶ Occipital Nerve Block
▶ Botulinum Toxin Injections
   for Headache

HOW TO PERFORM THE PROCEDURES
▶ Occipital Nerve Block
▶ Botulinum Toxin Injections for Headache

CONTRAINDICATIONS AND POTENTIAL COMPLICATIONS

The medical equivalent of epic novels has been written on the comprehensive management of headache. Per the mission of this book, only the basics of two commonly performed procedures used to treat headache will be discussed. These procedures are occipital nerve blocks (ONBs) and botulinum toxin injections. The goal is to add two main procedures to your armamentarium of treating occipital neuralgia and headache.

The greater occipital nerve is composed of sensory fibers that primarily originate from the C2 nerve root and to a lesser extent the C3 nerve root. The greater occipital nerve penetrates the nuchal fascia at the base of the skull. It tracks cephalad to innervate the medial portion of the posterior scalp (Fig. 26-1). The lesser occipital nerve also arises from a branch of the C2 nerve root or may originate from a combination of the

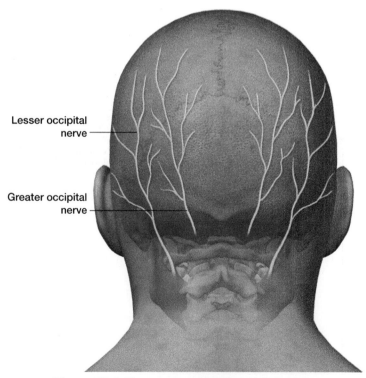

Lesser occipital
nerve

Greater occipital
nerve

Figure 26-1 The greater and lesser occipital nerves.

C2 and C3 nerve roots. It innervates the lateral portion of the posterior scalp and the pinna of the ear. Classically, the description of occipital nerve pain, occipital neuralgia, is a deep or burning pain with shock-like features over the occipital region. Injury to the occipital nerves can occur anywhere along their course from the cervical spinal roots to the tip of the nerve endings.

The trigeminal nucleus (origin of the trigeminal nerve) extends from the brainstem down to the upper cervical cord, where it comes into close approximation with the dorsal horns of the C1 and C2 nerve roots (remember, the occipital nerves originate from the C2 nerve root). This anatomic relationship is known as the trigeminal cervical complex (TCC) (Fig. 26-2). The TCC is thought to receive impulses from both the first division of the trigeminal nerve and nociceptive impulses from the greater occipital nerve.[1–5] Synaptic overlay at the trigeminocervical nucleus may allow for the referral of pain from the occipital nerve to any of the branches of the trigeminal nerve, with a propensity for the retro-orbital region.[5] This is a referred pain. Stimulation of the greater occipital nerve increases excitability of the dural connection to the trigeminocervical nucleus.[2] This explains how occipital neuralgia

can cause pain that reaches beyond the classical distribution of the occipital nerve. It may be that stimulation of the occipital nerve can cause headache mimicking that of a migraine.

Migraine is an episodic neurologic disorder that affects roughly 17% of women and 6% of men. The pain of migraine is thought to be mediated by trigeminal nerve afferents, which provide sensory innervation to the face and intracranial structures such as the dura and the cerebral vasculature (remember, brain tissue has no pain receptors). Although the exact cause is unknown, current hypotheses suggest that activation of the trigeminal nerve triggers a cascade of changes to the brain's dura and vasculature that leads to producing the migraine.

Research in humans has shown that an ONB, while effective for pain along the posterior scalp, may also lead to pain relief outside of the skin territory supplied by the nerve.[6,7] Again, ONBs temporarily reduce afferent nociceptive impulses to the trigeminocervical nucleus. This aberrant stimulation of trigeminal nerve innervated structures ceases, breaking the pain cycle. It has been hypothesized that an ONB leads to a "wind down" of central sensitization of migraine. ONBs are

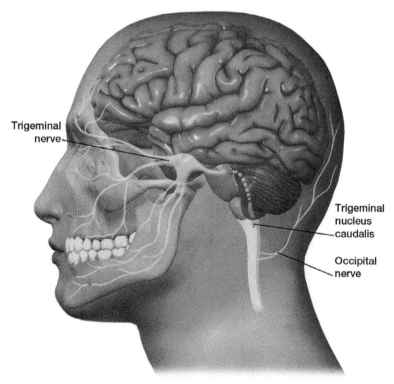

Figure 26-2 The trigeminal nucleus caudalis comes into close approximation with the dorsal horns of the C1 and C2 nerve roots, the C2 nerve root is the origin of the occipital nerves. This anatomical relationship is known as the trigeminal cervical complex (TCC). The TCC is thought to receive impulses from both the first division of the trigeminal nerve and nociceptive impulses from the greater occipital nerve.

also very beneficial for isolated occipital neuralgia when the direct skin territory supplied by the nerve is affected. Often palpating the nerve in the occipital groove elicits the pain. Open-label studies have found that, ONBs are potentially effective for the treatment of migraine, cluster headache, occipital neuralgia, and post-traumatic headache.

Dermatologists and plastic surgeons using botulinum toxin type A (Botox) to minimize hyperfunctional facial lines first reported that it prevented migraine headache. A number of patients receiving the injection for hyperfunctional facial lines indicated that it was also very helpful for their headaches, suggesting a possible association. These observations eventually led to a preliminary open-label study, which concluded that botulinum toxin is a beneficial therapeutic agent for both the acute and prophylactic treatment of migraine.[8] The toxin works by inhibiting the vesicular release of the neurotransmitter acetylcholine (ACh) at the neuromuscular junction, leading to muscle paresis or paralysis (Fig. 26-3).

Investigators originally theorized that botulinum toxin injections helped migraines by relieving muscle spasm and tension, which may be a trigger. A more contemporary understanding of migraine pathophysiology challenges this initial theory. The later theory refutes "muscle tension" as a likely trigger for migraine and observes that the prophylaxis of headache pain appears to outlast the paralysis of muscle in many patients. Also, some patients have reported that botulinum toxin is effective even when injected into areas not supplied by muscle (such as on the apex of the head). In addition, botulinum toxin is beneficial for migraine in acute episodes, taking effect within 1 to 2 hours, whereas muscle paralysis does not take hold for 3 days. Despite reports of improvement during acute attacks, botulinum toxin injections have a more robust body of evidence supporting their use as a prophylactic agent that sometimes improves over subsequent injections. Although the true mechanism by which botulinum toxin injections are effective for migraine prophylaxis is unclear, theories have suggested that they may exert a direct antinociceptive sensory block on trigeminal triggers of migraines.[9]

Additional mechanisms of action for botulinum toxin may involve antivasodilatory and anti-inflammatory properties. The toxin inhibits the release of nociceptive mediators, such as calcitonin gene-related peptide, substance P, and glutamate from peripheral termini of primary afferent nerves. By blocking the release of these neurotransmitters, the toxin blocks neurogenic inflammation, which in turn inhibits peripheral pain signals to the central nervous system. Clinical studies have reinforced its effectiveness. In a large randomized, double-blind, placebo-controlled trial of botulinum toxin A (PREEMPT), 1,384 patients with chronic migraine showed a significant reduction in headache days, improvement in functioning, and less disability as compared with placebo.[9]

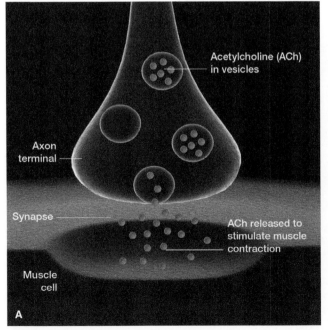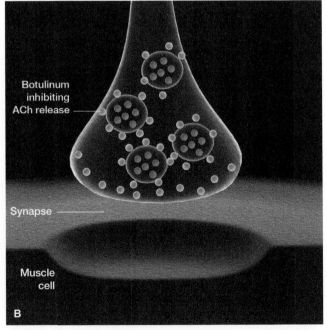

Figure 26-3 Botulinum toxin inhibiting the vesicular release of the neurotransmitter acetylcholine (ACh) at the neuromuscular junction. Its method of action for headache treatment seems to be unrelated to its muscle paralysis properties.

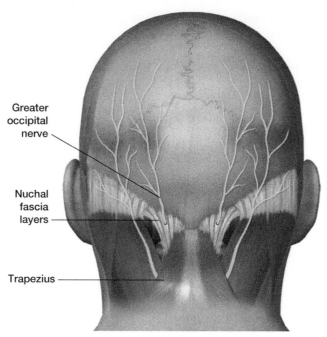

Figure 26-4 The greater occipital nerve lies at the base of the skull between the nuchal fascia layers and the trapezius muscle. The nerve is prone to flexion/extension injuries, as well as entrapment by spasm of the trapezius.

TABLE 26-1 The Three Primary Headache Types

Primary Headache Type	Description
Migraine	Headache lasting 4–72 h that has at least two of the following characteristics: Unilateral, pulsating, moderate to severe intensity, aggravated by physical activity. In addition, nausea or vomiting and/or photophobia and phonophobia should accompany it, and an aura may also precede it.
Cluster	Unilateral headache lasting 15–180 min with a periodicity of one every other day to eight per day that has one or more of the following characteristics: Conjunctival injection, lacrimation, nasal congestion, rhinorrhea, forehead and facial sweating, miosis, ptosis, and eyelid edema.
Tension	Muscle contraction headache, usually holocephalic.

WHEN TO USE

Occipital Nerve Block

ONBs are traditionally used in the treatment of occipital neuralgia, which may develop idiopathically or may be caused by trauma. The condition may involve unilateral or bilateral occipital nerves. The greater occipital nerve lies at the base of the skull between the nuchal fascia layers, as previously mentioned. Therefore, it is prone to trauma from flexion/extension injuries, as well as entrapment by spasm of the trapezius muscle (Fig. 26-4). If the head turns on impact, the injury may involve only one of the greater occipital nerves and may result in unilateral, rather than bilateral, symptoms.

ONBs may also be useful in both acute and prophylactic treatment of various primary headache disorders, including migraine, tension headache, and cluster headache. Table 26-1 provides a classic description of each of the three primary headaches.

Botulinum Toxin Injections for Headache

The US Food and Drug Administration (FDA) approved botulinum toxin type A, or Botox, in 2010 for headache prophylaxis in patients with adult chronic migraine who suffer headaches on 15 or more days per month, each lasting more than 4 hours. Botulinum toxin injections remain a very good option for the prophylaxis of migraine in patients who do not respond to other prophylactic medication therapy or simply do not want to take pills.

HOW TO PERFORM THE PROCEDURES

Occipital Nerve Block

An ONB is a safe and uncomplicated procedure that can be performed in an office setting. There is no standard protocol for this nerve block. A stepwise description of a commonly used protocol follows. The patient sits with the cervical spine flexed forward. Standing in back of the patient, the superior–lateral aspect of the occipital protuberance is palpated. From there the target site is 2 fingerbreadths laterally toward the side of pain or bilaterally if both sides are affected (Fig. 26-5). This is just medial to the occipital artery. Using a felt-tip marking pen, place an "X" on the skin at the intended target. The skin is prepped vigorously with alcohol. A 5-mL syringe should be filled with a mixture of a local anesthetic and steroid; an 18-gauge needle is used to draw up the medication. I use a mixture of 1 mL of 0.25% bupivacaine, 1 mL of 1% lidocaine, and 20 mg of Kenalog as my therapeutic agent. If bilateral injections are needed, 2 mL of 0.25% bupivacaine, 2 mL of 1% lidocaine, and 40 mg of Kenalog are drawn up into the same syringe and divided equally on both the left and right sides. After the medications are drawn up, the 18-gauge needle is removed from the syringe and a 1.5-in, 25-gauge needle is attached. The needle is then placed through the "X" marked on the skin at a very shallow angle, roughly 75 degrees pointing superiorly. The needle is advanced toward the target until its tip touches the periosteum of the

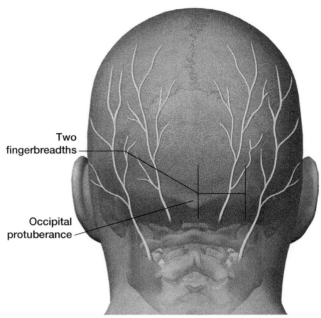

Figure 26-5 Target site for an occipital nerve block (ONB) is 2 fingerbreadths lateral to the occipital protuberance toward the side of pain.

underlying occipital bone. This is very superficial. The needle is then withdrawn 1 mm. After negative aspiration the therapeutic agent is injected, varying the needle angle in a fan-like motion (Fig. 26-6). The needle angle must be very shallow and directed laterally to involve the lesser occipital nerve and a number of superficial branches of the greater occipital nerve. Care should be taken to avoid medial injection toward the foramen magnum, which is the area of the cervical

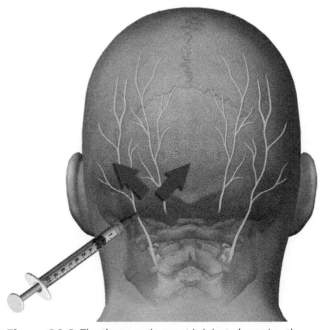

Figure 26-6 The therapeutic agent is injected, varying the needle angle in a fan-like motion.

cord and entrance to the brainstem. The needle is then withdrawn and pressure applied to the area.

Botulinum Toxin Injections for Headache

Botox (a common, commercially available form of botulinum toxin) is available in 200- and 100-unit vials. The recommended dose for treating migraine is 155 units, but in clinical practice anywhere between 100 and 200 units is used. The medication comes in a white powder contained in a sterile, vacuum-dried vial. To create an injectable solution it is necessary to add preservative-free 0.9% saline to the powder.

Using an 18-gauge needle, fill a 5-mL syringe with 4 mL of saline. Then puncture the latex vacuum-sealed, 200-unit Botox vial, which contains only the Botox powder. Allow the saline to be pulled into the vacuum-sealed, 200-mg Botox vial. Gently mix the Botox with the saline by rotating the vial so that the Botox powder fully dissolves. The solution should be clear, colorless, and free of particulate matter. Draw out your original 4 mL of volume back into the 5-mL syringe. Remove the 18-gauge needle and attach a 1-in, 30-gauge needle to your 5-mL syringe. In the resulting dilution, each 0.1 mL contains 5 units of Botox. Each injection will be 0.1 mL of solution (5 units of Botox), for a total of 31 small injections equaling 155 units (Table 26-2). In clinical practice, it is understood that each of your injections is not going to be exactly 0.1 mL of solution. Some practitioners will further divide the 4 mL of solution created into 0.5-mL syringes, each containing 25 units.

The effect of botulinum toxin type A on muscle strength depends on the volume injected, the size of the muscle, and individual patient variation. In general, 5 units are used for wrinkle lines, 25 to 50 units

TABLE 26-2 Botox Areas of Injection and Recommended Doses

Area	Recommended Dose
Frontalis (glabellar region)	20 units, divided into four sites
Corrugator	10 units, divided into two sites, one on each side
Procerus	5 units into one site
Temporalis	40 units, divided into eight sites, four on each side
Occipitalis	30 units, divided into six sites, three on each side
Cervical paraspinal muscle groups	20 units, divided into four sites, two on each side
Trapezius	30 units, divided into six sites, three on each side
Total dose	155 units, 31 sites

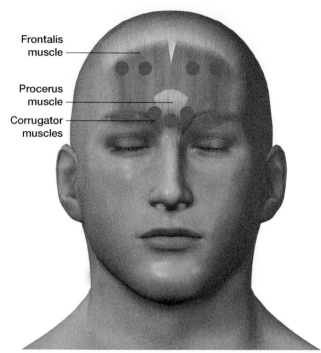

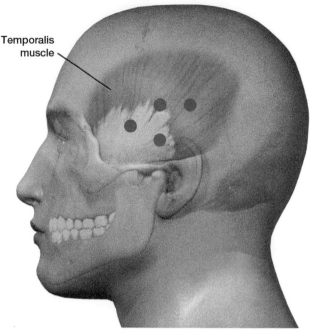

Figure 26-7 Four injections along the frontalis wrinkle line. One injection into each corrugator muscle. One injection into the procerus muscle.

Figure 26-8 Four injections into each temporalis muscle: Two injections where the hairline meets the scalp and two injections about an inch above the ear.

for smaller muscles, and 50 to 100 units for larger muscles. For example, a patient with cervical dystonia may require 200 units for paresis. The volume used for Botox injections for migraines is well below the volume needed to paralyze muscles like the trapezius, one of the muscles injected for the migraine Botox protocol, which receives only 15 units.

Insert the needle into the muscle with the bevel up, at approximately a 5-degree angle. The injection sites are as follows.

Frontalis (glabellar region): Four injections, each one along a frontalis wrinkle line for a total of 20 units (Fig. 26-7). The injections are made along a horizontal line, with the needle entering parallel to the wrinkle line and equally spread out.

Corrugator: A small pyramid muscle at the medial end of each eyebrow. The corrugator muscle draws the eyebrow medial and downward, producing vertical wrinkle lines. Each corrugator gets one injection of 5 units, for a grand total of 10 units (Fig. 26-7).

Procerus: A small pyramid muscle directly above the bridge of the nose. The muscle gets one injection containing 5 units (Fig. 26-7).

Temporalis: Two injections are done side by side where the hairline meets the scalp and two sites are located about an inch above the ear (Fig. 26-8), for a total of 20 units on one side. The same sites are repeated on the opposite side of the body, for a grand total of 40 units. To bring out this muscle, ask the patient to simulate chewing.

Occipitalis: Just lateral to the occipital groove, two sites are injected about 1 cm from each other, then one site just below these two sites to form what would look like a downward triangle. All of these sites receive a total of 15 units (Fig. 26-9). The same sites are injected on the opposite side for a grand total of 30 units.

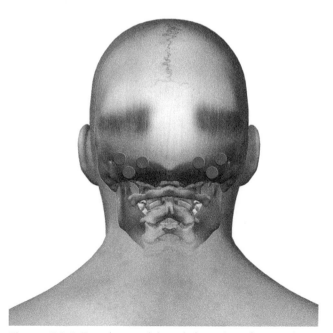

Figure 26-9 Two sites are injected about 1 cm from each other just lateral to the occipital grove and then a third just below to form a downward triangle.

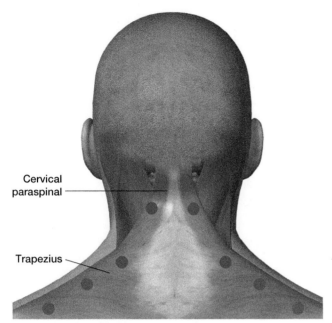

Figure 26-10 Two sites are injected for both the left and right cervical paraspinal muscles. Three equally spaced sites are injected along each trapezius.

Cervical paraspinal muscles: Two sites are injected for both the left and right cervical paraspinal muscles, for a grand total of 20 units (Fig. 26-10).

Trapezius: Three equally spaced sites are injected along the trapezius, which receives a total of 15 units. The same sites are repeated on the trapezius of the opposite side of the body, for a grand total of 30 units (Fig. 26-10).

The frontalis–glabellar region (Fig. 26-7) may be the best site for achieving the maximal therapeutic effect. Injection intervals are typically every 3 months. Many physicians will do an injection every 3 months for 1 year, then stagger the injections at greater intervals based on individual clinical response.

CONTRAINDICATIONS AND POTENTIAL COMPLICATIONS

Contraindications to both injections include systemic infection and infection of the skin where the needle is inserted.

Postblock ecchymosis is common after ONB. Manual pressure applied to the area immediately postblock decreases this. Postprocedure soreness is another frequent experience. It is critically important to keep the needle lateral to the occipital protuberance and just above bone to avoid improper needle placement.

Practice has shown that botulinum toxin injections are effective, safe, and well tolerated. The most common adverse events reported by patients treated with botulinum toxin injections for chronic migraine were neck pain and headache. A total of 1% of patients treated with botulinum toxin injections reported severe worsening of their headache compared with 0.3% of patients receiving placebo.[9] Individuals with known hypersensitivity to botulinum toxin should not receive it. It is recommended that pregnant women not receive botulinum toxin.

CASE STUDIES

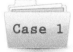

Case 1 A 26-year-old woman is seeing you for migraine. She has a strong family history of migraine; her mother and one of her sisters have migraines with similar symptoms. The woman herself has had significant headaches since the age of 14. They occur more than 15 times a month. They affect either side of her head; the pain is pulsating with an intensity that ranges from moderate to severe. The woman reports having tried "every medication." She is currently taking Topamax daily and uses Imitrex for abortive therapy when the headache becomes severe. She also takes Percocet 5/325 when the pain becomes very intense.

To decrease the severity and number of headache days, you offer the patient Botox injections for her chronic migraines. Her first response is, "Like the kind used for wrinkles?" You explain how dermatologists and plastic surgeons first discovered Botox to be helpful for migraine—that their patients with headaches kept coming back after they had Botox injections for hyperfunctional facial lines asking if there was a connection between the injection and improvement of their headache symptoms. You tell the patient that follow-up clinical research allowed the FDA to approve Botox injections for chronic migraine. You and the patient decide to proceed with a round of Botox injections into the designated sites to see if this helps her headaches. The patient follows up at 3 months and reports that although she still has migraines, the headaches are no longer as frequent or severe.

Case 2

A 37-year-old woman presents with a chief complaint of headache. She says that her headaches started about a year ago but have become more severe over the past 3 months. The patient believes she now has migraine headaches. The headaches always start on the right side. Photophobia and phonophobia may accompany them, but she denies any nausea or vomiting. There is no family history of headaches and no association with the menstrual cycle. In an attempt to alleviate the pain, she applies ice or heat to the back of her head.

On examination, she has tenderness along the path of the greater occipital nerve on the right side. The rest of the patient's neurologic examination is normal. After reviewing the diagnosis of occipital neuralgia with the patient, you talk about treatment options. You offer a neuropathic pain medication such as Lyrica (pregabalin) or Cymbalta (duloxetine hydrochloride) as well as a procedure such as an ONB. The patient asks how long she would have to take the medication if that is the treatment plan she chooses. You explain that you would probably keep her on the medication for at least 3 months to see how effective it is. The patient decides to have the nerve block rather than medication management.

REFERENCES

1. Bogduk N. Cervicogenic headache: Anatomic basis and pathophysiologic mechanisms. *Curr Pain Headache Rep.* 2001;5:382–386.
2. Bartsch T, Goadsby PJ. Stimulation of the greater occipital nerve induces increased central excitability of dural afferent input. *Brain.* 2002;125:1496–1509.
3. Bartsch T, Goadsby PJ. Increased responses in trigeminocervical nociceptive neurons to cervical input after stimulation of the dura mater. *Brain.* 2003;126(Pt 8):1801–1813.
4. Goadsby PJ, Bartsch T. On the functional neuroanatomy of neck pain. *Cephalalgia.* 2008;28(suppl 1):1–7.
5. Kerr FWL. Structural relationship of the trigeminal spinal tract to upper cervical roots in the solitary nucleus in the cat. *Exp Neurol.* 1981;4:134–148.
6. Caputi CA, Firetto V. Therapeutic blockade of greater occipital and supraorbital nerves in migraine patients. *Headache.* 1997;37(3):174–179.
7. Peres MF, Stiles MA, Siow HC, et al. Greater occipital nerve blockade for cluster headache. *Cephalalgia.* 2002;22(7):520–522.
8. Binder WJ, Brin MF, Blitzer A, et al. Botulinum toxin type A (BOTOX) for treatment of migraine headaches: An open-label study. *Otolaryngol Head Neck Surg.* 2000;123(6):669–676.
9. Aurora SK, Dodick DW, Turkel CC, et al. OnabotulinumtoxinA for treatment of chronic migraine: Results from the double-blind, randomized, placebo-controlled phase of the PREEMPT 1 trial. *Cephalalgia.* 2010;30(7):793–803.

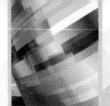

CHAPTER 27

Common Nerve Blocks

Nerves send sensory impulses to the brain for interpretation. These impulses travel in a regular pattern when the nervous system is working correctly. When a nerve is injured, this normally controlled transmission of neurologic impulses fails and the nerve fires aberrantly. This aberrant firing is interpreted by the brain as neuropathic pain. Injured nerves also develop an increased sensitivity to routine triggers such as mechanical, thermal, and chemical stimuli thus, not only are damaged nerves sending aberrant impulses interpreted as pain, but also there is an amplification of their activity in response to everyday triggers.

Many people mistakenly think of the term *nerve block* as a permanent block of a nerve's function. In clinical practice destruction of the nerve rarely occurs—rather, it is bathed in a local anesthetic solution that eventually wears off. For unknown reasons, pain relief via a nerve block can last longer than the life of the anesthetic injected. Nerve fibers sending pathological painful impulses to the central nervous system (CNS) become "trained" at aberrant transmission, in the same way that an athlete's muscles become highly trained at performing a task. The intensity and persistence of the pathologic signal is over and above what are appropriate functional levels. In addition, the CNS becomes trained at receiving these painful impulses; this is known as neuroplasticity. Neuroplasticity is the CNS ability to reorganize itself by forming new neural connections in response to new situations or to changes in their environment. Neuroplasticity takes place at both the transmitting and receiving ends, creating a powerful pathologic connection. This maladaptive pain signal can be broken with a nerve block. The block allows the continuous pain feedback loop to be broken, allowing the body to reset itself. The way that I explain this to my patients is that pain is transmitted along the neurologic system, similar to an electrical system. Like any electrical system, things can go haywire. So if an electrical gadget—such as your computer or phone—is not working properly, what is the first thing you do to try to fix it? You turn off and on the power. When the power comes back on, more often than not things return to normal. That is what we are trying to achieve with the nerve block; we are rebooting the system. Before the injection it is essential to discuss with patients; realistic expectations. Nerve blocks do not always provide prolonged pain relief and may need to be repeated to achieve maximal benefit.

In clinical practice, practitioners often add a steroid to the local anesthetic. The steroid suppresses the targeted nerve's response to inflammatory factors. This inflammatory response can aggravate a nerve, changing its normal firing pattern. Steroids also exert a membrane-stabilizing effect on injured nerve segments, reducing ectopic discharges from the affected nerve (Fig. 27-1).[1,2] The concentrated steroid dose delivered by needle directly to the level of pathology is in much lower quantities than would be needed via oral or intravenous administration.

In most nerve blocks a local anesthetics and steroid are used in combination. The local anesthetic is mixed in the same syringe as the corticosteroid solution. The primary corticosteroids on the market are listed in Table 27-1. There is no one particular steroid and local anesthetic combination that is a consensus choice. I use Kenalog, which is featured in the examples to follow. But if you decide to use Depo-Medrol or any other steroid, proper doses can easily be calculated: For

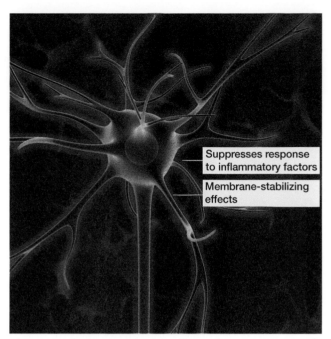

Figure 27-1 The physiological effects of steroids on injured nerves.

TABLE 27-1 Primary Corticosteroids for and Equivalent Doses

Trade Name	Generic Name	Equivalent Dose (mg)
Kenalog	Triamcinolone acetonide	40 (reference)
Depo-Medrol	Methylprednisolone acetate	40
Celestone	Betamethasone acetate	6
Decadron	Dexamethasone acetate	8

example, 40 mg of Kenalog is equivalent to 6 mg of Celestone (Table 27-1).

There are primarily two types of local anesthetics used for nerve blocks—lidocaine and bupivacaine—which both work by blocking fast voltage-gated sodium channels (Fig. 27-2). This prevents neuronal depolarization, blocking the painful nerve impulses that are sent to the brain. Dosages of 1% lidocaine and 0.25% bupivacaine are equivalent to each other,

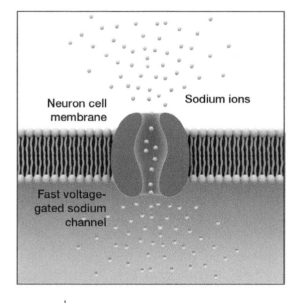

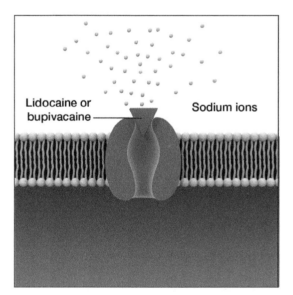

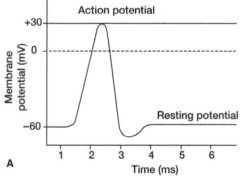

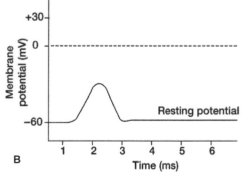

Figure 27-2 Lidocaine and bupivicaine block fast voltage-gated sodium channels, preventing neuronal depolarization. This blocks the transmission of pain. **A.** Sodium channel triggered action potential. **B.** Sodium channel action potential being inhibited by a local anesthetic.

TABLE 27-2 Lidocaine Versus Bupivacaine Onset and Duration of Action

Local Anesthetic	Onset of Action	Duration of Action (h)
Lidocaine 1%	45–90 s	1–2
Bupivacaine 0.25%	1–5 min	2–6

but differ in their time of onset and length of duration (Table 27-2).

WHEN TO USE

Peripheral nerve blocks can be extremely useful in providing pain relief. In some cases, a nerve block alone can provide significant relief. In other cases, a nerve block may allow a patient to fully participate in physical therapy, a key component of pain relief. Physical therapy, which may have been limited previously by intense levels of pain, now becomes a method of treatment.

Peripheral nerve blocks can also be diagnostic, helping to localize the pain generator—for example, if it is unclear if pain in the chest wall is coming from the intercostal nerves or deeper visceral structures. A diagnostic intercostal nerve block can help resolve this question.

HOW TO PERFORM THE PROCEDURE

The procedure is fully explained to the patient, all questions answered, and informed consent obtained. A "time out" is performed prior to the procedure including verbal confirmation of correct patient, procedure and procedural site.

Trigeminal Nerve Block: Ophthalmic (V1), Maxillary (V2), and Mandibular (V3) Branches

The trigeminal nerve is the fifth cranial nerve, responsible for sensory impulses originating from the face above the jaw line to the forehead. The trigeminal nerve has three branches: Ophthalmic (V1), maxillary (V2), and mandibular (V3) (Fig. 27-3). The ophthalmic, maxillary, and mandibular branches all originate from the base of the trigeminal nerve, the gasserian ganglion (Fig. 27-4). The pain of trigeminal neuralgia is most common in the maxillary (V2) and mandibular (V3) distributions. This sharp, electric pain radiates deep into the cheek, lips, and tongue, typically on one side of the face. It is described as brief episodes of stabbing and shock-like pain. Exacerbations often come in clusters, with complete remission between attacks.

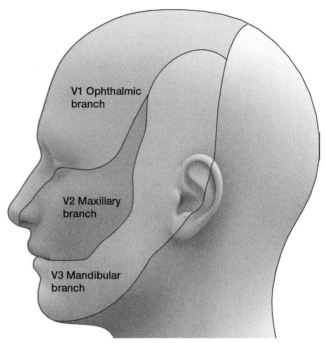

Figure 27-3 The trigeminal nerve has three divisions: Ophthalmic (V1), maxillary (V2), and mandibular (V3).

Rather than blocking the trigeminal (gasserian) ganglion, usually the branches of the trigeminal nerve that correlates to the patient's pain are blocked. A trigeminal (gasserian) block is technically challenging and carries substantial risk.[3,4] Remember, pain is most common in the maxillary (V2) and mandibular (V3) distributions of the trigeminal nerve in trigeminal neuralgia, thus often only these two branches need to be blocked. These nerve blocks may also be useful for atypical facial pain as well as pain generated by oral/facial cancer.

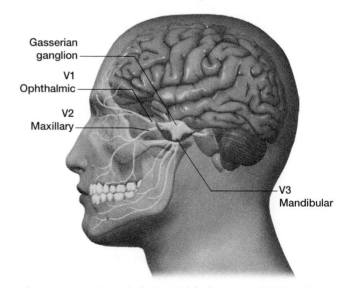

Figure 27-4 Trigeminal nerve with the anatomical locations of each branch.

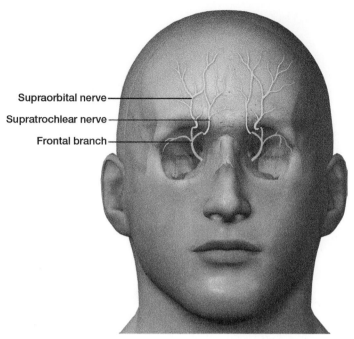

Figure 27-5 Frontal branch, a division of V1, dividing into the supraorbital and supratrochlear nerves. The supraorbital nerve supplies sensory innervation to the upper eyelid, forehead, and scalp. The supratrochlear nerve supplies sensory innervations to the upper nose and sends branches to the conjunctivae and the upper eyelid.

Trigeminal Nerve Block: Ophthalmic (V1) Branch: In clinical practice, branches of the ophthalmic (V1) branch of the trigeminal nerve are blocked, rather than the whole nerve, to treat pain around the eyes and nose. The ophthalmic nerve (the first division of the trigeminal nerve) splits into the lacrimal, frontal, and nasociliary branches. The frontal branch further divides into the supraorbital and supratrochlear nerves (Fig. 27-5). The supraorbital and supratrochlear nerves are the target of interest in an upper facial nerve block. The supraorbital nerve supplies sensory innervation to the upper eyelid, forehead, and scalp. The supratrochlear nerve supplies sensory innervations to the upper nose and sends branches to the conjunctivae and the upper eyelid.

Supraorbital and supratrochlear nerve block: The patient is placed in the supine position (face up). The primary landmark will be the bone of the superior orbit, in particular the supraorbital notch. The skin is then prepped with alcohol. A 3-mL syringe is filled with a mixture of a local anesthetic and a steroid; an 18-gauge needle is used to draw up the medication. I use a mixture of 2.5 mL of 0.25% bupivacaine and 20 mg of Kenalog as my therapeutic agent divided equally between the supraorbital and supratrochlear nerves. The 18-gauge needle is removed from the syringe once the medications have been drawn up, and a 1.5-in, 25-gauge needle is placed.

Push the eyebrow superiorly with your nondominant hand, which helps you to palpate the groove of the supraorbital notch, the site of the supraorbital nerve (Fig. 27-6). Using a felt-tip pen, place an "X" on the skin over the supraorbital notch. The needle is then placed through the "X," aiming at the bone. The needle is advanced till bone is felt, which should be at

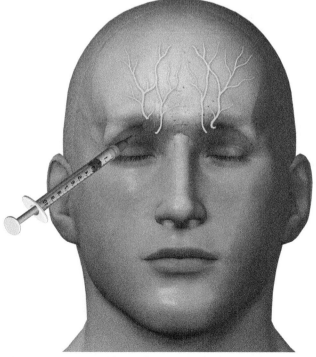

Figure 27-6 Nerve block of the supraorbital nerve at the supraorbital foramen.

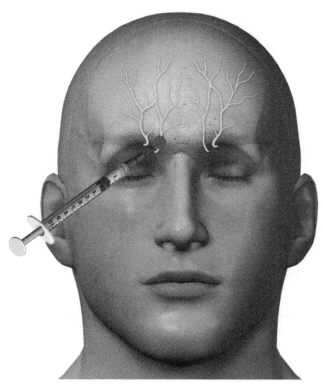

Figure 27-7 Nerve block of the supratrochlear nerve.

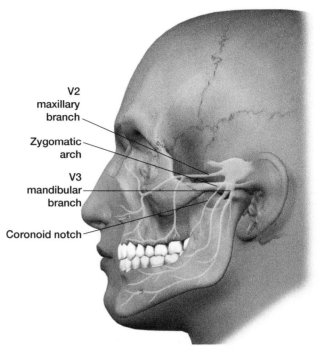

Figure 27-8 Coronoid notch view of the maxillary (V2) and mandibular (V3) branches of the trigeminal nerve. The coronoid notch approach can be used to block both the maxillary (V2) and mandibular (V3) branches of the trigeminal nerve.

a very shallow depth. The needle is withdrawn 1 mm after bone contact. The patient is instructed to verbalize any dysesthesias during the injection to prevent injection into the nerve itself. If dysesthesias are felt, the needle is repositioned prior to injection. After negative aspiration, the therapeutic agent is injected—in this case, 1.5 mL of your mixed local anesthetic and steroid solution.

The supratrochlear nerve can be accessed by redirecting the needle to the upper medial aspect of the superior orbital bone. This site is just lateral to the base of the nose (Fig. 27-7). By using a single entry site to block both nerves, the procedure is both more efficient and more comfortable for the patient. The same steps are performed as just described regarding injection of the therapeutic agent after negative aspiration. The needle is withdrawn and a bandage placed if needed.

Trigeminal Nerve Block: Maxillary (V2) and Mandibular (V3) Branches: The coronoid notch approach can be used to block both the maxillary (V2) and mandibular (V3) branches of the trigeminal nerve (Fig. 27-8). The patient is positioned on the fluoroscopic table in a supine position (face up). There is a slight groove under the zygomatic arch, the coronoid notch, which is your entry point. This can be located by palpation. After the notch is identified, the patient is asked to hold the mouth slightly open. Using a felt-tip marking pen, place an "X" just inferior to

the zygomatic arch (Fig. 27-9). The painful side of the face is draped and prepped in standard sterile fashion. The skin at the "X" is infiltrated with 2 to 3 mL of 2% lidocaine; use a 25-gauge needle to provide comfort during the procedure. The local anesthetic can be

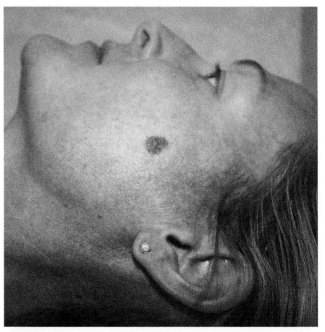

Figure 27-9 "X" on the skin showing needle entry site for a maxillary (V2) and mandibular (V3) nerve block, the coronoid notch approach.

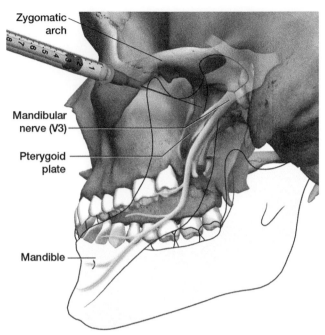

Figure 27-10 Needle touching the lateral pterygoid plate, the site of the mandibular nerve (V3).

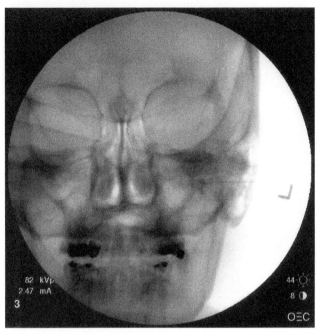

Figure 27-11 Proper contrast spread of trigeminal nerve block, V2 & V3 divisions.

drawn up with an 18-gauge needle before switching to a 25-gauge needle.

The fluoroscope is placed in the anteroposterior position. A 22-gauge, 2.5-in needle is advanced under fluoroscopy through the "X" in a perpendicular plane to the entry point on the skin till it comes in contact with the pterygoid plate, usually around 1.5 in deep (Fig. 27-10). This is the site of the mandibular nerve. After bone contact is made, the needle is withdrawn 1 to 2 mm. A 3-mL syringe with tubing containing contrast is connected to the needle. Tubing is used to enable you to see the contrast without having your hand obscure the image and protects your hand from radiation exposure. Inject the contrast, making sure it spreads properly (Fig. 27-11). Once proper contrast spread is seen, the 3-mL syringe containing the contrast is disconnected from the tubing. A 10-mL syringe with the therapeutic agent is connected to the tubing. I use a mixture of 2 mL of 0.25% bupivacaine and 20 mg of Kenalog as my therapeutic agent per division of the trigeminal nerve. Thus, if you are blocking both the maxillary (V2) and mandibular (V3) divisions, you would draw up 4 mL of 0.25% bupivacaine and 40 mg of Kenalog, dividing them equally over both nerves. The therapeutic agent is best drawn up before the procedure is started and placed on the sterile field, ready to go when needed. After negative aspiration, the therapeutic agent is then injected on to the mandibular nerve.

By redirecting the needle slightly anteriorly and superiorly from the pterygoid plate, the maxillary nerve (V2) can be found (Fig. 27-12). This is accomplished by "walking off" the pterygoid plate with the needle.

The term "walking off" refers to the action of tapping a needle against a bony structure as you move along it to determine where the edge is located. The maxillary nerve (V2) is roughly just superior and 1 cm past the pterygoid plate. After proper needle placement the same steps are performed as described previously regarding injection of the therapeutic agent after

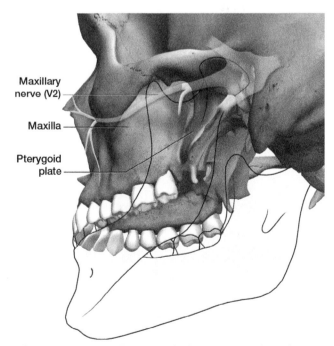

Figure 27-12 Maxillary nerve (V2) in relation to lateral pterygoid plate.

negative aspiration. The needle is withdrawn and a bandage placed if needed. Proper needle placement is of utmost importance—if the needle is advanced too far, it could enter the orbit. This can be closely monitored under fluoroscopy and easily prevented.

Median Nerve Block

Carpal tunnel syndrome (CTS) is one of the most common causes of pain in the hands. CTS may be unilateral or bilateral. It is caused by compression of the median nerve under the transverse carpal ligament (Fig. 27-13). It leads to an irritable electric sensation in the distribution of the median nerve. CTS presents with paresthesia, described as a painful electrical sensation in the palm, thumb, index, middle and part of the ring finger (Fig. 27-14). Upon waking, your patient may feel as if the hand is asleep; people tend to sleep with their wrist flexed, applying pressure to the median nerve for hours. In severe cases, it may lead to atrophy of the thenar eminence (muscle at the base of the thumb). Around 25% of patients will have long-term relief of their symptoms following a median nerve block for CTS.[5]

The patient is seated. The symptomatic hand should be placed on a table, palm up, and a chuck or towel placed under the wrist. Standing just lateral to the painful

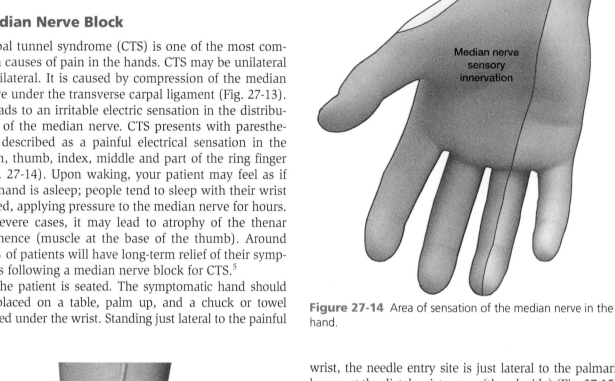

Figure 27-14 Area of sensation of the median nerve in the hand.

wrist, the needle entry site is just lateral to the palmaris longus at the distal wrist crease (thumb side) (Fig. 27-15). To aid in identification of the palmaris longus tendon, have the patient make a fist and simultaneously flex the

Figure 27-13 Carpal tunnel syndrome: Compression of the median nerve under the transverse carpal ligament (flexor retinaculum).

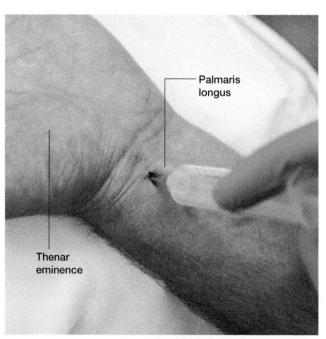

Figure 27-15 Anatomic entry point for a median nerve block. Needle entry is just lateral to the palmaris longus at the distal wrist crease (thumb side).

wrist. Using a felt-tip pen, place an "X" on the wrist at the skin entry site. The skin is prepped with alcohol. A 3-mL syringe is filled with a mixture of local anesthetic and steroid; an 18-gauge needle is used to draw up the medication. I use a mixture of 1.5 mL of 1% lidocaine and 20 mg of Kenalog as my therapeutic agent. The 18-gauge needle is removed once the medications have been drawn up, and a 1.5-in, 25-gauge needle is attached. The needle is placed at a 45-degree angle through the "X" that was placed on the skin. The needle is slowly advanced until the tip is just beyond the tendon. The patient is instructed to verbalize any dysesthesias during the procedure to prevent injection into the nerve itself. If dysesthesias are felt, the needle is repositioned prior to injection. After negative aspiration, the therapeutic agent is injected. The needle is withdrawn and a bandage placed if needed.

Suprascapular Nerve Block

The origin of the suprascapular nerve is the C5 and C6 nerve roots. After the C5 and C6 nerve roots come together to form the suprascapular nerve, the nerve passes inferiorly and posteriorly from the brachial plexus to the suprascapular notch (Fig. 27-16). It provides motor innervations to the supraspinatus and infraspinatus muscles. These muscles abduct the arm at the shoulder joint, functioning primarily during the first 10 to 15 degrees of movement. They provide sensory innervation to part of the shoulder joint and surrounding soft tissue. Suprascapular nerve blocks can be very helpful in alleviating shoulder pain.[6] The block allows for greater range of motion of the shoulder joint.

Suprascapular nerve blocks play a particularly interesting role in treatment of adhesive capsulitis, that is, frozen shoulder. This condition develops after a shoulder is injured or immobilized for an extended period of time. It is more common in people with diabetes, affecting 10% to 15% of people with the disease. In this condition, abnormal bands of fibrous tissue grow between the joint surfaces. Synovial fluid, which lubricates the joint, is lacking. Restricted range of motion and pain is characteristic. Arthrography shows diminished joint volume.

A suprascapular nerve block is a mainstay of interventional pain treatment for adhesive capsulitis (frozen shoulder) because there is little or no space to do an intra-articular shoulder injection. Physical therapy, which may have been limited previously by intense levels of pain, can now be used as a tool to regain shoulder function. This block is also good for suprascapular nerve entrapment. The nerve provides sensation to some parts of the shoulder ligaments, bursa, acromioclavicular joint, and sometimes skin of the upper arm. Suprascapular nerve entrapment occurs with compression by either the suprascapular ligament or a cyst (arising from the shoulder joint), which results in paralysis of the supraspinatus and infraspinatus. Suprascapular nerve entrapment is suspected if there is pain in the posterior aspect of the shoulder or weakness on abduction and/or external rotation.

To perform this procedure the patient lies on the fluoroscopic table in a prone position (face down). Drape the upper back on the side of the painful shoulder and prep it in standard sterile fashion. The fluoroscope is brought in to the anteroposterior position and the suprascapular notch brought into focus (Fig. 27-17).

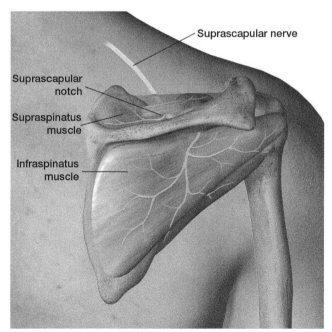

Figure 27-16 The suprascapular nerve at the suprascapular notch.

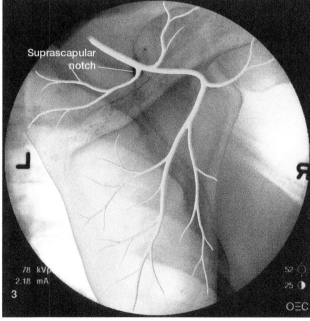

Figure 27-17 Fluoroscopic view of the suprascapular notch.

Using a sterile felt-tip marking pen, an "X" is placed at the scapula just below the notch. The skin at the "X" is infiltrated with 4 to 5 mL of 2% lidocaine, using a 25-gauge, 1.5-in needle to provide comfort during the procedure.

A 22-gauge, 3.5-in needle with a slight bend at the tip (the physician will typically slightly bend the end to help with steering) is then advanced under fluoroscopy through the "X" in a perpendicular plane to the skin and a parallel plane to the fluoroscope. The needle is advanced until it comes in contact with the scapula. After bone contact is made, the needle is gently "walked off" the scapula superiorly into the notch. The term "walking off" refers to the action of tapping a needle against a bony structure as you move along it to determine where the edge is located. The stylet of the needle is removed. A 3-mL syringe with tubing containing contrast is connected to the needle. Tubing is used to enable you to see the contrast being injected under live x-ray without having your hand obscure the image and protect your hand from direct radiation exposure. Inject the contrast, making sure it spreads properly (Fig. 27-18). Once proper contrast spread is seen, the 3-mL syringe containing contrast is disconnected from the tubing. A 10-mL syringe is filled with the therapeutic agent, a mixture of local anesthetic and steroid; an 18-gauge needle is used to draw up the medication. I use a mixture of 8 mL of 0.25% bupivacaine and 40 mg of Kenalog as my therapeutic agent. The therapeutic agent is best drawn up before the procedure is started and placed on the sterile field, ready to go when needed. The 10-mL syringe with the therapeutic agent is then connected to the tubing. After negative aspiration, the medication is injected. The needle is withdrawn and a bandage placed if needed.

Intercostal Nerve Block

The intercostal nerves originate from each of the 12 thoracic nerve roots. They branch anteriorly along the undersurface of each rib, providing sensory innervation to the chest (Fig. 27-19). It is traditionally taught that just under the ribs in the subcostal groove the intercostal vein, artery, and nerve are located in that order. The mnemonic is VAN—vein/artery/nerve. Cadaver studies have shown in actuality that there is tremendous variation in location from person to person.[7]

Intercostal nerve blocks are indicated in helping control the pain of herpetic neuralgia in a thoracic dermatome, in scar neuromas after thoracotomy, and after a rib fracture. They also have diagnostic indications, to help determine if pain is coming from the chest wall or from deeper visceral organs. Blockade should occur at the level of interest and one level above and below it. There is some degree of overlapping innervation from adjacent intercostal nerves. The intercostal nerves have no endoneural sheath; they travel as three or four separate bundles. This makes them easily amenable to blockade.

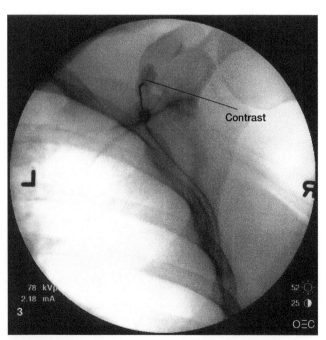

Figure 27-18 Proper contrast spread for a suprascapular nerve block.

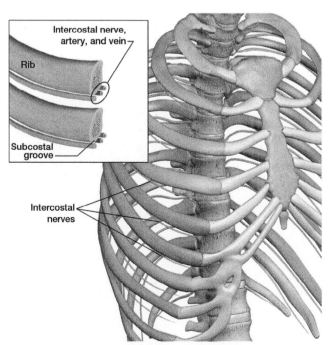

Figure 27-19 The intercostal nerves run along the undersurface of each rib in the subcostal groove.

In thin patients it is possible to perform this injection in the examination room. In larger patients whose ribs cannot be clearly palpated, it is best to complete the injection under fluoroscopy. When in doubt, do the injection under fluoroscopic guidance.

Intercostal Nerve Block in the Examination Room: The block may be performed with the patient in the prone, sitting, or lateral position. This discussion describes the seated procedure. The patient is sitting, leaning slightly forward. The arms should be forward, which pulls the scapulae laterally, facilitating access to the posterior rib angles. The intercostal nerve can be blocked anywhere proximal to the midaxillary line. The primary landmark is the angle of the rib 6 to 8 cm from midline (Fig. 27-20). At this point, the subcostal groove is the widest and the rib is relatively superficial. Standing behind the patient, start at the 12th rib and count up to the desired rib. Using a felt-tip marking pen, place an "X" over the center to bottom half of the desired ribs. The skin is prepped with alcohol. The skin just below the "X" is infiltrated with 1 to 2 mL of 2% lidocaine, using a 25-gauge needle to provide comfort during the procedure. A 10-mL syringe is filled with your therapeutic agent, a mixture of local anesthetic and steroid; an 18-gauge needle is used to draw up the medication. I use a mixture of 1.5 mL of 0.25% bupivacaine and 10 mg of Kenalog as my therapeutic agent, per intercostal nerve. Thus if three nerves are blocked, a mixture of 4.5 mL of 0.25% bupivacaine and 30 mg of Kenalog are drawn up into a single syringe, and each nerve receives a third of the mixture. The

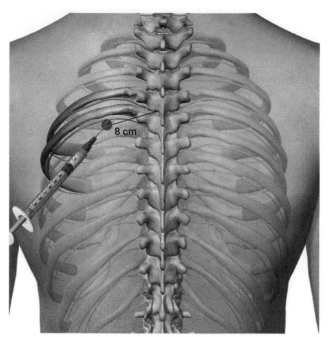

Figure 27-21 Needle placement for an intercostal nerve block: In the subcostal groove.

18-gauge needle is removed once the medications have been drawn up, and a 22-gauge, 1.5-in, short, beveled needle is attached to the 10-mL syringe containing the therapeutic agent.

When performing an intercostal nerve block, the needle is placed through the "X" that was marked on the skin. The needle is advanced until it comes in contact with the rib. After bone contact, the needle is slowly "walked off" the caudal aspect of the rib into the intercostal groove. The term "walking off" refers to the action of tapping a needle against a bony structure as you move along it to determine where the edge is located. By applying light pressure to the skin and pulling the skin down, you can direct your needle caudally. A subtle "pop" of the fascia of the internal intercostal muscle may be felt when you advance the needle into position. The needle is then tilted 20 degrees cephalad to point underneath the rib (Fig. 27-21). After negative aspiration, the therapeutic agent is injected. The needle is withdrawn and the same procedural steps followed for all levels to be blocked. A bandage is placed if needed.

Intercostal Nerve Block, Under Fluoroscopic Guidance: The patient lies on the fluoroscopic table in a prone position (face down). The back is prepped in standard sterile fashion. The fluoroscope is placed in the anteroposterior position. The ribs are identified under fluoroscopy. The primary landmark is the angle of the rib 6 to 8 cm from midline. At this point, the subcostal groove is the widest and the rib is relatively superficial. Using a metal marker and a sterile felt-tip marking

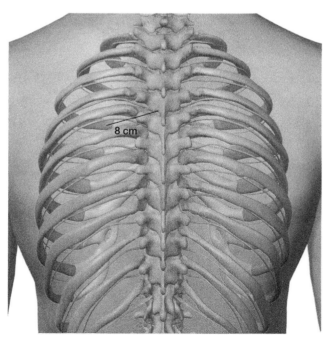

Figure 27-20 Intercostal nerve blocks are performed at the angle of the rib, 6 to 8 cm from midline.

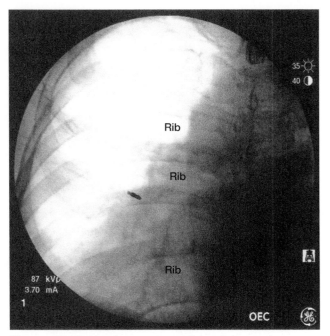

Figure 27-22 Needle entry target for an intercostal nerve block.

pen, place an "X" over the ribs of interest (Fig. 27-22). The skin just below the "X" is infiltrated with 1 to 2 mL of 2% lidocaine, using a 25-gauge needle to provide comfort during the procedure. A 10-mL syringe is filled with the therapeutic agent, a mixture of local anesthetic and steroid; an 18-gauge needle is used to draw up the medication. I use a mixture of 1.5 mL of 0.25% bupivacaine and 10 mg of Kenalog as my therapeutic agent per

intercostal nerve. Thus, for blockade of three nerves, draw up a mixture of 4.5 mL of 0.25% bupivacaine and 30 mg of Kenalog into a single syringe; place one-third of the mixture in each nerve. The 18-gauge needle is removed once the medications have been drawn up and the 10-mL syringe is placed on the sterile field.

A 22-gauge, 1.5-in, short, beveled needle is used for this procedure. The needle is placed through the "X" that was marked on the skin. The needle is placed perpendicular to the skin and parallel to the fluoroscope, then advanced until it comes in contact with the rib. After contacting the rib, the needle is slowly "walked off" the caudal aspect of the rib into the intercostal groove. The term "walking off" refers to the action of tapping a needle against a bony structure as you move along it to determine where the edge is located. A subtle "pop" of the fascia of the internal intercostal muscle may be felt. The needle is then tilted 20 degrees cephalad to point underneath the rib. The same steps are followed for each needle placed. A 3-mL syringe with tubing containing contrast is connected to the first needle. Tubing is used to enable you to see the contrast being injected under live x-ray without having your hand obscure the image and to protect your hand from direct radiation exposure. Inject the contrast, making sure it spreads properly in the subcostal groove (Fig. 27-23). Repeat these steps for all needles placed. Once proper contrast spread is seen, the 3-mL syringe containing contrast is disconnected from the tubing. A 10-mL syringe with the previously drawn up therapeutic agent is connected to the tubing and the therapeutic agent is injected. The needles are withdrawn and a bandage is placed if needed.

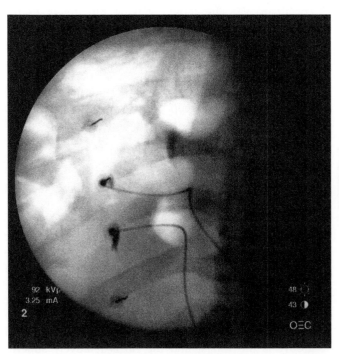

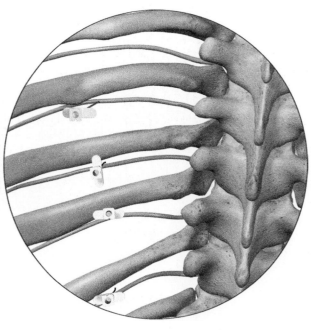

Figure 27-23 Fluoroscopic view of proper contrast spread for an intercostal nerve block.

Pelvic Nerve Block: Ilioinguinal, Iliohypogastric, and Genitofemoral Nerves

In a small number of patients an electric, burning groin pain develops after transverse lower abdominal procedures, hernia repairs, or hysterectomies. It is believed to occur because of an entrapment of a pelvic nerve or nerves in the sutures, mesh, or scar tissue. With the development of laparoscopic approaches to these procedures, the incidence of pelvic nerve entrapment has significantly decreased. Neuralgia may occur immediately after the procedure or up to several years.

There are three pelvic nerves that are most commonly affected: The iliohypogastric nerve, the ilioinguinal nerve, and the genitofemoral nerve. Because they run so closely to each other, one or more nerves may be involved. There is also overlap in the sensory supply of these nerves, making identification of which nerve is injured that much more difficult.

Nerve Block: Ilioinguinal, Iliohypogastric Nerves: For this block it is difficult to block each nerve individually, as they run very close together and their anatomic position can vary (Fig. 27-24). The patient is in the supine position (face up). Often a pillow is placed under the knees, as extending the legs can increase the patient's pain because of traction on these nerves. The primary landmark is the anterior-superior iliac spine (ASIS), which can be palpated. Use a felt-tip marking pen to place an "X" 2 cm medial and 2 cm cephalad to the ASIS (Fig. 27-25). The skin is then prepped with alcohol. The skin at the "X" is infiltrated with 3 to 4 mL of 2% lidocaine, using a 1.5-inch, 25-gauge needle to provide comfort during the procedure. A 20-mL syringe is filled with the therapeutic agent, a mixture of local anesthetic and steroid; an 18-gauge needle is used to draw up the medication. I use a mixture of 14 mL of 0.25% bupivacaine and 40 mg of Kenalog as my therapeutic agent. The 18-gauge needle is removed from the 20-mL syringe once the medications have been drawn up, and a 2.5-inch, 22-gauge needle is attached. You may need a 3.5-in needle for larger patients. The needle is placed through the "X" in a perpendicular plane to the skin. The patient is instructed to verbalize any dysesthesias during the procedure to prevent injection into the nerve itself. If dysesthesias are felt, the needle is repositioned prior to injection. Increased resistance is felt as the needle enters the external oblique muscle. A loss of resistance is noted as the needle passes through the external oblique muscle to lie between the external and internal oblique—a small "pop" is felt. After negative

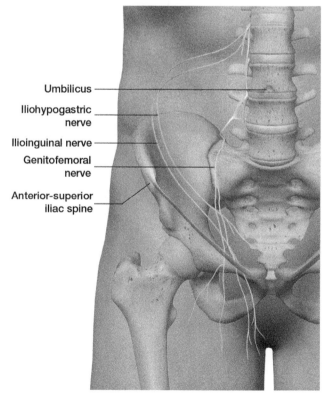

Figure 27-24 Ilioinguinal, iliohypogastric, and femoral branch of the genitofemoral nerve.

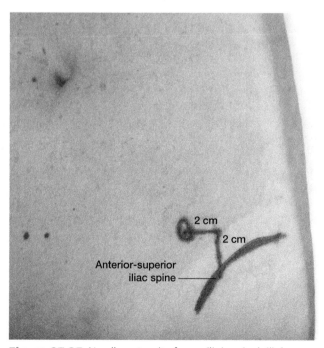

Figure 27-25 Needle entry site for an ilioinguinal, iliohypogastric, nerve block. Two centimeters medial and 2 cm cephalad to the anterior-superior iliac spine (ASIS).

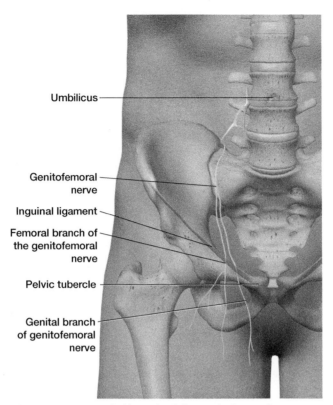

Umbilicus

Genitofemoral
nerve

Inguinal ligament

Femoral branch of
the genitofemoral
nerve

Pelvic tubercle

Genital branch
of genitofemoral
nerve

Figure 27-26 Genital branch of the genitofemoral nerve.
The primary landmark is the lateral aspect of the pubic tubercle on the painful side.

aspiration, 7.5 mL of therapeutic agent is injected at that site as well as medially and laterally. The needle is inserted further, once again using loss-of-resistance technique, until it passes between the internal oblique and the transverse abdominus—a second small "pop" is felt. After negative aspiration, the remaining 7.5 mL is injected at that site as well as medially and laterally. Because the exact location of the nerve is not known and varies from person to person, this is a "field block": The whole area is saturated with the therapeutic agent. The needle is withdrawn and a bandage placed if needed.

Spillover of medication may occur, which could lead to blockade of the femoral nerve and quad weakness until the local anesthetic wears off.

Nerve Block: Genitofemoral Nerve: The primary landmark is the lateral aspect of the pubic tubercle on the painful side (Fig. 27-26). Standing lateral to the location of the pain, use a felt-tip marking pen to place an "X" just lateral to the pubic tubercle and below the inguinal ligament (Fig. 27-27). The skin is prepped with alcohol. The skin at the "X" is infiltrated with 3 to 4 mL of 2% lidocaine, using a 25-gauge needle to provide comfort during the procedure. A 10-mL syringe is filled with the therapeutic

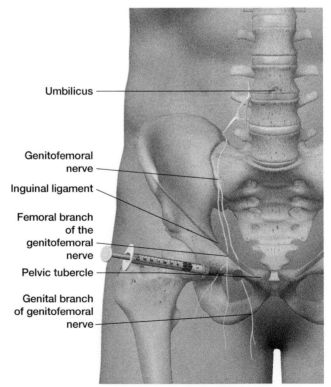

Umbilicus

Genitofemoral
nerve

Inguinal ligament

Femoral branch
of the
genitofemoral
nerve

Pelvic tubercle

Genital branch
of genitofemoral
nerve

Figure 27-27 Needle entry site for a genitofemoral nerve block is just lateral to the pubic tubercle and below the inguinal ligament.

agent, a mixture of local anesthetic and steroid; an 18-gauge needle is used to draw up the medication. I use a mixture of 6 mL of 0.25% bupivacaine and 40 mg of Kenalog as my therapeutic agent. The 18-gauge needle is removed once the medications have been drawn up, and a 2.5-in, 22-gauge needle is placed through the "X." The patient is instructed to verbalize any dysesthesias during the procedure to prevent injection into the nerve itself. If dysesthesias are felt, the needle is repositioned prior to injection. After negative aspiration, the therapeutic agent is injected in a fan-like motion. Because the exact location of the nerve is not known and varies from person to person, this is a "field block": The whole area is saturated with the therapeutic agent. The needle is withdrawn and a bandage placed if needed.

Lateral Femoral Cutaneous Nerve Block

The lateral femoral cutaneous nerve is purely sensory, derived from the L2 and L3 nerve roots. It

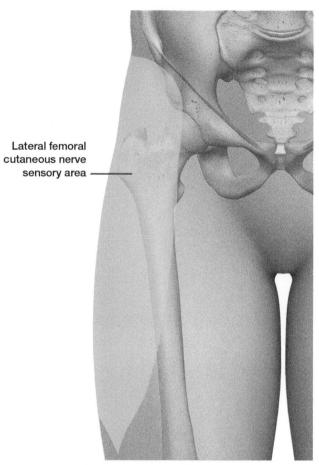

Figure 27-29 Sensory area covered by the lateral femoral cutaneous nerve.

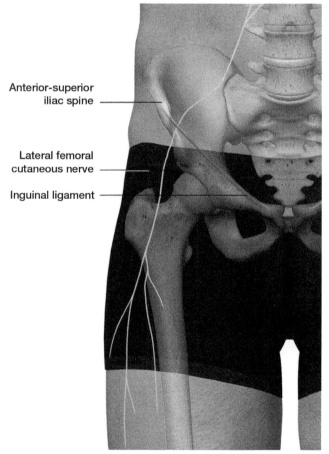

Figure 27-28 The lateral femoral cutaneous nerve. The lateral femoral cutaneous nerve is purely sensory, derived from the L2 and L3 nerve roots.

passes just medial and inferior to the ASIS. This is where it is accessed for a nerve block (Fig. 27-28). The nerve then passes underneath the inguinal ligament and enters the thigh. It supplies the anterolateral aspect of the thigh starting just below the hip (Fig. 27-29).

Patients complain of anterior and lateral thigh burning and/or tingling pain. The symptoms are primarily unilateral but can occur bilaterally. When the nerve becomes compressed or irritated, it causes pain in the anterior lateral thigh, commonly referred to as meralgia paresthetica. The word *meralgia* is derived from the Greek word *meros,* meaning thigh, and also meaning pain. Paresthetica refers to paresthesia, an abnormal sensation of the body such as numbness, tingling, or burning. A lateral femoral cutaneous nerve block can help with the symptoms and help to alleviate compression in some cases.

The patient lies in the supine position (face up). The primary landmark is the ASIS, which can be palpated. Standing lateral to the painful thigh, use a felt-tip marking pen to place an "X" 2 cm medial and 2 cm

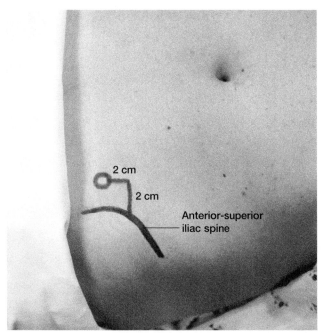

Figure 27-30 Needle entry site for a lateral femoral cutaneous nerve block. Two centimeters medial and 2 cm caudad to the ASIS.

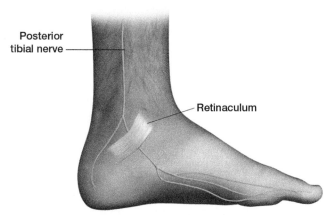

Figure 27-31 Posterior tibial nerve passing through the tarsal tunnel.

caudad to the ASIS (Fig. 27-30). The skin is then prepped with alcohol. The skin at the "X" is infiltrated with 3 to 4 mL of 2% lidocaine, using a 1.5 in, 25-gauge needle to provide comfort during the procedure. A 10-mL syringe is filled with a mixture of local anesthetic and steroid; an 18-gauge needle is used to draw up the medication. I use a mixture of 7 mL of 0.25% bupivacaine and 40 mg of Kenalog as my therapeutic agent. The 18-gauge needle is removed once the medications have been drawn up, and a 2.5-in, 22-gauge needle is attached to the 10-mL syringe and placed through the "X." The patient is instructed to verbalize any dysesthesias during the procedure to prevent injection into the nerve itself. If dysesthesias are felt, the needle is repositioned prior to injection. Resistance is encountered as the needle advances until a "pop" is felt as the fascia lata is penetrated by the needle. After negative aspiration, the therapeutic agent is injected. The needle is directed medially and laterally in a fan-wise motion, delivering the therapeutic agent. Because the exact location of the nerve is not known and varies from person to person this is a "field block": The whole area is saturated with the therapeutic agent. The needle is then withdrawn and a bandage placed if needed.

Posterior Tibial Nerve Block

Tarsal tunnel syndrome is an entrapment neuropathy of the posterior tibial nerve in the tarsal tunnel. The tibial nerve passes into the foot through the tarsal tunnel, located posterior to the medial malleolus (Fig. 27-31). In the tunnel, the posterior tibial nerve splits into three separate nerves. One nerve continues to the heel; the other two (medial and lateral plantar nerves) continue to the bottom of the foot. In tarsal tunnel syndrome, the nerve becomes trapped as the area under the flexor retinaculum becomes too small. This condition is analogous to CTS of the wrist. Pain radiates from the tarsal tunnel into the foot. Patients often describe this pain as a shooting, electric pain radiating from the medial malleolus into the big toe and the three adjacent toes.

The patient lies in the supine position (face up) with the leg externally rotated to expose the medial malleolus. A chuck or towel is placed under the ankle. The practitioner stands just medial to the painful side. The insertion site is posterior to the medial malleolus. Using a felt-tip pen place an "X" over the insertion site (Fig. 27-32). The skin is prepped with alcohol. A 3-mL syringe is filled with the therapeutic agent, a mixture of local anesthetic and steroid; an

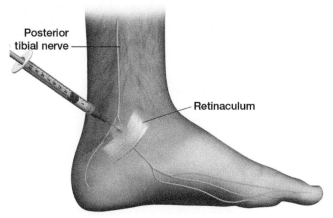

Figure 27-32 Needle entry site for a posterior tibial nerve block.

18-gauge needle is used to draw up the medication. I use a mixture of 1.5 mL of 1% lidocaine and 20 mg of Kenalog as my therapeutic agent. The 18-gauge needle is removed once the medications have been drawn up, and a 1.5-in, 25-gauge needle is placed through the "X" on the skin at a 45-degree angle with the bevel of the needle pointed inferiorly. The patient is instructed to verbalize any dysesthesias during the procedure to prevent injection into the nerve itself. If dysesthesias are felt, the needle is repositioned prior to injection. The injection is deep to the superficial fascia. The needle is advanced toward the medial malleolus until bone is felt, then withdrawn 1 to 2 mm. After negative aspiration, the therapeutic agent is injected. The needle is withdrawn and a bandage placed if needed.

CONTRAINDICATIONS AND POTENTIAL COMPLICATIONS

Contraindications include systemic infection and infection on the skin where the needle is to be inserted. For all these injections, although rare, there is always a chance of infection, hematoma, and nerve damage.

Trigeminal nerve block: The chances for hematoma increase because the region is highly vascular. Temporary weakness of the muscles of mastication may also occur.

Intercostal nerve block: With an intercostal nerve block, pneumothorax (collapsed lung) may occur because the intercostal nerves are intimately located next to the pleura. The incidence is less than 1%, but is higher in patients with chronic obstructive pulmonary disease. It is essential to weigh the benefits of the procedure carefully against the possibility of a pneumothorax.

CASE STUDIES

 Case 1 A 52-year-old woman presents with trigeminal neuralgia of the right side of her face, which she has had for the past 5 years. Most days, she has mild pain, which she describes as electric and stabbing. Over the past 6 months, the pain has increased in both frequency and intensity, disrupting the quality of her life. The woman takes Lyrica (pregabalin) 150 mg po bid. (She has been on Tegretol [carbamazepine] in the past).

The pain is in the maxillary (V2) and mandibular (V3) divisions of the trigeminal nerve. Imaging, which has always been negative, is once again negative. Your patient and you decide that the best course of action would be a trigeminal nerve block in hopes of resetting the pathologic firing of the trigeminal nerve. The patient undergoes a V2 and V3 nerve block under fluoroscopic guidance. She reports an excellent response, and her symptoms abate. After 2 months of no symptoms, you start to wean her off Lyrica and she eventually stops taking it. After going 3 months without an attack, she has an episode, and you put her back on Lyrica.

 Case 2 A 41-year-old overweight man presents to your office with a chief complaint of sciatica. He reports that he has been having pain in his right leg. Recently, the pain became so intense that he went to the emergency department, where he received pain medication and had x-rays of his lumbar spine. You look up the report and the x-rays are normal. The patient reports no pain in his left leg and no back pain, just a burning, electric pain in his right leg that does not go past the knee. No particular event is associated with original initiation of the pain. It has been of gradual onset and steadily increasing in severity. He has no change in bowel or bladder function.

On examination, the patient has full strength, with normal reflexes and sensation intact to light touch. He grabs the top lateral aspect of the thigh and says that is the location of the pain. Based on history and examination, he has pain in the region of the lateral femoral cutaneous nerve. You diagnose meralgia paresthetica. In the office that day, after obtaining informed consent, you perform a lateral femoral cutaneous nerve block. The patient reports an immediate reduction in his pain. He enrolls in a workout program at his local YMCA with the goal of losing weight as this is most likely a compressive neuropathy.

REFERENCES

1. Marshall LL, Trethewie ER, Curtain CC. Chemical radiculitis: A clinical, physiological and immunological study. *Clin Orthop Relat Res.* 1977;129:61–67.
2. Devor M, Govrin-Lippmann R, Raber P. Corticosteroids suppress ectopic neural discharge originating in experimental neuromas. *Pain.* 1985;22:127–137.
3. Fraioli B, Esposito V, Guidetti B, et al. Treatment of trigeminal neuralgia by thermocoagulation, glycerolization, and percutaneous compression of the gasserian ganglion and/or retrogasserian rootlets: Long-term results and therapeutic protocol. *Neurosurgery.* 1989;24(2):239–245.
4. Taha JM, Tew JM Jr, Buncher CR. A prospective 15-year follow up of 154 consecutive patients with trigeminal neuralgia treated by percutaneous stereotactic radiofrequency thermal rhizotomy. *J Neurosurg.* 1995;83(6):989–993.
5. Gelberman RH, Aronson D, Weisman MH. Carpal-tunnel syndrome: Results of a prospective trial of steroid injection and splinting. *J Bone Joint Surg Am.* 1980:62(7):1181–1184.
6. Rohof OJ. Pulsed radiofrequency of the suprascapular nerve in the treatment of chronic intractable shoulder pain. In: Raj PP, ed. *2nd World Congress of WIP.* Istanbul: Blackwell Science; 2001.
7. Hardy PA. Anatomical variation in the position of the proximal intercostal nerve. *Br J Anaesth.* 1988;61(3):338–339.

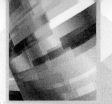

CHAPTER 28

Discogenic Pain: Lumbar Discography

WHEN TO USE

HOW TO PERFORM THE PROCEDURE

CONTRAINDICATIONS AND POTENTIAL COMPLICATIONS

A vertebral disc is built like a jelly doughnut. The inner jelly part is the nucleus pulposus and the outer layer is the anulus fibrosus (Fig. 28-1). Intervertebral discs have been a suspected source of spine pain, and in 1947 investigators identified a nerve supply to the disc. Nerve innervation of a vertebral disc is limited to the outer third of the anulus fibrosus. A healthy disc has a high water content and acts as a cushion between two vertebral bodies. As a disc loses water content over time, it shrinks and becomes prone to developing cracks and tears in the anulus fibrosus. Radial tears in the innervated layer of a vertebral disc, the anulus fibrosus may be a source of low back pain (Fig. 28-2). In fact, 39% of people with chronic low back pain have degenerative discs.[1] However, a number of people who have degenerative discs on imaging have no pain. Simply having degenerative discs on imaging is not enough to diagnose discogenic pain. Degenerative disc(s) on imaging, focal low back pain,

and pain that cannot be explained by other reasonable causes combined lead to the diagnosis of degenerative disc disease.

Provocative discography is a diagnostic test for discogenic pain, helping pinpoint the disc(s) in which the pain originates. The role of discography is to distinguish a symptomatic disc from similarly degenerative ones on the basis of pain reproduction. A needle is inserted into the nucleus pulposus and contrast is slowly injected under pressure, which stresses the disc. Typically, a disc will not produce pain when stressed with less than 50 pounds per square inch (psi) of pressure. During the discography procedure, the patient remains awake and alert while contrast is slowly injected. The patient reports whether the stress put on the disc during the injection reproduces the pain usually experienced. This is analogous to palpation for tenderness. This is a functional diagnostic test; thus although a patient may have three

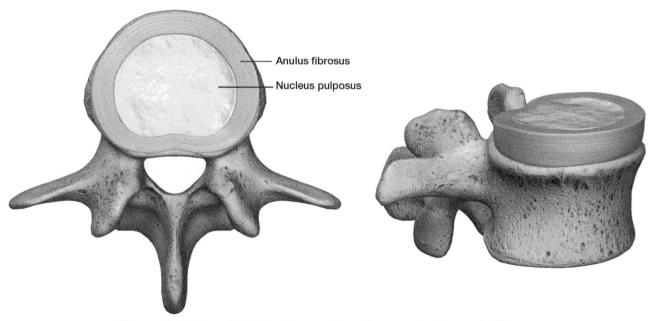

Anulus fibrosus

Nucleus pulposus

Figure 28-1 Intervertebral disc: Inner nucleus pulposus and outer annular fibrosus.

Figure 28-2 Radial tear in the anulus fibrosus. Radial tears in the innervated layer of a vertebral disc, the anulus fibrosus, are thought to be a source of low back pain.

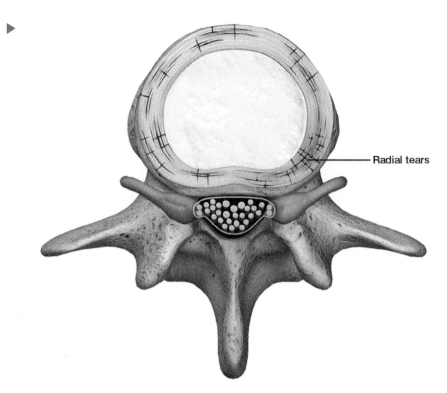

— Radial tears

degenerative discs on imaging and significant back pain, discography may reveal only one of the three degenerative discs that is actually a source of low back pain. Vanharanta et al.[2] found that concordant pain (pain equivalent to the patient's normal back pain) reproduced on discography correlated with the extent of annular disruption. This means that the more symptomatic the disc, the more dramatic the response would be on discography.

WHEN TO USE

For focal back pain of suspected discogenic origin, it is appropriate to prescribe rest and physical therapy for a few weeks in patients who do not have progressive pain

or significant neurologic deficit. If the pain does not improve and imaging reveals degenerative discs, it is appropriate to present interventional and surgical options. A series of epidural steroid injections is reasonable treatment option. If the patient does not respond. Discography is an interventional diagnostic test (not therapeutic), which can lead to surgical treatment if results are positive. A patients who refuse future surgical options such as fusion and artificial disc replacement (ADR) should not undergo this invasive diagnostic procedure. There is no point in obtaining the results of an interventional diagnostic test if you cannot act on the results.

Spine surgeons often obtain the results of provocative discography to help determine if a patient would benefit from an ADR or spinal fusion. In 2004, the Food

Figure 28-3 Artificial disc replacement. **A:** The CHARITE total disc replacement is composed of three parts; two cobalt-chromium alloy endplates and a sliding ultra-high-molecular-weight polyethylene (UHMWPE) core. **B:** Disc replacement at the L4 to L5 level. (A, from Bridwell KH, DeWald RL. *The Textbook of Spinal Surgery,* 3rd ed. Philadelphia, PA: Lippincott Williams & Wilkins; 2011,484; B, from Cox JM. *Low Back Pain: Mechanism, Diagnosis, and Treatment,* 7th ed. Philadelphia, PA: Lippincott Williams & Wilkins; 2011,469.)

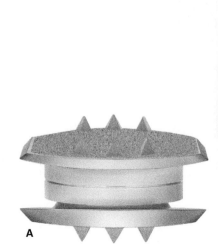

A

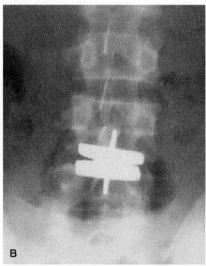

B

and Drug Administration (FDA) approved ADR which entails replacement of the painful disc with an artificial disc (Fig. 28-3). At this time, however, ADR does not have an excellent track record like knee and hip replacement. A spinal fusion fuses vertebral bodies in an attempt to alleviate pain and instability on the theory that removing the painful disc will stop pain. In patients undergoing fusion for low back pain, 89% derived significant relief when discography had revealed disc disease and pain reproduction, whereas only 52% derived relief when morphologic changes of the disc were seen but no pain reproduction was produced during discography.[3] It is possible to fuse multiple levels if multiple discs are involved. Discography helps avoid fusion at a level where the disc is abnormal on imaging but functionally not producing pain.

HOW TO PERFORM THE PROCEDURE

It is important to explain the procedure to the patient completely, answer all questions, and obtain informed consent. (The practitioner should be sure to emphasize that this is a diagnostic, not a therapeutic, procedure. It is essential to clarify that discography will not

provide pain relief and is, on the contrary, used to elicit pain.)

The patient should receive preoperative antibiotics; 2 g of cefazolin sodium (Ancef) is appropriate. The use of intravenous antibiotics before the procedure begins may prevent the occurrence of discitis after the procedure.

It is necessary to perform discography under fluoroscopic guidance (live x-ray) for accuracy and safety. After arrival in the fluoroscopy suite, the patient lies on the fluoroscopy table in the prone position (face down). A "time out" is performed prior to the procedure including verbal confirmation of correct patient, procedure and procedural site. Noninvasive hemodynamic monitors and pulse oximetry are placed.

The skin over the low back is prepped with betadine and drapes are placed over the area in standard sterile fashion. The fluoroscope is placed in the anteroposterior (AP) position. The fluoroscope is then tilted if necessary in a cephalad to caudad motion to "square up" the endplates of the vertebral bodies (Fig. 28-4). The disc of interest is visualized and the fluoroscope is rotated obliquely, away from the person performing the procedure. The fluoroscope

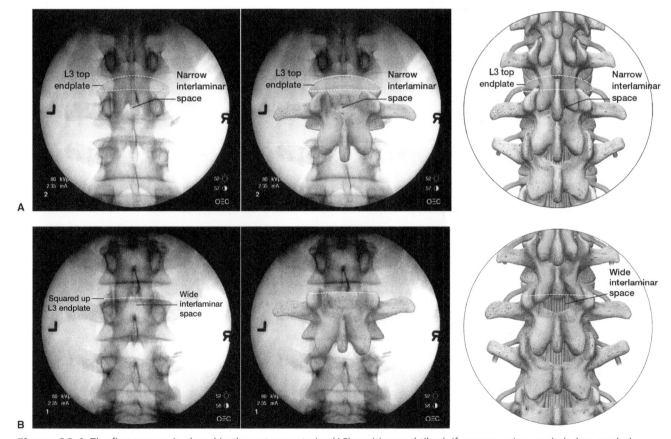

Figure 28-4 The fluoroscope is placed in the anteroposterior (AP) position and tilted, if necessary, in a cephalad to caudad motion to "square up" the endplates of the vertebral bodies. **A.** In the first panel of pictures the top of the L3 vertebral body is slanted which narrows the entry window into the disc. **B.** In the second panel of pictures the angle of the camera has been adjusted in a cephalad position to "square up" the top of the L3 vertebral body which widers the entry window into the disc.

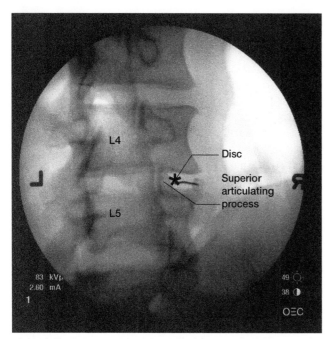

Figure 28-5 The camera should be in the oblique view so that the superior articulating process divides the vertebral body in half. An "X" is placed on the skin just lateral to the superior articulating process.

is rotated enough so that the superior articulating process divides the vertebral body in half. The posterior oblique angle is the position that allows best access to the disc. Using a metal marker and a felt-tip marking pen, an "X" is placed on the skin just lateral to the superior articulating process (Fig. 28-5).

The skin and subcutaneous tissue is anesthetized with 2% lidocaine using a 1.5-in, 25-gauge needle.

After the skin is anesthetized, a double-needle approach is usually taken to help gain sterile access to the disc. A 2-in, 18-gauge introducer needle is placed through the "X" in a perpendicular fashion to the skin and parallel to the fluoroscope. This is the position along an oblique path to the disc. A smaller needle – 5-in, 22-gauge – is then fed through the larger needle to the intradiscal space. The needle is advanced until resistance is felt in the oblique view. Entering the disc through the anulus fibrosus is often described as feeling similar to a needle entering an orange (Fig. 28-6). The camera is then rotated to the lateral position, which allows the interventionalist to know the depth of the needle. The needle is advanced anteriorly and medially to the anterior third of the disc. Once this is accomplished, the camera is rotated to the AP position. The needle should be in the center of the disc in the AP view. If the needle is lateral to midline on the side that was entered, the approach is not shallow enough. Once proper placement is confirmed, the same steps are followed for all discs to which the operator needs to gain access. Usually a needle is placed into the suspected symptomatic disc as well as into the discs on the level above and below. The most common locations for needle placement are the L3/L4, L4/L5, and L5/S1 discs. Because the iliac crest can obscure the oblique entrance to the L5/S1 disc, this level is the most technically difficult to place.

The stylets of the 5-inch, 22-gauge needles are then removed. The stylet is used to prevent tissue from collecting within the needle. A discmonitor with tubing is connected to one needle at a time as the disc undergoes testing (Fig. 28-7). Tubing is used so you can see the

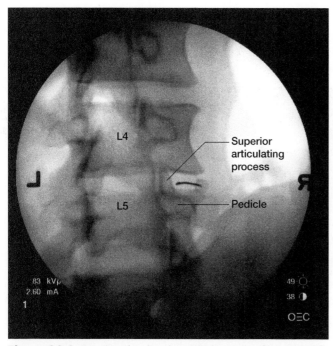

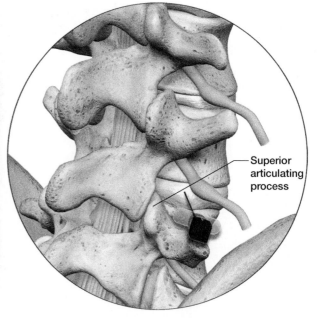

Figure 28-6 Entering the disc through the anulus fibrosus is often described as a feeling similar to a needle entering an orange.

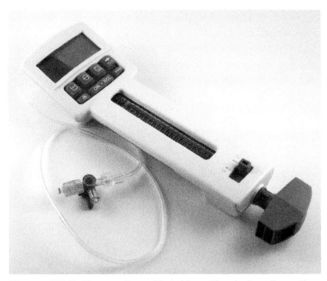

Figure 28-7 Discmonitor with tubing. The device allows the doctor to determine how many pounds per square inch (psi) is being applied at any time while pressurizing the disc.

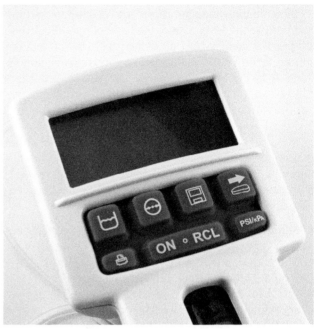

Figure 28-8 Face of the discmonitor providing digital readout.

contrast injected under live x-ray without having your hand obscure the image and to protect your hand from radiation exposure. Contrast is injected in a controlled manner, using the line-pressured discmonitor that has a digital readout (Fig. 28-8). This allows the interventionalist to know how many psi are being applied to the disc as the contrast is slowly being injected. Opening pressure is recorded at the first sight of contrast (Fig. 28-9). The patient is then asked to verbalize when pain is felt and whether it is the kind normally experienced – that is, concordant pain – or whether it is different. In a healthy disc the patient may feel no pain as the pressure is slowly increased to 50 psi over opening pressure. Once the discs have been fully tested, a local anesthetic can be injected into any painful disc to relieve postprocedural discomfort.

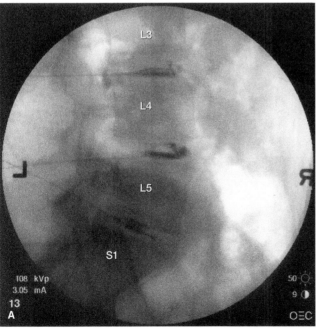

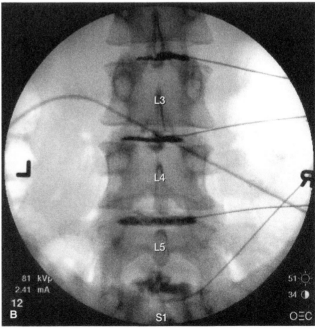

Figure 28-9 Lateral and posterior views (**A, B**) of a discogram.

The following data are recorded: Whether the patient had pain at the level tested, the level of pain 0 to 10 on a visual analog scale, at what pressure the patient started feeling pain, and whether the pain was concordant. It is important to remember that healthy discs can be painful when stressed above 50 psi over opening pressure; thus discs should not be stressed above this level.

It is crucial to test multiple levels, because without an asymptomatic control disc, it is impossible to determine the validity of the test. Discography is positive if it satisfies the following International Spine Interventional Society (ISIS) criteria:

- Stimulation of the target disc reproduces concordant pain.
- The pain that is reproduced is registered as at least a 7 on a 10-point visual analog scale.
- The pain that is reproduced is produced at a pressure less than 50 psi over opening pressure.
- Stimulation of an adjacent disc provides negative control.

With a provocative discogram, there is the potential for false-positive results. This can occur for a number of reasons. One potential cause is needle placement into the annular layer rather than the nucleus pulposus. An annular injection is painful in a healthy disc. Another potential cause is discography performed without a line pressure discmonitor: Clinicians sometimes simply inject the contrast using a syringe, crudely gauging pressure with the amount of pressure applied by their thumb. Lack of equipment to monitor exact pressure often results in pressure greater than 50 psi, which causes pain in a disc that is healthy. Psychological factors also influence results, which makes patient selection crucial (see When Not to Use and Potential Complications).

After the procedure, the patient has a CT scan so that the disc can be imaged while it still contains contrast. Postdiscography CT allows the detection of annular pathology.

CONTRAINDICATIONS AND POTENTIAL COMPLICATIONS

Patient selection is crucial in discography, as it is in most diagnostic interventional procedures. Potential candidates must understand that the prerequisites for discography are being able to tolerate the procedure physically and being able to cooperate in providing responses. Patients must be able to clearly differentiate between the pain caused by having a needle in their back and the possible pain caused by pressurizing a disc in an attempt to reproduce the normal pain. If a patient cannot provide reasonable feedback during the procedure, he or she is not a suitable candidate.

It is important to note that discography is strictly a diagnostic procedure. If the results of the test will not influence the treatment plan, the interventional procedure is not warranted. Contraindications include infection, coagulopathy, and pregnancy. Discography is rarely performed in the cervical spine.

The most feared complication is discitis. The disc is prone to infection because of its avascular nature. Clinical symptoms usually occur 2 to 4 weeks after the procedure and include pain, limited lumbar motion, and fever. Two measures have reduced the incidence of discitis: Aseptic technique and prophylactic antibiotics.

CASE STUDY

A 61-year-old man complains of low back pain. The pain, which he has had for the past 2 years, does not spread to his legs. He has low back pain every day, which affects his activities of daily living. He has just completed a 6-week course of physical therapy which was moderately helpful. He has also tried using nonsteroidal anti-inflammatory drugs and muscle relaxants, and when the pain becomes significant, he takes a Percocet 10/325. Recent imaging – magnetic resonance imaging (MRI) of the lumbar spine – shows degenerative discs at L3/L4, L4/L5, and L5/S1 to varying degrees with minimal facet changes, no disc herniations or nerve root compression.

The patient receives a referral to a pain management specialist. After reviewing treatment options – which included more physical therapy, further medication changes, potential interventional procedures, and possible surgery – the patient elects to proceed with a series of epidural steroid injection. After two injections, the patient has minimal change in his pain. The patient states that if one or more of the degenerative discs is the source of his pain, at this point he wants them surgically removed. The patient understands that based on his MRI and his continued pain, his surgical options may include a three-level fusion. The discogram will show how many levels clinically cause pain. The risks, benefits, and alternatives to a discogram are reviewed with the patient and he decides to have the procedure. Table 28-1 presents discogram results.

TABLE 28-1 Discogram Results for 61-year-old Male with Low Back Pain of 2 Years Duration

Disc Level	Opening Pressure (psi)	Pressure at Which Pain is Felt	Pain Level at 50 psi	Concordant
L3/L4	12	None	None	No pain
L4/L5	17	31	9/10	Concordant
L5/S1	15	28	10/10	Concordant

The postdiscography CT scan shows extensive annular tears at L4/5 and L5/S1. The patient plans to see a spine surgeon for an evaluation of a two-level fusion at L4/5 and L5/S1.

REFERENCES

1. Bogduk N, Twomey L. *Clinical Anatomy of the Lumbar Spine.* 3rd ed. New York, NY: Churchill Livingstone; 1997.
2. Vanharanta H, Sachs BL, Spivey MA, et al. The relationship of pain provocation to lumbar disc deterioration as seen by CT/discography. *Spine (Phila Pa 1976).* 1987;12:295–298.
3. Colhoun E, McCall IW, Williams L, et al. Provocation discography as a guide to planning operations on the spine. *J Bone Joint Surg Br.* 1988;70:267–271.

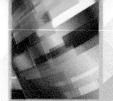

CHAPTER 29

Spinal Cord Stimulation

Since 15 BC electricity has been used to treat pain. Ancient Roman physicians used the torpedo fish, also known as electric ray, to treat headaches and gout. Over time the advancement of using controlled electricity to treat pain has led to the spinal cord stimulator. The development of the spinal cord stimulator centered around the gate control theory of pain published by Wall and Melzack in 1965. It holds that pain transmission to the brain occurs through the "gate," in the substantia gelatinosa in the dorsal aspect of the spinal cord (Fig. 29-1). At the "gate" both large myelinated fibers (pressure, touch, and vibration) and thin pain transmitting fibers, (unmyelinated C fibers and lightly myelinated A-delta fibers) synapse

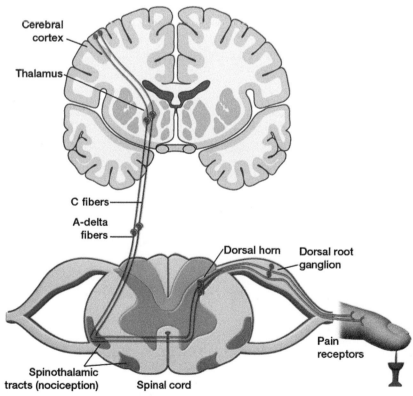

Figure 29-1 Pain transmitted from a body part to the dorsal aspect of the spinal cord up to the brain for interpretation.

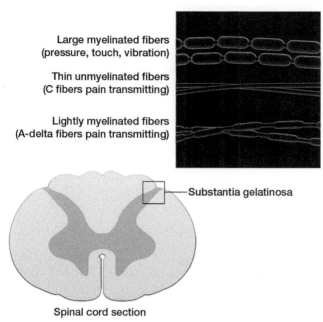

Large myelinated fibers
(pressure, touch, vibration)

Thin unmyelinated fibers
(C fibers pain transmitting)

Lightly myelinated fibers
(A-delta fibers pain transmitting)

Substantia gelatinosa

Spinal cord section

Figure 29-2 Multiple sensory impulses synapse at the substantia gelatinosa in the dorsal horn of the spinal cord.

(Fig. 29-2). Through the "gate" only one message can pass at a time and the passage of large myelinated fibers are preferred over thin fibers.[1] A spinal cord stimulator activates these large myelinated fibers (mechanoreceptors) as well as polysynaptic interneurons (PSINs) effectively closing the "gate" on the smaller pain fibers (Fig. 29-3). The PSINs when activated fire back on the dorsal horn blocking pain receptors from synapsing. The greater the activity of larger myelinated fibers (mechanoreceptors) and PSINs

there is to the activity of thin pain fibers, the less pain sensation is felt. The goal is to activate the specific set of large myelinated fibers (mechanoreceptors) and PSINs that overlap the areas of pain. It is possible to do this without causing discomfort or motor effects. Think about it this way. If a bee stings you a common response is to start rubbing the area where you feel the piercing sharp pain. Essentially what you are doing is activating mechanoreceptors by creating a sense of vibration over the area, which overrides the painful sensation trying to get through the "gate."

This is the main theory, but the exact mechanism of spinal cord stimulation is not completely understood. Spinal cord stimulation may alter pain as well by modulating the descending pathways. After ascending pathways send pain signals to the brain, descending pathways are activated to complete the loop and alter pain transmission as it enters the spinal cord. This effect may occur through GABAergic interneurons. Spinal cord stimulation is also known to inhibit sympathetic outflow. This leads to an increase in blood flow and a reduction of oxygen demand in ischemic tissue. Interestingly cerebrospinal fluid levels of vascular endothelial growth factor which is thought to modulate neuronal transmission and promote chronic neuropathic pain are reduced by spinal cord stimulation in patients with failed back surgery syndrome.

The flexible, catheter-style leads of the spinal cord stimulator never physically touch the spinal cord. Instead they enter the posterior epidural space. The epidural space is the outermost space in the spinal canal, lying outside the dura mater inside the surrounding vertebrae (Fig. 29-4). It is the same location in which a

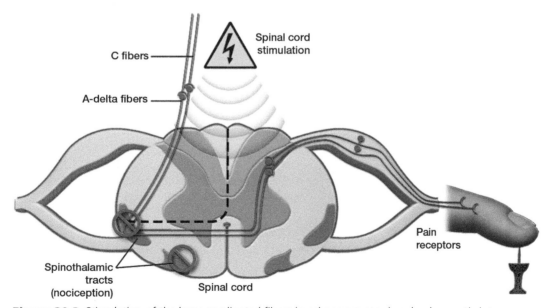

C fibers

Spinal cord
stimulation

A-delta fibers

Pain
receptors

Spinothalamic
tracts
(nociception)

Spinal cord

Figure 29-3 Stimulation of the large myelinated fibers (mechanoreceptors) and polysynaptic interneurons (PSINs) in the dorsal horn of the spinal cord blocks unmyelinated and lightly myelinated fibers from transmitting a pain signal up to the brain through the spinothalamic tract.

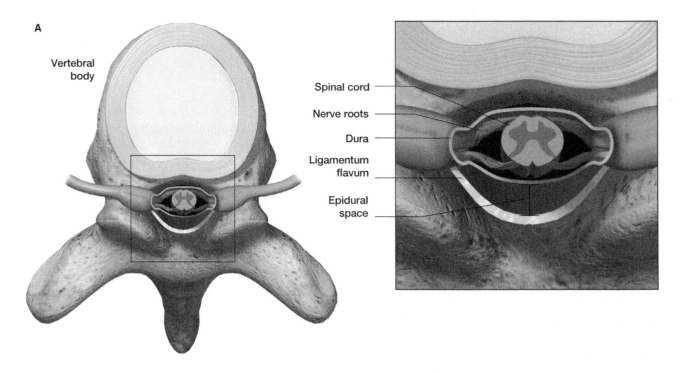

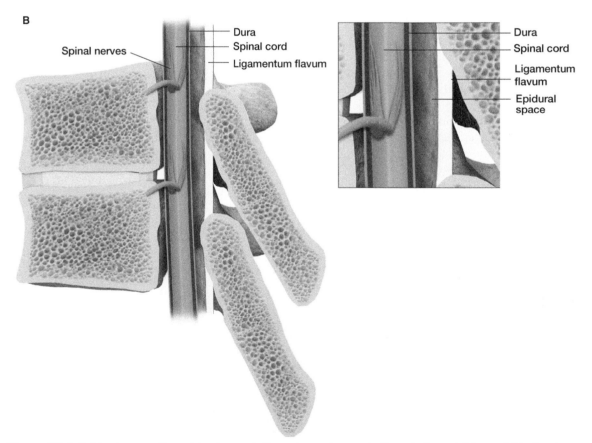

Figure 29-4 Epidural space. The epidural space is the outermost space in the spinal canal, lying outside the dura mater inside the surrounding vertebrae. **A.** Axial view of the epidural space. **B.** Sagital view of the epidural space.

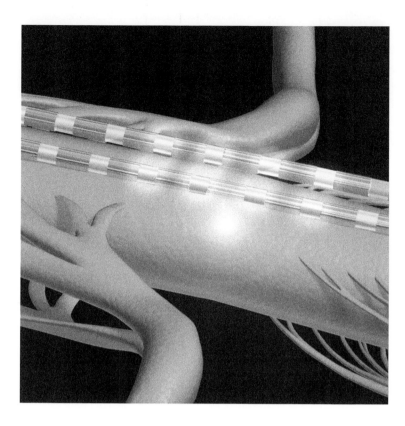

◀ **Figure 29-5** Stimulation of the large myelinated mechanoreceptors and polysynaptic interneurons (PSINs) in the dorsal horn of the spinal cord. The leads are cylindrical polyurethane flexible catheters with multiple evenly spaced electrode contacts.

catheter is placed to deliver anesthesia to the expectant mother during childbirth. Controlled electric current is driven to the back of the spinal cord to stimulate the large myelinated fibers of the dorsal horn (Fig. 29-5).

An analogy I give to my patients to help them understand the purpose of the spinal cord stimulator is that the heart runs on electricity and when it malfunctions a pacemaker is used to correct it. The nervous system runs on electricity as well and when it malfunctions, it too can be corrected using a pacemaker. Like the heart pacemaker the spinal cord stimulator system consists of two catheter-style leads and a battery that sits under the skin. In fact, many of the same companies that manufacture the heart pacemaker also make the pacemaker for pain. The leads are cylindrical polyurethane flexible catheters with multiple evenly spaced electrode contacts. The battery is currently about the size of a silver dollar (Fig. 29-6).

WHEN TO USE

Much of the original work implementing spinal cord stimulation was done by spine surgeons who were not seeing positive results with repeat surgery for patients who did not respond to the first operation. The first spinal cord stimulator was placed in 1967 for failed back surgery syndrome—when a patient has spine surgery and continues to have significant pain despite proper surgical correction. Other indications beyond failed back surgery syndrome include: Complex regional pain syndrome (formerly known as reflex sympathetic dystrophy),[2] cervical and lumbar radiculopathy, arachnoiditis, peripheral neuropathy, and intractable pain from postherpetic neuralgia. It is primarily used for neuropathic pain, not nociceptive pain (pain from bone, joints, organs). Spinal cord stimulation is more effective in treating extremity (in a limb) than axial pain, thus for people with back and leg pain, leg pain is more responsive to stimulation than back pain. In Europe, spinal cord stimulation is often used to treat ischemic pain arising from peripheral vascular disease in the

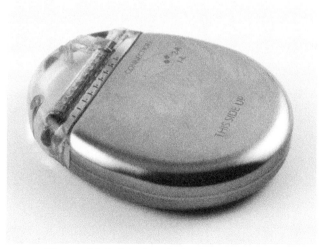

Figure 29-6 Spinal cord stimulator generator.

Figure 29-7 Spinal cord stimulation increasing blood flow ▶ into a limb by creating a sympathetic block allowing a para-sympathetic-induced vasodilation.

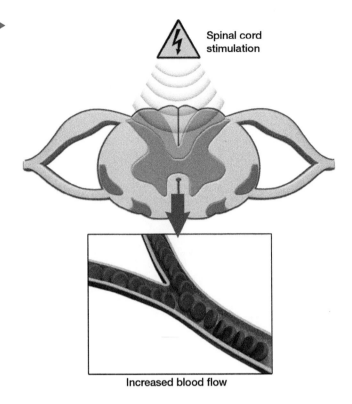

Increased blood flow

lower extremities. The sympathetic block created by the stimulation allows for parasympathetic-induced vasodilation. It has been shown that spinal cord stimulation improves perfusion pressure and red blood cell flow velocity, and may improve the possibility for limb salvage (Fig. 29-7).[3] Spinal cord stimulation is a tertiary treatment for pain and should be entertained when less invasive measures have been tried first.

Before implantation of a permanent system, patients first undergo a spinal cord stimulation trial to determine if full implantation is appropriate. The trial involves placement of flexible catheter-type leads into the posterior epidural space under fluoroscopic guidance (Fig. 29-8). This requires no knife, because an introducer needle provides access to the epidural space. A local anesthetic such as lidocaine is necessary to ensure patient comfort.

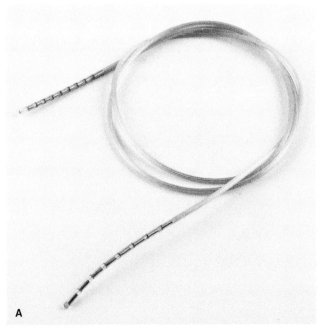

A

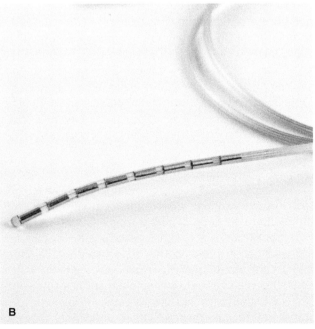

B

Figure 29-8 **A.** Spinal cord stimulator flexible catheter lead. **B.** Magnified view of the contacts at the tip of the lead.

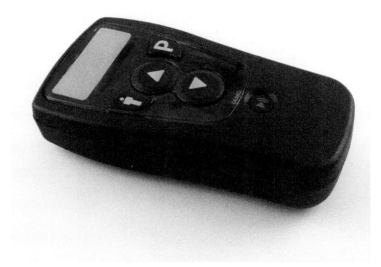

Figure 29-9 Handheld spinal cord stimulator remote control features, which include turning the device on and off, varying intensity, and choosing from multiple stimulation programs.

The practitioner simply feeds the leads into the posterior epidural space via the introducer needle, adjusting them under fluoroscopic guidance until the patient verbally reports that the stimulation covers the area of pain and there is no aberrant stimulation. A stitch or a StayFIX® pad anchors the leads to the skin. After the practitioner connects the leads to a small connection wire, it is necessary to dress the area in standard sterile fashion, usually with a 4 × 4 bandage and Tegaderm. The connection wire plugs into an outside generator that sits in a pouch that the patient wears. A handheld device (Fig. 29-9) controls stimulation features, which include turning the device on and off, varying intensity, and choosing from multiple stimulation programs. The patient then goes home shortly after the procedure.

The trial period offers the unique opportunity for the patient to experience what life is like with the implant before deciding to have it permanently. There is essentially no other surgical procedure allowing the patient to try it out first. Once you get a new hip or new knee, the procedure is not reversible. A spinal cord stimulator trial is like "leasing with an option to buy." During this phase, the patient is able to assess the utility of the spinal cord stimulator under everyday conditions, activities, and posture. The patient makes adjustments to the stimulator settings via the handheld device to obtain the best possible coverage. The two primary restrictions are no showering

(sponge baths are allowed) and no lifting of heavy objects greater than 10 pounds. The trial typically lasts for 3 to 7 days. After the trial period, the patient returns to the office and the trial leads are removed. To remove the leads simply release the stitches and apply light traction to the leads and they should slip out. The trial is considered positive if the patient has at least 50% pain relief, no significant side effects, and would like to progress to implantation.

HOW TO PERFORM THE PROCEDURE

Trial—Lower Body Pain

The procedure is fully explained to the patient, all questions answered, and informed consent obtained. The patient is given preoperative antibiotics; I use 2 g of Ancef. The patient is brought to the fluoroscopy suite and placed on the fluoroscopic table in the prone position (face down). One to two pillows are placed under the abdomen, which opens up access to the epidural space between the lumbar vertebrae. A "time out" is performed prior to the procedure including verbal confirmation of correct patient, procedure and procedural site. Noninvasive hemodynamic monitors and pulse oximetry are placed. The skin is prepped with betadine and drapes are placed over the area and fluoroscope in standard sterile fashion. The fluoroscope is placed in the anteroposterior (AP) position, then tilted

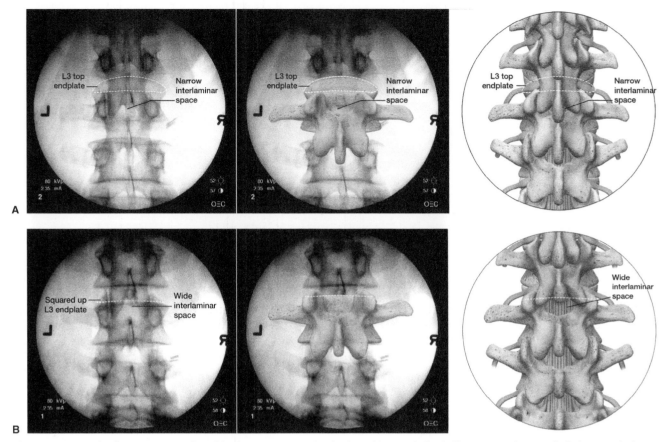

Figure 29-10 The fluoroscope is placed in the anteroposterior (AP) position and tilted, if necessary, in a cephalad to caudad motion to "square up" the endplates of the vertebral bodies. **A.** In the first panel of pictures the top of the L3 vertebral body is slanted which narrows the entry to the interlaminar space. **B.** In the second panel of pictures the angle of the camera has been adjusted in a cephalad position to "square up" the top of the L3 vertebral body which widens the entry to the interlaminar space making the procedure easier to perform.

if necessary in a cephalad to caudad motion to "square up" the endplates of the vertebral bodies (Fig. 29-10).

Needle entry into the epidural space between the laminae of T12 and L1 is optimal. Based on the patients individual anatomy, an epidural space above or two below T12–L1 may be chosen. Needle angle should be 45 degrees or less when entering the epidural space so the leads will be at an angle that will allow them to glide along the posterior epidural space. To accomplish this the needle needs to enter the skin not above the epidural space you are targeting but a level or two below it. The touhy needle should be introduced paramedianly and advanced medially so as to enter at the mid line. For example, using a metal marker and a felt-tip marking pen, an "X" is placed on the skin overlying the right L2 lamina (Fig. 29-11). The skin and subcutaneous tissue are anesthetized with 2% lidocaine using a 1.5-in, 25-gauge needle. After the skin and subcutaneous tissue are anesthetized. A 3.5 22 gauge spinal needle is used to numb the predetermind path of the tuohy needle. This provides an extra layer of patient

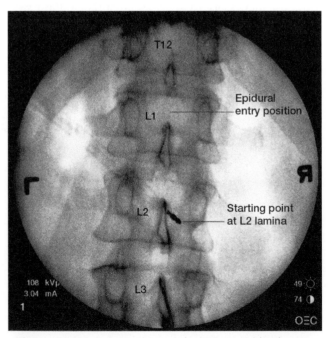

Figure 29-11 Entry position at the T12–L1 epidural space.

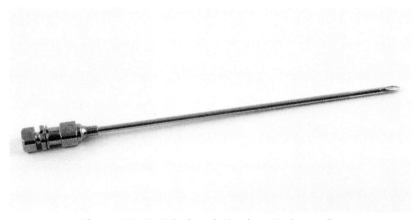

Figure 29-12 Spinal cord stimulator Tuohy needle.

comfort. Next an 18 gauge needle is used to make a puncture at the skin level to decrease surface tension for the more dull like styleted touhy needle. The styleted Tuohy needle (Fig. 29-12) is placed through the "X" in a perpendicular fashion to the skin and parallel to the fluoroscope. The needle is advanced cephalad until bone contact is made with the right L1 lamina, the lamina above the entry point at L2. Once the lamina is contacted, the needle is slightly retracted and advanced superiorly and medially toward the center of the T12–L1 epidural space (Fig. 29-13). The needle then enters the ligamentum flavum, a typically thick

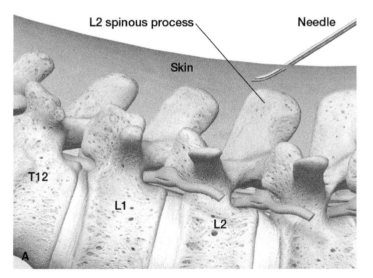

▶ **Figure 29-13** Needle path to properly enter the epidural space for a spinal cord stimulator lead. The path of the needle on its way to the epidural space needs to be shallow, roughly 45 degrees or less; therefore, the needle needs to enter the skin not above the epidural space you are targeting but a level or two below it. **A.** Needle position at the start of the procedure over the L2 lamina. **B.** Final needle position entering the T12–L1 posterior epidural space.

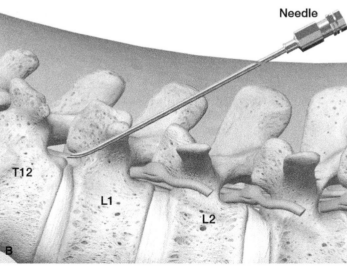

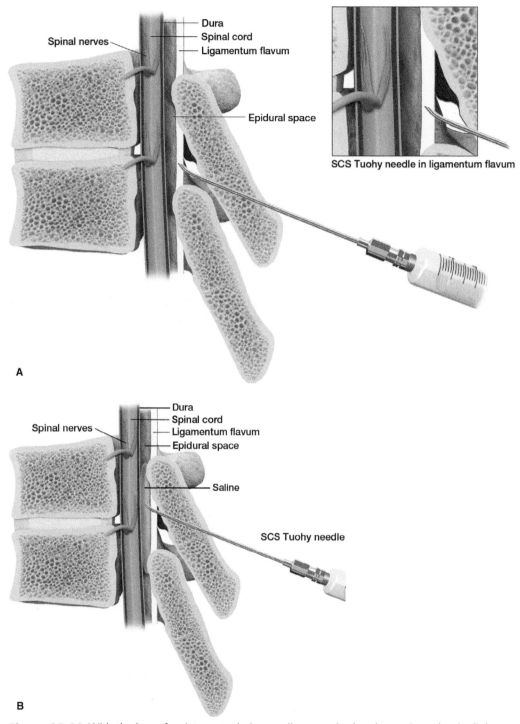

Spinal nerves
Dura
Spinal cord
Ligamentum flavum
Epidural space
SCS Tuohy needle in ligamentum flavum

A

Spinal nerves
Dura
Spinal cord
Ligamentum flavum
Epidural space
Saline
SCS Tuohy needle

B

Figure 29-14 With the loss-of-resistance technique, saline stays in the glass syringe despite light pressure being applied to it as the bevel of the needle is up against the ligamentum flavum. As the needle pushes through the ligamentum flavum preservative free saline is sucked into the epidural space by negative pressure indicating proper position.

ligament that "grabs" the needle as you enter it. At this point the stylet of the Tuohy needle is removed and a glass syringe is attached to the needle. I fill the glass syringe with 2 mL of preservative saline; some doctors use air. When the needle is in the ligamentum flavum, the saline stays in the syringe despite applying light pressure to the plunger. As the needle advances past the ligamentum flavum the preservative free saline is sucked into the epidural space by negative pressure indicating proper position (Fig. 29-14). This is known as the loss-of-resistance technique.

Needle position is confirmed in the lateral fluoroscopic view. Aspiration is performed, which should be negative for blood and cerebrospinal fluid. When all

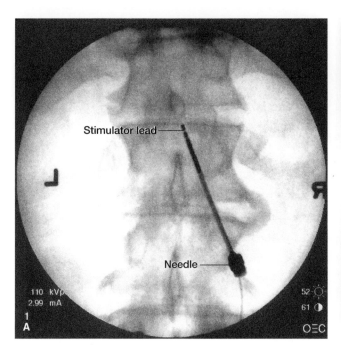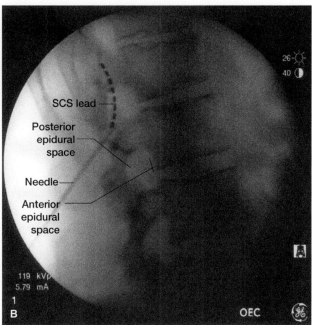

Figure 29-15 Spinal cord stimulator lead entering the epidural space in **A.** AP view, **B.** Lateral view.

these checkpoints are confirmed, a spinal cord stimulator lead is fed through the Tuohy needle into the epidural space under live fluoroscopy (Fig. 29-15). If the needle is properly positioned, the lead will travel cephalad without resistance as it is advanced. The lead may tend to drift laterally as it is advanced under live fluoroscopy in the epidural space and should be steered to stay midline. Keep in mind the slanted shape of the epidural space. If you enter the space too laterally the lead will have a tendency to fall off into the 'gutter' and then into the anterior epidural space. The lead is advanced to a predetermined level based on the patient's pain (Table 29-1). Always advance the lead slowly each patients epidural space will vary in size. Patients with less space may feel electrical sensations as the lead is advanced. Once the lead is in position take a lateral fluoroscopic view to ensure placement is in the posterior aspect of the epidural space. For most trials the interventionalist will repeat the same steps just described and advance a second lead to the predetermined height so that two leads lie side by side (Fig. 29-16). This can be done using an ipsilateral approach or a contralateral approach.

During this process the patient is awake and alert. Once the leads are brought into position, the steering caps are removed from the leads. The leads are then connected to sterile connection box that has wires that are plugged into a computer. When stimulation is slowly turned on, the doctor asks the patient where the stimulation is felt. The amplitude, pulse width and frequency are adjusted till the patient verbally reports excellent coverage. The computer helps the interventionalist adjust the leads so that they are properly placed.

If adjusting the settings on the computer does not result in ideal stimulation, it may be necessary to adjust the leads to the spinal segment above or below the current level. For example, the spinal level that correlates to the right leg is slightly different from patient to patient. The patient should report no aberrant stimulation in areas other than where pain is experienced. Once the patient is completely happy with the stimulation, the leads are disconnected from the computer and the stylets are removed. The leads are then anchored to the skin with a stitch or a StayFIX® pad or both. A final fluoroscopic picture is needed, which can be used as a reference for the permanent implantation or if leads migrate.

Trial—Upper Body Pain

For the corresponding conditions that affect the upper body, the same steps are taken to place the leads in the cervical posterior epidural space. A pillow is placed under the chest to help open the interlaminar space. Because of the decreased diameter of the cervical epidural space, only one lead may be needed. The typical entry level is T1–T2. For cervical lead placement your needle angle can be between 45–55 degrees and still

TABLE 29-1 Proper Level for Lead Placement—Lower Body Pain

Area of Pain	Common Lead Placement Target
Chest wall	T1–T2
Back and legs	T7–T9
Legs	T10
Pelvis	L1 (A lower entry point is needed)

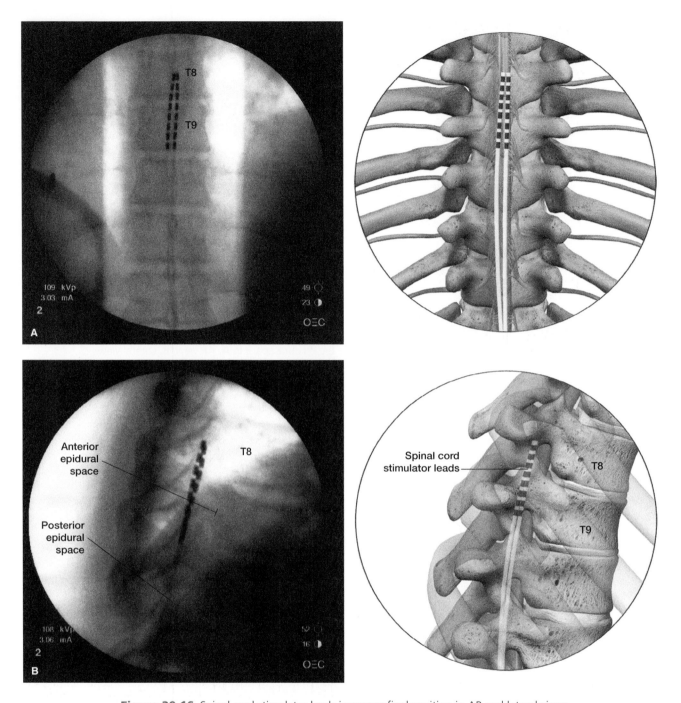

Figure 29-16 Spinal cord stimulator leads in proper final position in AP and lateral views.

have the lead advance up the posterior epidural space this is due to the natural curvature of the spine. The leads are advanced to a predetermined level based on the patient's pain (Table 29-2).

Full Implant

It is necessary to complete full implantation in the operating room.

TABLE 29-2 Proper Level for Lead Placement—Upper Body Pain

Area of Pain	Common Lead Placement Target
C2	Neck and shoulder to hand
C4	Forearm to hand

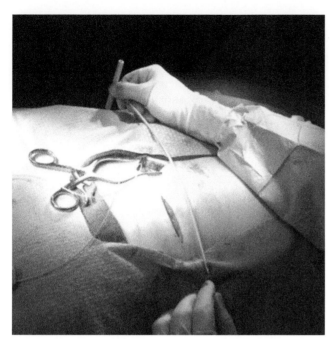

Figure 29-17 A tunneling rod is used to bring the leads from the midline incision to the gluteal pocket.

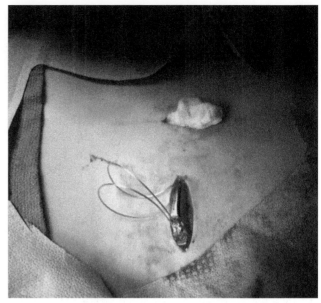

Figure 29-18 Battery pocket.

The incision site should be over the epidural space a level below the predetermined epidural entry position. For example if you plan to enter the epidural space at T12–L1 the incision should be over L1–L2. The skin at the predetermined incision site is anesthetized. A midline incision approximately 2 cm is then made. The skin is then dissected down to the level of the supraspinal ligament using both sharp and blunt dissections. Homeostasis is maintained with electro–cautery. Through the incision the same steps that were performed for the trial are used to place the leads into the posterior epidural space. After proper position has been confirmed. The Tuohy needles are removed over the leads while the leads are maintained in place. A lead anchor is then fed over each lead into your midline incision. The stylets of the leads are removed. Lead placement is rechecked in AP and lateral views to make sure the leads have not moved. Once confirmation has occured the anchors are secured to the supraspinatus ligament and locked around the lead. At this point proper lead placement is checked for the last time under fluoroscopy. Attention is then drawn to the predetermined gluteal site, an incision approximately 5 cm long is made after the skin is anesthetized. Via careful dissection, a pocket for the battery is created at a depth no deeper than 2 cm (just under the skin). The goal is to create a pocket that matches the size of the battery. A battery template provided in the kit can be used to confirm proper pocket size. A tunneling rod is used to bring the leads from the midline incision to the gluteal pocket. The tunneling rod is introduced to the midline incision, where the leads sit, and tunneled to the flank along a preanesthetized tunneling track to the battery

pocket (Fig. 29-17). The tunneling rod is removed and the outside plastic hallow sheath that covered it is left in place. The leads are slipped through the hollow conduit in the flank to the battery pocket. The plastic conduit is then removed. The leads are attached to the battery. At this point an electrical diagnostic check is done to confirm the signal from the battery is properly transmitted to the lead contacts. If the connection fails often the leads are not inserted deep enough into the battery. Once a proper connection is confirmed. The leads are locked into place using the torque wrench provided in the kit. Both the midline incision and battery pocket are fully washed out. The battery is then placed into the pocket (Fig. 29-18). A generous coil of lead wire into the gluteal space is left to allow for changes in posture. Both the gluteal and midline incisions are properly closed and dressed. I use 10 mL of 0.5 bupivacaine injected around both the midline incision and battery pocket for postoperative pain control. The patient is then brought to the recovery room, closely monitored for an hour or so, and allowed to go home. The patient is usually seen in the office within a week of implantation. I do not allow my patients to lift anything greater than 10 lb for at least 6 weeks after surgery.

Larger paddle leads can be inserted by a spine surgeon in some advanced cases, which are beyond the scope of this book.

CONTRAINDICATIONS AND POTENTIAL COMPLICATIONS

Patients should not be treated with a spinal cord stimulator trial/implantation if manifesting any of the following conditions:

- Systemic infection
- Known allergy to stimulator material

- Untreated major psychological comorbidities
- Drug abuse problems
- Inability to provide proper feedback during the trial phase
- Extreme epidural scarring, spondylosis, or scoliosis that interferes with lead advancement

It is generally accepted that all patients should receive psychological clearance before undergoing spinal cord stimulator trial/implantation. The crucial issues are whether the patient has any major psychological disorders that would interfere with a proper trial and whether the patient is psychologically capable of having a device implanted. It is essential that the patient understands that the trial period may result in no pain relief.

Potential complications resulting from stimulator implantation include postoperative infection, hema-toma, inadvertent dural puncture and subsequent spinal headache. Potential device-related complications include generator failure and electrode fracture, both of which are rare. The most common reported adverse event is lead migration. There will always be slight lead migration, as the leads shift scar within the epidural space until they scar down. The exact rate of symptomatic lead migration is unknown as reprogramming of stimulation often allows the physician to recapture proper stimulation. However, further surgery may be needed to correct lead migration.

Postoperatively, magnetic resonance imaging is contraindicated for patients with a spinal cord stimulator, just as it is for those with a heart pacemaker. However, computed tomography is acceptable. The spinal cord stimulator poses no problems for airport security checks. Patients should not scuba dive deeper than 10 m.

CASE STUDY

A 54-year-old man complains of pain that radiates down his right leg to his thigh and down his left leg to his toes. The pain is electric, constant, and worse with activity. The spinal surgery he underwent 2 years ago only partially helped alleviate the pain. Postoperative images are appropriate, showing a good decompression with no neuro-compressive lesions. Before surgery, the man underwent a series of epidural steroid injections, which had no effect. Since surgery, he has had another round of epidural steroid injections. He is participating in physical therapy and takes Percocet and amitriptyline. He states that the pain disrupts his daily life and that he would eventually like to be off pain medication.

You refer the patient to a pain management specialist trained in spinal cord stimulation. In a trial, he has a positive response, a 75% reduction of his pain. So he has a spinal cord stimulator implanted. The patient is able to obtain partial coverage over the right leg and full coverage over the left leg. The patient's pain is significantly reduced; he is able to stop taking all narcotics but takes amitriptyline to help with residual pain.

REFERENCES

1. Melzack R, Wall PD. Pain mechanisms: A new theory. *Science.* 1965;150:971–979.
2. Kemler MA, Barendse GA, van Kleef M, et al. Spinal cord stimulation in patients with chronic reflex sympathetic dystrophy. *N Engl J Med.* 2000;343:618–624.
3. Jacobs MJ, Jörning PJ, Beckers RC, et al. Foot salvage and improvement of microvascular blood flow as a result of epidural spinal cord electrical stimulation. *J Vasc Surg.* 1990;12(3):354–360.

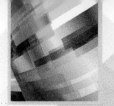

CHAPTER 30

Programmable Intrathecal Pain Pump

WHEN TO USE

HOW TO PERFORM THE PROCEDURES
▶ **The Trial**
▶ **Full Implantation**
▶ **Pump Refills**

CONTRAINDICATIONS AND POTENTIAL COMPLICATIONS

There are several ways of delivering pain medication. Typical routes of administration are oral, transdermal, intramuscular, intravenous, and epidural. Programmable intrathecal pain pumps were developed to treat pain on a tertiary level. They deliver medication via a catheter directly to the intrathecal space, the fluid-filled space between the thin layers of tissue that cover the brain and spinal cord. The intrathecal administration of centrally acting agents bypasses the blood–brain barrier, resulting in much higher concentrations of medication in the cerebrospinal fluid (CSF).

Inadequate methods for treatment of cancer pain helped stimulate the development of the programmable intrathecal pump. Some cancer patients with painful forms of the disease require escalating doses of opioids for proper pain control. At a critical point in their cancer-related pain management, the standard administration of escalating pain medications causes systemic side effects with or without pain relief. The equivalent dose of opioids needed to control pain becomes overwhelming, causing sedation, nausea, severe constipation, and emesis. The rationale in the development of the programmable intrathecal pump is that it can deliver a fraction of the systemically needed medication directly to the central nervous system (CNS), achieving the same level of pain control with less drug-induced side effects. The equivalent dose of morphine given intrathecally is only 1/300 the amount given orally in a 24-hour period. Intrathecal administration can allow for much more effective pain control.

The pump delivers a continuous infusion of medication directly to the CNS that can be adjusted according to analgesia and/or side effects (Fig. 30-1). The solution usually infused is morphine but fentanyl or Dilaudid can be used as well, to which an adjuvant medication can be added. The most common adjuvant

medication used is the local anesthetic bupivacaine (a longer-acting local anesthetic). Ziconotide and clonidine are used as well. Adding adjuvant drugs to the opioid solution can enhance the treatment regimen, acting synergistically.

WHEN TO USE

Intrathecal pain pumps are reserved for patients who have failed conservative treatment with medications and primary pain procedures. Intrathecal analgesia is appropriate for approximately 5% to 10% of cancer patients.[1]

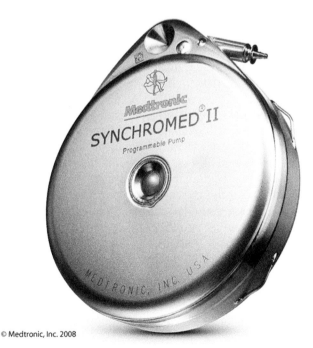

© Medtronic, Inc. 2008

Figure 30-1 Implanted programmable pump for intrathecal administration of medication.

A randomized clinical trial comparing the impact of adding intrathecal analgesia to medical management with that of medical management alone in patients with refractory cancer pain found that intrathecal therapy improved pain scores, reduced the incidence of drug-related toxicity, reduced reliance on systemic analgesia, improved survival rates, and also improved the quality of life of both the patients and their caregivers.[2]

As with most procedures, proper patient selection helps predict success. For best results, it is essential that patients have chronic pain, defined as lasting longer than 3 to 4 months; be expected to live more than 3 months; have pain that is not relieved by optimal medical management; and have no untreated psychopathology that impedes treatment success. In clinical practice, a number of interventional pain management physicians have stopped using programmable intrathecal pumps for conditions other than cancer. Several complications related to the procedure, device, and its maintenance over time often outweigh the theoretical advantages of programmable intrathecal pain pump use in noncancer-related pain. There is frequently a continued need for oral medications. By the time these complications arise in cancer patients they have succumbed to the disease.

There is one other indication for programmable intrathecal pumps. Investigators have found that these pumps are clinically beneficial in patients with severe spasticity (e.g., cerebral palsy) when oral administration of muscle relaxants has failed. The pumps contain the muscle relaxant baclofen rather than an opioid.

HOW TO PERFORM THE PROCEDURES

The Trial

Before implantation of a permanent system, patients first must undergo a screening trial of intrathecal opioids to see if full implantation is appropriate. The response to the acute administration of intrathecal opioids is thought to predict the treatment's long-term efficacy. The goal is to see if the patient has pain relief and if relief occurs without side effects that would contraindicate the therapy. There is no proven method of performing these trials, but the following discussion briefly describes two of the most common. One method consists of giving the patient a bolus of medication; after gaining access to the intrathecal space, the practitioner performs a lumbar puncture and injects a bolus dose of drug of interest. Another method, more extensive method which is commonly used, involves placement of an intrathecal catheter under fluoroscopic guidance. The practitioner then connects the catheter to a bag of premixed opioid solution and often an adjuvant medication, typically bupivacaine. The patient is admitted to the hospital, medication infusion occurs over time, with titration until pain relief occurs. The trial is considered positive if the patient has at least 50% pain relief without side effects. This method allows the provider to determine if intrathecal therapy will be successful and what dose of medication is needed to provide pain relief before implanting the full system. There is no standard length for the duration of the screening trial, but the norm is 2 to 4 days.

For the trial the procedure is fully explained to the patient, all questions answered, and informed consent obtained. The patient is given preoperative antibiotics; 2 g of Ancef (cefazolin sodium) or 1 g vancomycin if the patient has a penicillin or cephalosporin allergy. The patient is brought to the operating room and placed on the fluoroscopic table in the prone position. Special care is taken to pad all pressure points. A "time out" is performed prior to the procedure including verbal confirmation of correct patients procedure and procedural site. Noninvasive hemodynamic monitors, pulse oximetry, and a nasal cannulus are placed. The skin of the back is prepped with antiseptic solution; drapes are placed over the area in standard sterile fashion. The fluoroscope is positioned in the anteroposterior (AP) position. The fluoroscope is then tilted if necessary in a cephalad to caudad motion to "square up" the endplates of the vertebral bodies (Fig. 30-2).

Using a metal marker and a felt-tip marking pen, an "X" is placed on the skin overlying the right lamina at L4 for a right paramedian approach. (A left paramedian approach can be used if that is easier for the operator.) The skin and subcutaneous tissue are anesthetized with 2% lidocaine using a 1.5-in, 25-gauge needle. After the skin and subcutaneous tissue are anesthetized, the styleted Tuohy needle that comes in the kit is placed through the "X" using a 45-degree angle, oblique paramedian insertion technique. The Tuohy needle is advanced to the intrathecal space at L2–L3, a level above where the skin was entered (Fig. 30-3). When the needle reaches the ligamentum flavum, the ligamentum flavum will grab the needle. At that point, remove the stylet and slowly advance the needle. When the needle reaches the intrathecal space, CSF will start dripping out, confirming proper needle placement (Fig. 30-4). Needle position is further confirmed on AP and lateral fluoroscopic views. A specially designed radiopaque intrathecal catheter is fed through the Tuohy needle into the intrathecal space. The tip of the catheter is designed so that it can be seen under fluoroscopy. The catheter is most commonly advanced to the level of the T9 vertebral body, under live fluoroscopic guidance. Based on the individual's anatomy, technically it may be more feasible to place the catheter at a different level. Once proper placement is confirmed, an adapter (included in the kit) is attached to the tip of the catheter. CSF should be returned easily via the catheter when aspirating with a 3-mL syringe. Aspiration should be negative for vascular flow. Proper placement is further confirmed with injection of contrast, allowing visualization of

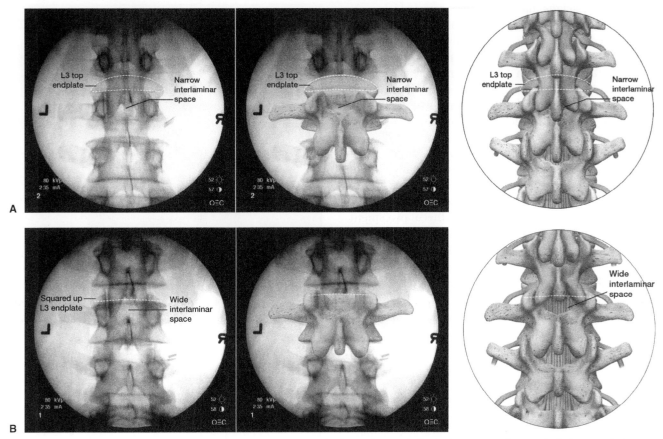

Figure 30-2 The fluoroscope is placed in the anteroposterior (AP) position and tilted, if necessary, in a cephalad to caudad motion to "square up" the endplates of the vertebral bodies. **A.** In the first panel of pictures the top of the L3 vertebral body is slanted which narrows the entry to the intralaminar space. **B.** In the second panel of pictures the angle of the camera has been adjusted in a cephalad position to "square up" the top of the L3 vertebral body which widens the entry to the intralaminar space making the procedure easier to perform.

proper intrathecal spread under fluoroscopy. For the intrathecal trial, the adapter is then removed so that the Tuohy needle can be carefully slipped over the properly situated intrathecal catheter. The catheter is then secured to the skin with a bandage and the adapter is reattached.

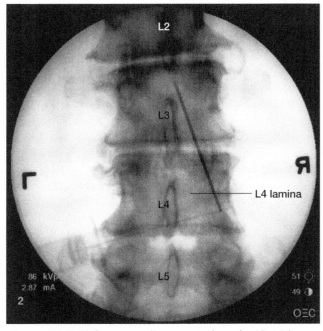

Figure 30-3 Right paramedian approach to the L2–L3 intrathecal space.

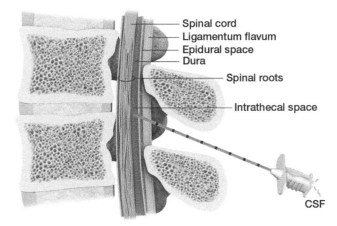

Figure 30-4 Touhy needle in the intrathecal space with CSF dripping out confirming proper needle placement.

Some physicians have switched from placing the catheter in the intrathecal space to placing it in the epidural space when performing trials for possible pump insertion. The procedure is technically less difficult in the epidural space, with a lower complication profile. Although the intrathecal catheter trial placement is optimal, as it mimics what the patient eventually may receive, it is believed that the epidural trial still provides important information relative to possible side effects and efficacy of pain. If the epidural trial is positive, the catheter will be placed intrathecally for full implantation. The amount of medication used during the epidural trial will be reduced by a ratio of 10:1 to account for the full-implantation intrathecal placement. See Chapter 17, Epidural Catheter Analgesia for instructions on how to properly place an epidural catheter.

Full Implantation

For full implantation, the intrathecal catheter placement procedure is the same as a trial except that the patient is placed in the lateral decubitus position. The skin on the back, as well as the flank and abdomen, is prepped with antiseptic solution. The fluoroscope is rotated so that an AP picture can be taken in the lateral decubitus position (Fig. 30-5). The same steps are followed as outlined in the trial to place the intrathecal catheter. A midline incision approximately 2 cm is made after the skin and subcutaneous tissue is anesthetized at the level of the Tuohy needle. The Tuohy needle is left in place to protect the catheter. The skin is then dissected using both sharp and blunt dissections. Homeostasis is maintained with cautery. Expose an area of the fascia that is large enough to place the anchor. A purse-string suture is then placed around the Tuohy needle (Fig. 30-6). A purse-string suture is a continuous circular suture that closes the surrounding tissue around the Tuohy needle as it is pulled together. The Tuohy needle is carefully withdrawn over the intrathecal catheter while the catheter is maintained in place. The

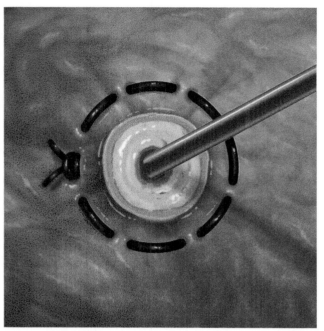

Figure 30-6 Purse-string suture being tightened around the touhy needle. A purse-string suture is a continuous circular suture that closes the surrounding tissue around the Tuohy needle as it is pulled together.

tissue pressure applied by the purse-string suture should be sufficient to prevent any CSF leak or minimize it, but not stringent enough to collapse the catheter. Once again, many physicians will reattach the adapter to the distal end of the catheter and confirm proper CSF return by aspirating gently. The catheter is then placed into the flexible anchor (provided in the kit). The wing-shaped anchor looks like a monarch butterfly. The anchor wings come together to close around the catheter; while doing this, grasp the catheter near the fascial exit site to prevent its dislodgement. Once the catheter is snapped into the center of the anchor by bringing the anchor wings together, the anchor is sutured into the fascia via the islets in the anchor, using nonresorbable sutures. Careful attention should be paid to this part of the procedure to avoid catheter kinking or torsion. After the catheter is anchored it should be checked again to make sure that CSF is easily returned, ensuring that the catheter is patent. At this point the fluoroscope can be removed from the operating area, providing more room to work.

Attention is now drawn to the abdomen: The skin is anesthetized over the site of the predetermined pocket location with 2% lidocaine. The provider should be standing facing the abdomen rather than reaching over the patient. The predetermined site is the lower abdominal quadrant that is face up at about the level of the umbilicus. An incision is made and a pocket created to fit snugly around the pump. The typical incision is 4 to 6 in. Homeostasis is maintained with cautery.

After the pump pocket is created, a tunneling rod is introduced to the midline incision, where the catheter

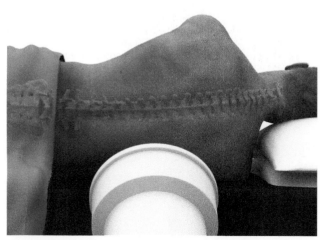

Figure 30-5 Patient in the lateral decubitus position, fluoroscope rotated to make an AP view.

sits, and tunneled to the flank along a preanesthetized tunneling track to the predetermined pump pocket in the abdomen. The tunneling rod is bent before using it so that it naturally curves along the flank. The tunneling rod is removed and the outside plastic hollow sheath that covered it is left in place. The catheter is slipped through the hollow conduit to the pump pocket. The plastic conduit is then removed.

The sealed pump in the kit contains normal saline. The normal saline in the chambers of the pump must be completely removed. A needle is placed through the self-sealing reservoir septum and 10 mL of normal saline should easily be aspirated. The pump is then filled by slowly injecting the preordered medication. The catheter is connected to the pump via the rubber pump connector (Fig. 30-7). The connector has three parts – the first is a strain-relief sleeve with a connector pin that is slipped into the intrathecal catheter. The pin should be advanced until the catheter is against the closest large ring. The second section is the catheter interface, which connects the strain-relief pin and sleeve to the sutureless connector. The last part, the sutureless connector, is attached directly to the pump. Position the catheter port of the pump at the pump pocket site in line with the opening of the sutureless pump connector. Guide the sutureless pump connector until the connector fully covers the catheter port. The connector snaps into place. Confirm proper attachment by tugging as if to remove the connector from the pump. The connector should be firmly attached. Next, fill the catheter with 1 to 2 mL of preservative-free 0.9% normal saline via the catheter access port, just superior to the reservoir septum, using the supplied 24-gauge needle and a 10-mL syringe filled with preservative-free normal saline. The pump is then primed, that is, it moves the medication slowly through its system to prevent leaving air pockets and an improper bolus dose.

The pump pocket and midline back incision are fully irrigated, and the pump is placed into the pocket. The pump should be placed with the septum side facing the skin and any excess catheter placed behind the pump to prevent damage to the catheter during refilling. The pump should be no more than 2.5 cm beneath the skin. The pump is anchored to the subcutaneous fascia using the assigned anchor loops on the pump. If the pocket is snug enough, anchoring the pump down is not needed. The pocket is closed and properly dressed. The patient is transported to the recovery room and admitted to the hospital for postoperative pain control and monitoring. Postoperatively, the patient typically wears a soft abdominal binder for 4 to 6 weeks.

Pump Refills

The pump is refilled with medication percutaneously via a self-sealing septum, placed just underneath the skin. Using a specially designed needle, the pump can be refilled by placing the needle through the skin into the septum of the pump. Tubing attached to a sterile syringe is connected to the needle and the pump is aspirated to remove any unused medication. Then a preordered syringe containing the patient's medication is connected to the tubing and the pump if filled. Refilling pumps is necessary an average of every 3 months, but this varies greatly depending on the infusion rate and concentration of the medication. It is possible for the practitioner to adjust the rate of infusion using a handheld computerized device.

To refill the pump the patient lies in the supine (face up) position on the examining table. The skin above the pump is prepped with antiseptic solution. The pump refill kit is opened and the drape is placed over the prepped skin. The pump template is removed from the kit and placed on the skin as you palpate the pump. Match up the template with the pump that lies beneath it. Often the pump will not be lying flush with the skin; to aid in properly matching the template, hold the sides of the pump when possible so that it is parallel to the skin. Once this is accomplished place the needle, provided in the kit, through the skin via the opening in the template (Fig. 30-8). The needle should pass through

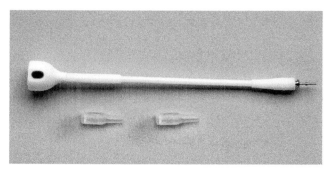

Figure 30-7 The catheter is connected to the pump via the rubber pump connector.

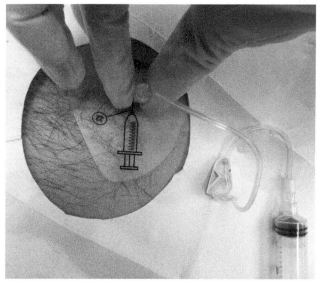

Figure 30-8 Pump refill: Pump template with needle entering the septum of the pump.

superficial tissue, then through the rubber septum, and finally into the reservoir of the pump tapping up against the metal back of the reservoir. The needle should be attached to the rubber tubing in the kit. The syringe provided in the kit is attached to the tubing and the remaining medication in the pump is fully aspirated. If you are not able to aspirate unused medication, you are not in the reservoirs. By analyzing the pump using the computerized handheld controller before the refill, you will know how much fluid to expect to be left in the pump. The leftover pump medication is properly discarded.

If the amount of fluid returned is significantly different than what is expected, the pump needs to be fully interrogated. This is a rare occurrence, but one of the most common causes is a granuloma formation at the tip of the catheter in the intrathecal space. In this case, the amount of medication traveling through the catheter is restricted and a significantly greater amount of fluid will be extracted from the reservoir than what is expected.

After the proper amount of medication is returned, the syringe containing the new medication is attached to the medication filter; the filter is attached to the rubber tubing after the syringe containing the leftover medication is disengaged. The new medication is slowly injected into the pump. Commonly, I will inject 2 to 3 mL of the medication, then make sure that I can withdraw the medication back to reconfirm proper

placement rather than inject the complete full volume at first. After the pump is filled, the needle is discarded and the pump setting is adjusted using the handheld computerized device to reflect the new reservoir volume.

CONTRAINDICATIONS AND POTENTIAL COMPLICATIONS

Contraindications to pump implantation include systemic infection, active intravenous drug use, and known allergy to the pump material or the medication recommended for treatment. Implantation should take place only if the patient has a positive trial.

There are three types of potential complications from pump implantation: Surgical, device-related, and drug-related. Potential surgical complications include postoperative infection, hematoma, improper placement of the catheter, and CSF leaks. Potential device-related complications include granuloma formation at the tip of the catheter (which stops free flow of fluid), catheter fracture, catheter kinking, and pump failure (the last is rare). Potential drug-related complications, which primarily result from human error, include inappropriate programming of the device, missing the septum during refill, and infusion of the incorrect medication or improper concentration of the correct medication.

CASE STUDY

You have been treating a 68-year-old man with multiple myeloma for the past year. He complains of pain in multiple parts of his body. You have followed the World Health Organization analgesia ladder to help control his pain, escalating the medication for symptomatic relief. During this time, the man visits a pain management specialist for a consult and to see if a procedure to aid in proper pain control is possible. The patient is currently taking OxyContin (oxycodone) 60 mg q8h, naproxen 500 mg bid, and Percocet (oxycodone and acetaminophen) 10/325 one tab q4–6h prn, and he has recently received a pamidronate

infusion. The patient reports that the medication moderately helps with the pain but makes him very drowsy and very constipated. His wife adds that his quality of life has completely diminished over the last 6 months.

The pain specialist recommends a trial of intrathecal opioids. The patient undergoes a 3-day trial in the hospital with intrathecal catheter placement for morphine and bupivacaine infusion, experiencing a substantial decrease in his pain, without side effects. Ten days later, the patient has implantation of a permanent pump. The patient lives for another 13 months with good pain management before succumbing to the myeloma.

REFERENCES

1. Paice JA, Penn RD, Shott S. Intraspinal morphine for chronic pain: A retrospective, multicenter study. *J Pain Symptom Manage.* 1996;11(2):71–80.

2. Smith TJ, Staats PS, Deer T, et al. Randomized clinical trial of an implantable drug delivery system compared with comprehensive medical management for refractory cancer pain: Impact on pain, drug-related toxicity, and survival. *J Clin Oncol.* 2002;20(19):4040–4049.

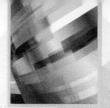

CHAPTER 31

Percutaneous Lumbar Disc Decompression

WHEN TO USE	CONTRAINDICATIONS AND POTENTIAL COMPLICATIONS
HOW TO PERFORM THE PROCEDURE	

A vertebral disc is built like a jelly doughnut. The inner jelly part is the nucleus pulposus and the outer layer is the anulus fibrosus (Fig. 31-1). The anulus fibrosus can become weak, which causes the nucleus pulposus to herniate into it and sometimes through it. This herniation of disc material out of its normal position causes compression and irritation of the adjacent nerve root (Fig. 31-2). This irritation is termed radicular pain. When a nerve root is irritated, it sends an aberrant signal up to the brain, which is interpreted as pain along the entire nerve. For example, when the L5 nerve root is irritated, it sends an aberrant signal up to the brain, which tricks the brain into thinking pain is not just at the nerve root but along the course of the entire L5 nerve. People often describe this sensation as a burning, electric, sharp pain that can be constant or intermittent. It starts in the lower back/buttocks and radiates down one leg or both.

Most disc herniations (90%) occur in the disc that lies between the fourth and fifth lumbar vertebral bodies (L4–L5) and the disc that lies between the fifth lumbar vertebral body and the sacrum (L5–S1). This is a matter of physics, because the greatest range of motion in the spine is at the L4–L5 and L5–S1 levels.

Practitioners use several measures for treatment for radiculopathy caused by a herniated disc. Earlier chapters discuss these techniques.

- Fluoroscopically guided epidural steroid injections. The steroids decrease inflammation at the site of injury.
- Medication. First-line agents include antiseizure and/or antidepressant medications used for neuropathic pain.
- Physical therapy. This can alleviate pressure on the spine by strengthening core muscles and increasing flexibility.

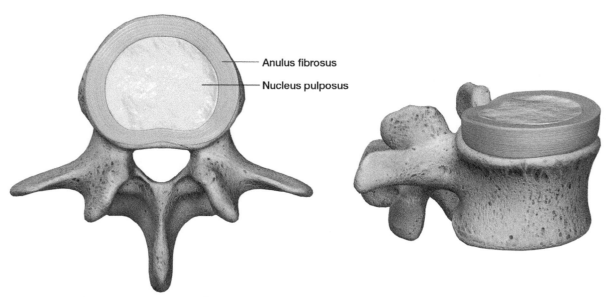

Figure 31-1 Anatomy of a vertebral disc. Inner nucleus pulposus and outer anulus fibrosus.

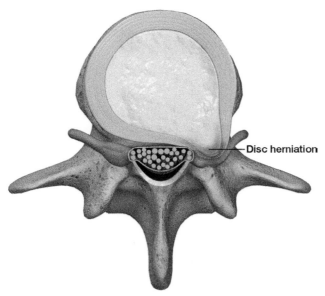

Figure 31-2 Irritation of a nerve root caused by a herniated disc.

- Spinal cord stimulation. Electrical current is used to alter pain perception.

The development of interventional pain management, however, has led to an explosion of techniques that attempt disc decompression with minimally invasive approaches.

One interventional technique used to treat radicular pain focuses on decreasing the amount of nucleus pulposus tissue. The goal is to decrease the amount of internal disc pressure by removing some of the nucleus pulposus, which allows the disc to implode back to its original form (Fig. 31-3). The objective of the

procedure is to relieve pressure on the affected nerve root without damaging surrounding tissue and to minimize postoperative complications. Pressure transducers placed in the disc have recorded a significant drop in intradiscal pressure after nucleus pulposus extraction.[1] A list follows of historical interventional procedures aimed at reducing intranuclear disc pressure.

Nucleoplasty: A needle with a radiofrequency tip is placed into the center of the nucleus pulposus. Using radiofrequency energy (heat), nucleus pulposus tissue is ablated in a controlled manner. The temperature at the tip of the radiofrequency needle decreases significantly in the tissue not immediately adjacent to the tip during the ablation.

Chemonucleolysis: A needle tip is placed into the center of the nucleus pulposus, and chymopapain – a proteolytic enzyme – is injected into the nucleus pulposus. The enzyme degrades nucleus pulposus tissue. The downside of this procedure is that it is difficult to predict how much material the enzyme will digest. If the enzyme is released outside the nucleus pulposus, it could possibly cause neurologic damage.

Percutaneous Laser Discectomy: This is similar to nucleoplasty, but rather than using heat from a radiofrequency tip a laser is used to vaporize a portion of the nucleus pulposus. Heat transfer from the procedure remains a significant concern.

Reimbursement for these historical lumbar disc decompression procedures, in which there is no physical removal of disc material, is no longer covered. In these procedures it is also unclear how much disc material is removed, if any. Mechanical percutaneous lumbar disc decompression with nuclear extraction has become a mainstay of minimally invasive disc

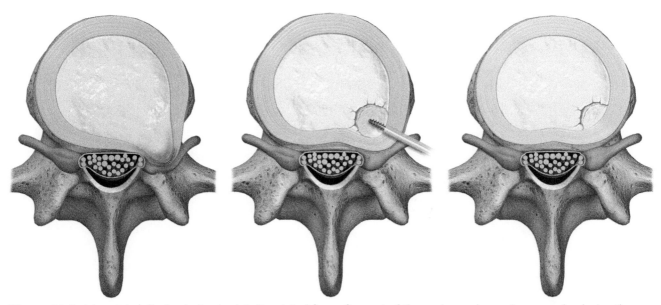

Figure 31-3 A herniated disc imploding back to its original form after part of the nucleus pulposus is removed reducing the amount of internal disc pressure.

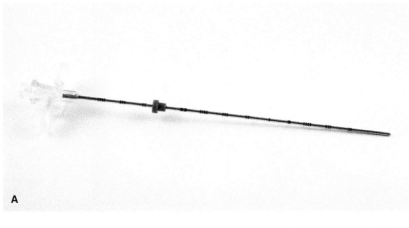

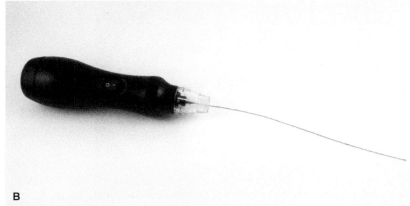

Figure 31-4 A. Introducer needle. **B.** Auger which is inserted into the introducer needle once the introducer needle is placed into the nucleus pulposus.

decompression. This procedure involves insertion of an introducer needle into the nucleus pulposus. A smaller needle with an augerlike device that rotates at high speeds passes through this introducer needle (Fig. 31-4). The auger is turned on and disc material is physically extracted.

WHEN TO USE

Mechanical percutaneous lumbar disc decompression is appropriate for patients with back and/or leg pain of at least 3 months' duration who have (1) failed to respond to conservative treatment, including fluoroscopically guided epidural steroid injections, and (2) a contained disc herniation (no radiologic evidence of free or extruded disc fragments). The disc height must be at least 60% of the original height. If disc compression has resulted in more than a 60% reduction in height, the introducer needle can not be properly placed into the disc.

Mechanical percutaneous lumbar disc decompression has several advantages. It is an outpatient, minimally invasive procedure requiring only a local anesthetic for comfort – the patient goes home usually an hour after the procedure. A physician whose practice includes a fluoroscopy suite can perform the procedure in the office. In addition, it causes minimal postprocedure complications and does not create scar tissue. If the procedure is unsuccessful, the patient can undergo traditional surgical discectomy. Trying mechanical percutaneous disc decompression first will not influence the results of follow-up surgical decompression.

However, it is important to note that controlled studies have found that percutaneous lumbar mechanical disc decompression is inferior to traditional surgical discectomy. In properly chosen candidates, traditional surgical discectomy may have an 80% to 95% success rate, well above that of percutaneous lumbar disc decompression.

HOW TO PERFORM THE PROCEDURE

The procedure is fully explained to the patient, all questions answered, and informed consent obtained. The patient is given preoperative antibiotics; I use 2 g of Ancef. The patient is brought to the fluoroscopy suite and placed on the fluoroscopic table in the prone position (face down). A "time out" is performed prior to the procedure including verbal confirmation of correct patient, procedure and procedural site. Noninvasive hemodynamic monitors and pulse oximetry are placed. Light sedation can be used, but

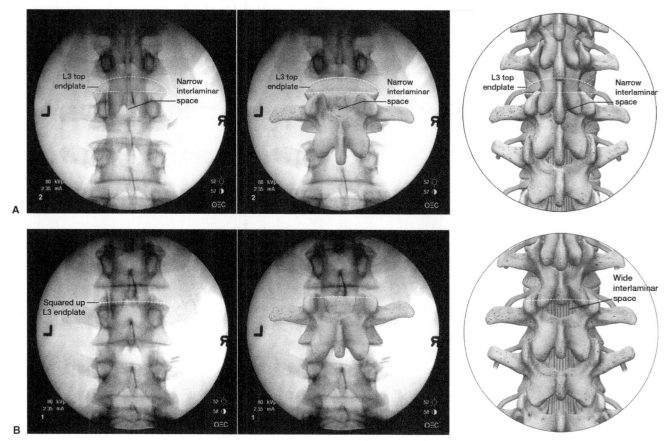

Figure 31-5 The fluoroscope is placed in the anteroposterior (AP) position and tilted, if necessary, in a cephalad to caudad motion to "square up" the endplates of the vertebral bodies. **A.** In the first panel of pictures the top of the L3 vertebral body is slanted which narrows the entry window into the disc. **B.** In the second panel of pictures the angle of the camera has been adjusted in a cephalad position to "square up" the top of the L3 vertebral body which widens the entry window into the disc space.

many practioners only use a local anesthetic the patient must remain awake to inform the operator if the needle makes contact with the nerve root as it is being carefully guided into the center of the disc.

The skin over the low back is prepped with betadine and drapes are placed over the area in standard sterile fashion. The fluoroscope is placed in the anteroposterior (AP) position. The fluoroscope is then tilted if necessary in a cephalad to caudad motion to "square up" the endplates of the vertebral bodies (Fig. 31-5). The disc of interest is visualized and the camera is rotated obliquely, away from you. The fluoroscope is rotated enough so that the superior articulating process divides the vertebral body in half (Fig. 31-6). This angle is the position that allows the best access to the disc. Using a metal marker and a felt tip marking pen, an "X" is placed on the skin at the needle entry position. This position is just lateral to the superior articulating process.

The skin and subcutaneous tissue is anesthetized with 2% lidocaine using a 1.5-in, 25-gauge needle. There are many percutaneous lumbar disc decompression kits on the market. All kits come with two main parts: an introducer needle with a stylet and an auger. The introducer needle is placed through the "X" in a

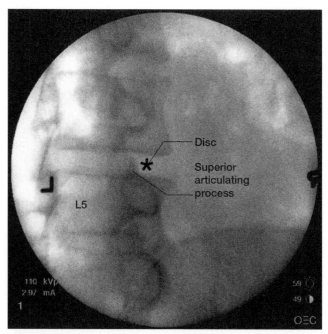

Figure 31-6 Oblique fluoroscopic view allows for visualization of the proper needle entry path to the vertebral disc. The fluoroscope is rotated enough so that the superior articulating process divides the vertebral body in half.

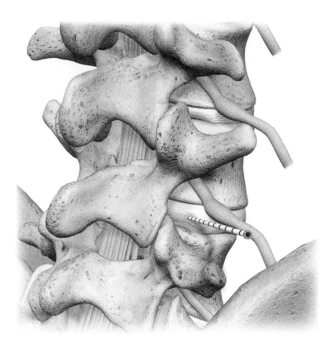

Figure 31-7 Needle position in the oblique view. The introducer needle is advanced until resistance is felt at the anulus fibrosus.

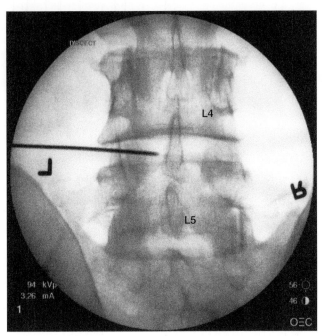

Figure 31-9 Proper needle position in the anteroposterior view.

perpendicular fashion to the skin and parallel to the fluoroscope. This is the position along an oblique path to the disc. The introducer needle is advanced until resistance is felt at the anulus fibrosus, in the oblique view (Fig. 31-7). Entering the disc through the anulus fibrosus is often described as feeling similar to a needle entering an orange. The camera is then rotated to the lateral position, which allows the interventionalist to know the depth of the introducer needle. The needle should then be advanced further to the middle of the disc (Fig. 31-8), keeping on a medial plane. Once this is accomplished, the camera is rotated to the AP position. The needle should be toward the center of the disc in the AP view (Fig. 31-9). If the needle is far lateral to midline on the side that was entered, the approach was not shallow enough, which is a common mistake. Because the iliac crest can obscure the oblique entrance to the L5/S1 disc, this level is the most challenging.

Once proper placement is confirmed, the stylet of the introducer needle is removed. The stylet is used to prevent tissue from collecting within the needle while entering the disc. The auger is placed into the introducer needle and locked into place (Fig. 31-10). The camera is rotated back to the lateral view so that needle depth can be monitored while removing disc material. The device is then activated, enabling the contained auger to extract part of the nucleus pulposus. The device is turned on for 30 seconds at a time and then turned off to prevent overheating the disc.

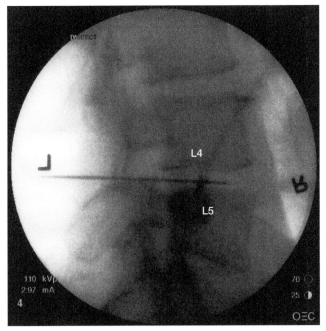

Figure 31-8 Proper needle position in the lateral view.

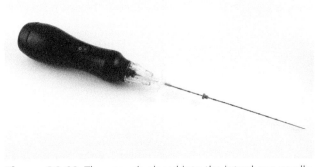

Figure 31-10 The auger is placed into the introducer needle and locked into place.

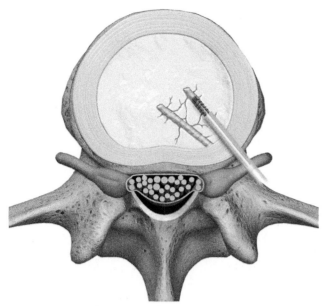

Figure 31-11 Channels made with the auger through the nucleus pulposus for extraction.

Under a lateral view, the needle should be adjusted to make channels through the disc to help with extraction, taking great care not to violate the posterior anulus fibrosus (Fig. 31-11). There is no set amount of disc material that needs to be extracted. Because of the potential for loss of disc height and lack of evidence that removing a larger amount is more beneficial, it is generally accepted to remove between 1 and 3 mL. The auger is then disengaged from the introducer needle and slowly withdrawn. Nuclear material is measured on the auger shaft. The auger can be reinserted, and often is, if more nuclear material needs to be extracted. After 1 to 3 mL of nuclear material is extracted, the introducer needle is removed and a bandage is placed.

CONTRAINDICATIONS AND POTENTIAL COMPLICATIONS

Patient selection is crucial. Patients who are poor candidates include those with a free or extruded disc fragment. Contraindications are evidence of progressive neurologic deficit; disc height that is less than 60% of the original height; any form of spine instability; and infection, coagulopathy, and pregnancy.

Discitis is the most feared complication. The disc is prone to infection because of its avascular nature. Two measures have reduced the incidence of infection: Aseptic technique and prophylactic antibiotics. Patients receive intravenous antibiotics prophylactically 30 to 60 minutes before the procedure begins.

CASE STUDY

Case

A 41-year-old man has back pain that radiates down the posterior lateral aspect of the right leg. He has had these symptoms for at least 2 years. He is currently taking Lyrica, has had a fluoroscopically guided epidural steroid injection every 3 months for the past year, and has also tried physical therapy.

A magnetic resonance imaging scan reveals a disc herniation at L4/L5 to the right that is compressing the nerve root. There are no free fragments or extruded disc material. You offer the patient a surgical consultation to have the herniated disc removed. However, the patient refuses surgery and wants to know if there are other options. You fully explain the mechanical percutaneous lumbar disc decompression procedure, emphasizing that compared with traditional surgical discectomy, the results are inferior. The patient still refuses surgery.

The patient undergoes the decompression procedure in the fluoroscopy suite. The practitioner removes 2 mL of nuclear material. After an uneventful procedure, the patient is released 1 hour later. Unfortunately, his pain does not improve significantly and he later opts for traditional discectomy.

REFERENCE

1. Castro WH, Jerosch J, Rondhuis J, et al. Biomechanical changes of the lumbar intervertebral disc after automated and nonautomated percutaneous discectomy: An in vitro investigation. *Eur Spine J.* 1992;1(2):96–99.

PART IV

Multimodal Approach to Pain

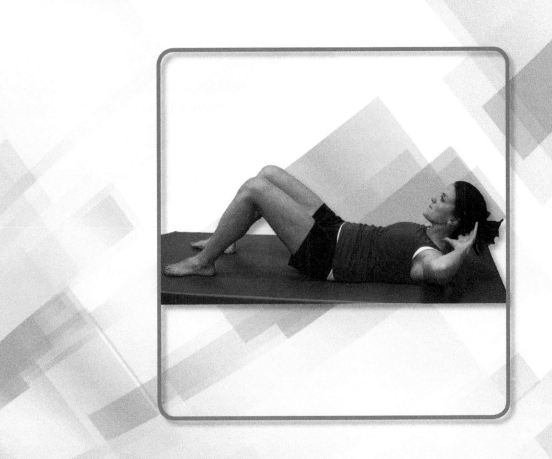

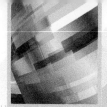

CHAPTER **32**

Physical Therapy

Physical therapy is used to preserve, enhance, or restore physical function and movement. The mainstays of this therapy include balance, endurance, stretching/range of motion, and strengthening. The goal is to alleviate current painful symptoms and prevent future pain. To accomplish this, the physical therapist acts as a motivator, challenger, and educator. Functional goals and targeted exercises are based on the patient's specific complaints. Physical therapists use a number of exercises, as well as devices, in treating patients. Patients are taught proper form and technique in performing these exercises, which helps to facilitate maximal response. Along with alleviating pain, physical therapy has been shown to improve mood and quality of life. The techniques are often useful in combination with other forms of pain management including injection therapy, medication, and surgery.

Physical therapists emphasize lifestyle modification, because environmental factors can maintain and in some cases enhance pain. Lifestyle modifications include alteration in posture and improvement in body mechanics to minimize mechanical stress during daily activities. Nutritional guidance may also be appropriate.

Acute painful conditions can resolve during the set time the patient is working with the physical therapist. For chronic pain conditions, the patient will need to learn how to take an active role in self-care and transition to a structured home physical therapy program. In the current health care climate, patients are no longer seen as passive recipients of therapy. Patients are expected to take an active role in their well-being and to learn to perform their own physical therapy routine after being properly educated – much like insulin-dependent diabetics who learn how to check blood

sugar, change their diet, and administer insulin after being taught the basics.

WHEN TO USE

Chronic pain patients often try to protect the area that hurts by avoiding movement that exacerbates the pain. This in turn causes a negative series of events to occur that results in deconditioning: Muscle disuse, atrophy, and loss of contractile strength. Tendons and ligaments lose tensile and insertion strength as well as tissue elasticity. In the absence of movement and weight-bearing, there is minimal remodeling of tissue which is necessary to maintain proper integrity. Vital structures are then subject to rapid tearing, even with minor stresses. Physical therapy breaks this vicious cycle of deconditioning and pain.

Wolff law, developed by anatomist/surgeon Julius Wolff, states that bone in a healthy person will adapt to the loads to which it is exposed. Connective tissue and muscle responds to mechanical loading the same way bone does. This is why people lift weights to maintain and increase muscle strength. To remain healthy, muscle and connective tissue demands regular mechanical loading. Exercise is crucial to the health of articular cartilage because it ensures the passage of synovial fluid over articular surfaces. This critical movement of synovial fluid over cartilage provides nutrients and removes waste; otherwise, waste products build up and articular surfaces degenerate (Fig. 32-1). It is essential that the synovial lined load-bearing joints, of the spine, the hips and knees, receive appropriate filtration. Interestingly, the spine's intervertebral discs are also heavily dependent on the same sort of movement. Lumbar spine movement facilitates

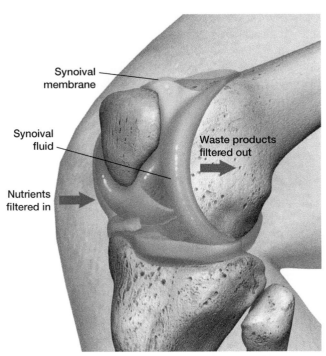

Figure 32-1 Synovial fluid filtering over cartilage tissue which provides nutrients and takes away waste products.

Labels in figure:
Synoival membrane
Synoival fluid
Nutrients filtered in
Waste products filtered out

critical fluid exchange between the discs and their nutritional source, the interstitial fluid surrounding the spine. Joint stiffness and pain are caused by deterioration and inflammation of the lining of the synovial joints.

Physical therapy is effective in returning patients to work and in decreasing sick time and medication use. It is especially important to start physical therapy quickly if a patient is too debilitated to work. Less than 50% of people who are disabled by their pain for more than 6 months ever return to work.[1]

HOW TO USE

During the initial consult, the physical therapist establishes a baseline of the patient's pain and functional status. The patient and therapist then define endpoints and a time frame to achieve goals, for example, they may decide that at the end of the program the patient should be able to walk on the treadmill for 10 minutes and lift 15 lb from knee to chest eight times. The patient should reach these goals through a series of exercises that gradually increase in intensity.

Balance

Proper balance is often a problem for people with chronic painful conditions. It can lead to falls and difficulty walking. Balance exercises are crucial to many physical therapy routines. Patients may require a device to aid in balance, such as a four-prong cane. Instruction on proper use of the device is part of physical therapy.

Endurance

One of the mainstays of physical therapy is endurance, which improves the patient's cardiovascular status. Working muscles may require energy faster than the body can deliver. This is especially true in deconditioned individuals, who have a decreased oxygen supply available to working tissue. The deprivation of oxygen leads to the early formation of lactate in muscles with use. In those cases, the working muscles generate energy anaerobically. When oxygen is limited, the body does not produce energy aerobically but proceeds to its next best option, temporarily converting pyruvate into a substance called lactate, allowing energy production to continue.

A side effect of high lactate levels is an increase in the acidity of the muscle cells, along with disruption of other metabolites, causing both pain and fatigue. This is one reason why patients have soreness when they start physical therapy. Endurance training increases capillary density, decreasing the diffusion distance from blood to muscles (Fig. 32-2). The positive change in the oxygen supply available allows for more efficient muscle dynamics with less production of lactic acid. Endurance exercises are key in becoming conditioned. If your patient is not keen on traditional physical therapy because they think it is too much, start with aqua therapy. I have had a number of patients decline physical therapy; starting it is just too much for them. When I suggest an alternative, aqua therapy – physical therapy in the pool, a number of patients are willing to try. These are often the patients who need it the most.

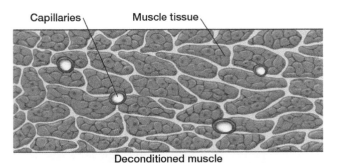
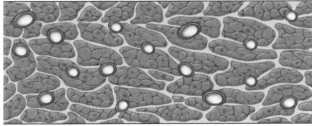

Figure 32-2 Increased capillary density decreases the diffusion distance from blood to muscles. This leads to a positive change in the oxygen supply available allowing for more efficient muscle dynamics with less production of lactic acid.

Labels in figures:
Capillaries
Muscle tissue
Deconditioned muscle
Normal muscle

Stretching/Range of Motion

Stretching is a generic term used to encompass therapeutic exercises designed to lengthen pathologically shortened soft tissue structures, leading to an increase in range of motion. Stretching helps to maintain functional ability, and it prevents muscle spasm and contractures. Range of motion exercises can be either passive (the therapist guides the patient, helping with the work of motion involved in the stretching maneuver) or active (the patient physically participates in the stretching maneuver). It is best to begin stretching after muscles are warm and the body temperature has increased. Stretching exercises are most effective when the patient holds the force applied to the body (e.g., a certain position) just beyond a feeling of pain and needs to be held for at least 10 seconds.

Strengthening

Strengthening prevents muscle atrophy and improves functionality. Strength training increases both the number and size of skeletal muscles and mitochondria. For strengthening, weights and resistance bands are often useful. Strengthening can also help control the patient's weight because it speeds up metabolism. On average, strength training can increase the resting metabolic rate by 7%.

Low Back Exercises

The number one chronic pain condition that sends patients to physical therapy is low back pain. The exercises used specifically for low back pain are geared at reducing pressure on the spine. They include low back strengthening exercises, stretching of the hip flexors, and abdominal muscle exercises. These exercises help to reduce axial loading on the spine's facet joints and decrease neural foraminal stenosis, which can lead to sciatica. The remainder of this section describes some primary low back exercises.

Lower Back Strengthening Exercises (Fig. 32-3)

- **Straight-leg raises.** Lie on the back on the ground or on an exercise mat, with the hands underneath the buttocks. The back should remain on the ground. Extend the legs. Lift them about 2 ft, keeping the knees straight, and then slowly lower the legs. Both legs can be elevated together or one at a time.
- **Supine scissor kicks.** Lie on the back on the ground or on an exercise mat, with the hands underneath the buttocks. The back should remain on the ground. Extend the legs, and alternately lift the legs in the air – lower one and then raise the other in quick succession.
- **Standing knee raise.** Hold on to a sturdy object and keep the back straight. Bend the knee and lift the foot off the ground. Raise the bent knee to waist level or as high as possible without going higher than waist level. Hold this position for a few seconds. Do a set of ten and switch to the opposite leg.

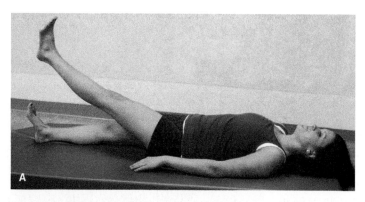
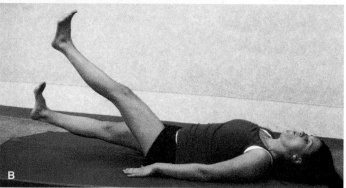
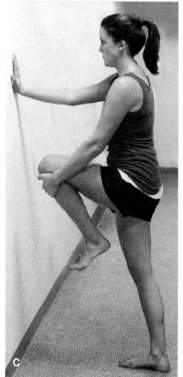

Figure 32-3 Lower back strengthening exercises. **A:** Straight-leg raise. **B:** Supine scissor kick. **C:** Standing knee raise.

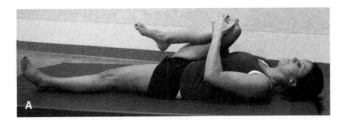

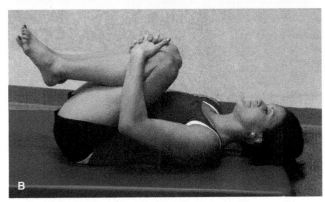

Figure 32-4 Hip flexion exercises. **A:** Single knee to chest. **B:** Double knee to chest.

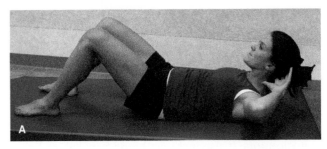

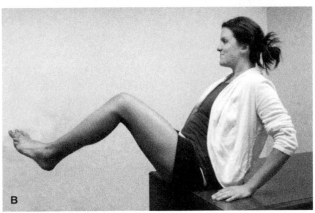

Figure 32-5 Abdominal strengthening exercises. **A:** Abdominal crunch. **B:** Half V sit-ups.

Hip Flexor Stretching (Fig. 32-4): The hip flexors function to lessen the angle between the upper leg and the torso. Tightness in the hip flexors leads to an inability to extend the hip sufficiently during walking, increasing stress on the lumbar spine.

- **Single knee to chest.** Lie on the back on the floor or on an exercise mat with knees bent and feet flat on the floor. Slowly pull the right knee toward the shoulder and hold 5 to 10 seconds. Lower the knee and repeat with the other knee.
- **Double knee to chest.** Lie on the back on the floor or on an exercise mat with knees bent and feet flat on the floor. Slowly pull both knees toward the shoulders and hold 5 to 10 seconds. Lower the legs and repeat.

Abdominal Strengthening Exercises (Fig. 32-5): Abdominal strengthening improves the mechanical efficacy of the spinal muscular support system. Abdominal muscle groups become contiguous with the thoracolumbar fascia, which sheathes the bundles of erector spinae muscles (Fig. 32-6). Abdominal muscles assist and enhance the role of the erector spinae.

- **Abdominal crunch with feet on the floor.** Lie flat on the back on the floor with knees bent. Point the arms straight up toward the ceiling with the hands grasped together. Lift the shoulders toward the ceiling. The shoulders should be only a couple of inches off the mat when the exercise is complete. Hold that position for a second, then go back to starting position, and repeat. Keep the back as straight as possible.

- **Half V sit-ups.** Sit about halfway onto a flat bench with the hands holding onto it right behind the buttocks. Extend the legs so that they are completely straight, then bring them back to the chest.

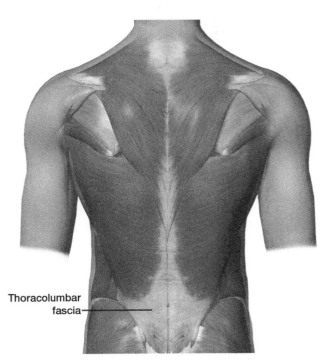

Thoracolumbar fascia

Figure 32-6 Thoracolumbar fascia. Abdominal muscle groups become contiguous with the thoracolumbar fascia.

OTHER MODALITIES

Heat

Therapeutic heat is a commonly used adjuvant to the previously described exercises. Heat increases the extensibility of collagen tissue, decreases joint stiffness, and improves muscle spasm. Heat relieves pain by stimulating thermoreceptors and decreasing activation of nociceptors. It also increases blood flow, which helps resolve inflammatory infiltrates and edema.

Therapeutic Ultrasound

The application of ultrasound involves using a round-headed wand or probe that is in direct contact with the patient's skin. Gel is used on all surfaces of the probe head to assist in transmission of the ultrasonic waves and reduce friction. Ultrasound is high-frequency sound waves above the range of human hearing. Original benefits were linked to tissue heating which leads to increased blood flow, reduction in muscle spasm, and increased extensibility of collagen fibers. Theoretical benefits include the stimulation of physiological processes, such as tissue repair, but this remains unclear.

Transcutaneous Electrical Nerve Stimulation

A transcutaneous electrical nerve stimulation (TENS) unit is a small, battery-powered, portable electrical device used to treat pain (Fig. 32-7). It has two to four

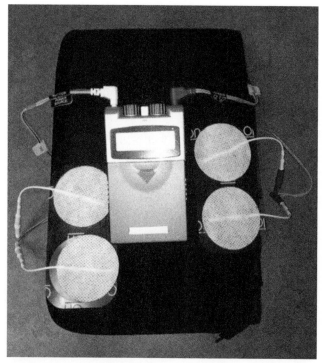

Figure 32-7 TENS unit.

leads connected to sticky pads which are positioned over the skin to cover or surround the painful area. The location of the pad varies, even for patients with similar conditions. The TENS unit delivers a low-voltage electrical impulse to the padded surface electrodes in a series of alternating electrical current impulses. The larger impulses are postulated to activate large myelinated fibers. Large nerve fiber stimulation is thought to block small pain-transmitting fibers. Some experts also believe that TENS unit activates the release of natural endorphins at the level of the pituitary by using alternating low-frequency pulses.

When the TENS unit is turned on, a light tingling sensation should be felt over the area where the pads are placed. The signal intensity also know as pulse width (duration of the pulse) produced from the TENS device can be adjusted, the goal being to produce paresthesia without muscle contraction. At initial use, the patient adjusts the settings to find the most comfortable effective sensation. TENS is virtually side effect free. The unit can be attached to the patient's belt for ease of use. TENS should not be used in patients with cardiac pacemakers or a history of cardiac dysrhythmia.

COMPLIANCE

Some patients stop going to physical therapy after one or two sessions, or never go. It is imperative that chronic pain patients understand that they are likely to experience soreness and fatigue with exercise when starting physical therapy. Their muscles have lost both strength and endurance because of inactivity. An increase in soreness after physical therapy is to be expected and does not equal a new injury. Setting up proper expectations when the referral is made begins with the physician educating the patient about what to expect. If the patient is extremely deconditioned, aqua therapy might be the appropriate starting point.

Physical therapy can be crucial in a multimodal approach to pain but is useless if the patient does not comply. It is difficult to assess patients' compliance because they often do not admit noncompliance. The medical literature on compliance cites many factors that are associated with noncompliance, with differing degrees of magnitude. Patients with chronic illness seem to be less compliant than patients with acute illness. This may be because patients with an acute illness can expect recovery, thus are motivated to be compliant with their regimen, versus the nature of chronic pain seeming insurmountable.

One noteworthy factor is an external locus of control, which leads patients to believe that health and illness hardly depend on their own behavior. Instilling hope can be achieved by emphasizing a positive outcome. This sets up the groundwork for your patient to comply with physical therapy. "This can help your pain," is a very powerful statement. It gives the patient an internal locus of control, from which the patient's actions determine the extent of recovery from illness. It is crucial to emphasize to your patients with chronic pain that the only way to get their muscles and joints working properly is with physical therapy. I often say, "We need to pump blood into the area that hurts you and pump waste products, that have been building up, away. No medication or injection I have to offer you can do this." The physical therapy regimen itself is a major determinant of success. Complex regimens lead to more noncompliance than simple ones.

CASE STUDIES

Case 1

A 58-year-old woman with chronic lumbar back pain from spinal stenosis, facet arthropathy, and lumbar radiculopathy has been your patient for a year. She initially took Percocet 5/325 one tablet twice a day as needed, and her pain level was suitable. About 3 months ago, she began taking an increased dose, three times a day as needed, because of increased pain. Today she is asking for the Percocet to be increased to four times a day.

After reviewing the patient's case and physical examination, it is clear that she has become more deconditioned. She has little endurance, is tight in the hip flexors, and has poor muscle tone. Rather than perpetuating a negative cascade of events, you do not prescribe an increase in narcotic dosage. Instead, you identify and explain the problem of deconditioning and make a referral to physical therapy. You tell the patient that it is normal to feel sore during the first month of physical therapy because there has been deconditioning with prolonged disuse of the spinal joints and muscles. The patient's physical therapy course is approved for two times a week for 8 weeks.

You see the patient 1 month later and ask how the physical therapy is going. The patient says that she never went. At this point, it is imperative to instill confidence in the patient and help her understand that back pain improves with physical therapy. Convince the patient that there is realistic hope that with the help of physical therapy, she can participate in some of the activities she previously enjoyed. During the initial physical therapy consult, the physical therapist and patient set specific goals for the 8-week period, including improving flexibility of the hamstrings from 45 degrees to 70 degrees in straight-leg raising, improving endurance on the treadmill from 3 minutes to 15 minutes, and improving posture. After 8 weeks, the goal is to have motivated and educated the patient sufficiently to continue these exercises properly at home.

Case 2

A 42-year-old man, a bond trader, has axial low back pain. He says it is a deep, dull, and achy pain that is worse with prolonged sitting or standing. The pain is also bad when he is on the trading floor and in constant, stressful motion. His physical examination and magnetic resonance imaging scan are normal.

The patient requests to be treated without medication. He knows he needs to lose some weight and says that with his duties of his current job, he just does not have time to go to physical therapy. Trigger point injections performed in the office have been helpful, but his back still bothers him by the end of the work day. He asks for another mode of treatment. At this point, you recommend a TENS unit. You explain how it works – that he can apply the pads to his back, attach the unit under his shirt to his pants, and wear it at work. On his follow-up, the patient is very happy. He says that he applies the TENS unit at mid-day, leaves it on until the market closes, and then slips it back in his desk. The patient reports significant pain relief with the device.

REFERENCE

1. Waddell G. Biopsychosocial analysis of low back pain. *Ballieres Clin Rheumatol.* 1992;6:523.

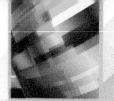

CHAPTER 33

Complementary Treatments

ACUPUNCTURE   THERAPEUTIC MASSAGE

COGNITIVE BEHAVIORAL THERAPY   HYPNOSIS

BIOFEEDBACK

Complementary medicine is defined as medical interventions not routinely taught at American medical schools. Although there have been great strides in conventional pain management over the past two decades, there are significant inadequacies, causing many patients to seek other options for controlling their pain. This chapter describes complementary treatments that do not involve physical therapy, oral medications, injections, or surgical procedures.

ACUPUNCTURE

Acupuncture is a form of traditional Chinese medicine established sometime between 4,000 and 5,000 years ago ("acus" means needle and "puncture" means penetration). According to traditional Chinese medicine, our body is balanced with a system of properly distributed energy called "gi" (pronounced *chee*). The flow of life energy – gi energy – circulates along our body in lines called "meridians" (Fig. 33-1). The gi energy that

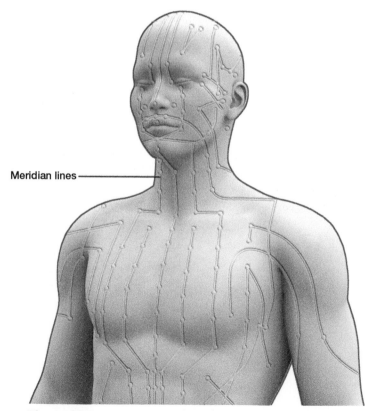

Meridian lines

Figure 33-1 Acupuncture: The flow of gi along meridian lines.

exists in the meridian lines is balanced, as is the energy of nature, according to the Chinese yin yang principle. An imbalance in energy is thought to be the cause of illness. Acupuncture aims at establishing and maintaining appropriate flow through these meridians.

In the United States, more than 3,000 physicians use acupuncture to treat a variety of conditions, including headache, musculoskeletal pain, nausea, and addiction. Patients usually undergo acupuncture sessions two to three times per week for a period of at least 3 to 6 weeks. When performed by well-trained practitioners, acupuncture carries minimal risk.

There are approximately 360 classic acupuncture points. Interestingly, greater than 70% of these points correlate with myofascial trigger points. Practitioners place the acupuncture needles along different meridian lines. The selection of needle placement depends on the underlying pathology. Recent Western studies suggest that acupuncture may have multiple effects on the body. Research has shown that acupuncture releases endogenous opioids – the same ones that are released with running, known to cause "runner's high." In one study, naloxone, an opioid antagonist, partially reversed the analgesia caused by acupuncture. Acupuncture may also activate large myelinated nerve fibers. According to the gate control theory, the stimulation of large myelinated fibers causes inhibitory effects on pain-transmitting unmyelinated fibers. In addition, acupuncture may lead to alterations in the hypothalamus, modifying the limbic system response to pain.

COGNITIVE BEHAVIORAL THERAPY

Pain is a complex experience that is influenced not only by its underlying pathophysiology, but also by an individual's cognition, affect, and behavior. Cognitive behavioral therapy (CBT) attempts to alter the psychological principles governing pain. Our attitudes, beliefs, and expectations determine our emotional and behavioral reactions to painful situations.[1] Irrational beliefs and distorted attitudes toward oneself, one's environment, and the future perpetuate depression and pain.

There are three pillars of CBT. The first component is helping the patient understand that cognition and behavior can affect the perception of pain. The second component is training – patients are taught the pain control techniques of relaxation, imagery, and self-coping. In relaxation training, exercises are used to decrease muscle tension, reduce emotional distress, and divert attention from pain. In imagery training, patients are taught to meditate on pleasant imagery to divert attention away from severe pain episodes. In self-coping training, how the patient interprets information is modified. Self-defeating thoughts such as "I will never get better" and "there is nothing I can do" are transferred into the healing thoughts "I am learning to cope and heal myself" and "I am learning how I can help myself."[2] Patients learn to gain a feeling of control over their pain. The third component involves applying what is learned in training to daily situations, including pain flares and other challenges.

CBT is typically carried out in small group sessions of three to six patients that are held weekly for 8 to 10 weeks. The groups are typically led by a psychologist.

BIOFEEDBACK

Biofeedback is the practice of providing information to the patient about unconscious physiologic processes such as heart rate and muscle tension. This form of therapy involves instrumentation that tracks specific physiologic indicators of tension in the body. The most common form of biofeedback involves using electromyographic (EMG) feedback from the affected region. The patient is able to see the electrical activity in muscle tissue. Patients are able to monitor muscle spasm and overactivity. With this information, the patient learns to control voluntarily a normally nonvoluntary aspect of physiology that may be linked to the pathogenesis of a given disease. Biofeedback is thought to be most helpful in low back pain and headache related to myofascial spasm.

THERAPEUTIC MASSAGE

Massage therapy which is often used for pain relief and muscle relaxation involves the rubbing, stroking, and kneading of soft tissue for therapeutic reasons. Typical forms include acupressure (Shiatsu), Swedish massage, reflexology, and myofascial release. Massage releases muscle tension and promotes relaxation. Physiologically, it improves blood circulation to the muscle. Improved circulation enhances tissue perfusion and oxygenation. This allows for the removal of lactic acid and other toxins from muscle tissue. Therapeutic massage may also help alleviate the pain caused by fibrous scar tissue.

HYPNOSIS

Hypnosis, defined as a state of focused concentration, uses an altered level of consciousness to harness the power of suggestion. It causes a relaxed state of mind, in which an individual is open to reasonable suggestion. The goal is to provide positive behavior changes to treat a number of painful conditions. Some experts propose that the hypnotic state may increase patients' control over autonomic nervous system functions ordinarily considered beyond conscious control. An induction can take several seconds or up to 10 minutes or longer. Contraindications to hypnosis include psychiatric illnesses such as schizophrenia and manic depression.

CASE STUDY

Case

A 47-year-old woman with clinically debilitating rheumatoid arthritis suffers from chronic pain in her wrists, fingers, knees, feet, and ankles. She has had bilateral knee replacements. She is taking methotrexate as a disease-modifying agent as well as long-acting morphine (MS-Contain) 60 mg twice a day and Percocet 10/325 once a day as needed for pain. The patient's pain level has been stable with this medication regimen.

During today's interview, however, it is clear that the patient is unhappy. Her answers are short, and her affect is flat. A simple and proven screening test for depression is to directly ask a patient if he or she is depressed. When you ask the patient, she replies that she is not depressed, she is frustrated by the prospect of not getting any better. She goes on to say that although the medications take the edge off the pain, she still has pain every day and wishes she did not even have to take pain medication. You explain that there is a way to help better control her pain and give her an improved sense of control. You explain the basics of CBT. The patient is excited and encouraged.

REFERENCES

1. Domar AD, Friedman R, Benson H. Behavioral therapy. In: Warfield CA, ed. *Principles and Practice of Pain Management.* New York, NY: McGraw-Hill; 1993: 437–444.

2. McIndoe R. A behavioural approach to the management of chronic pain: A self management perspective. *Aust Fam Physician.* 1994; 23(12):2284–2292.

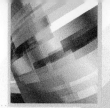

CHAPTER **34**

Chiropractic Treatment

MANIPULATION AND MOBILIZATION

Chiropractic care is a form of integrative medical treatment concerned with mechanical disorders of the musculoskeletal system. D.D. Palmer founded chiropractic treatment in Davenport, Iowa in 1890. His son B.J. brought it to prominence in the early part of the 20th century. The World Health Organization defines chiropractic as a health care profession concerned with the diagnosis, treatment, and prevention of disorders of the neuromusculoskeletal system and study of the effects of these disorders on general health.

The basis of chiropractic discipline is the philosophy that spinal joint dysfunction interferes with the body's overall function. There is a belief that spine health and general health are related in a fundamental way. This relationship between spine health and general health is mediated through the nervous system, as per this theory.[1] Vertebral misalignment, which Palmer called subluxation (Fig. 34-1), causes altered spinal nerve vibration (Fig. 34-2), that can be too tense or too slack, affecting the tone (health) of the organ attached to that particular spinal nerve. As per chiropractic teaching, vertebral subluxation is thought to interfere with the "innate intelligence" exerted via the human nervous system and is believed to be a primary underlying risk factor for many diseases such as diabetes, coronary artery disease, and hypertension.

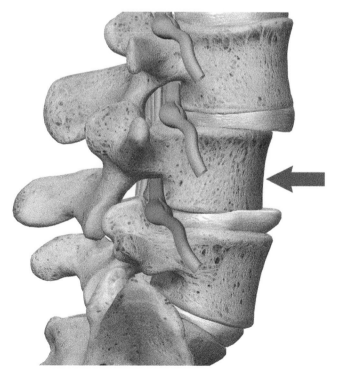

Figure 34-1 Vertebral subluxation.

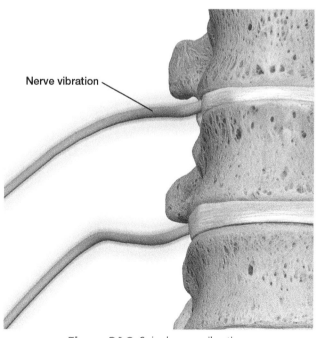

Figure 34-2 Spinal nerve vibration.

Chiropractic treatment sessions involve manual therapy of the spine, joints, and soft tissue. Therapeutic care also emphasizes a variety of lifestyle modifications – including diet and nutritional programs – as well as self-care and coping strategies for the patient experiencing pain.

Chiropractors divide themselves into two groups, "straights" and "mixers." The "straight" philosophy, taught by D.D. Palmer, considers vertebral joint subluxation to be the primary cause of all disease. The focus of straight chiropractors is to detect and correct vertebral subluxation via manual adjustments and not mix other types of traditional medical management. A survey of North American chiropractors in 2003 revealed that 62% believed vertebral subluxation significantly contributed to disorders of the internal organs (heart, lung, or stomach).[2] Mixers, who are now the majority of chiropractors, incorporate mainstream medical evidence. They believe subluxation to be just one of many causes of disease.

Chiropractic schools usually offer 2-year programs, completion of which bestows the candidate the degree of Doctor of Chiropractic Medicine (DC). Chiropractors are not licensed to write medical prescriptions or perform procedures in the United States. Their license to order laboratory tests (blood work) or imaging (x-rays, CT scans, MRIs) varies by state. A chiropractor may refer a patient to a specialist.

Chiropractic treatment remains a valuable tool for patients seeking integrative medicine options. At any given time, the percentage of the population that makes use of chiropractic care falls between 6% and 12%.[3] The most common reason for referral to a chiropractor is back or neck pain.

MANIPULATION AND MOBILIZATION

Most treatment involves manipulation of the spine, joints, and soft tissue. The two main types of therapeutic interventions are manipulation and mobilization.

- Spinal manipulation is usually a manual maneuver during which a joint complex is taken past the normal range of motion, but not as far as to dislocate the joint, in an attempt to increase its range of motion. Often there is a thrust, which is a sudden force that causes an audible release. Most chiropractors use a manipulation table to gain mechanical leverage during treatment (Fig. 34-3).
- Mobilization involves low-velocity passive motion to cause movement and stretching of the muscles and joints with the goal of increasing range of motion.

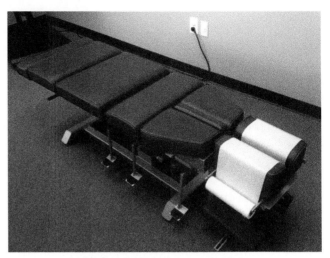

Figure 34-3 Manipulation table.

Some chiropractors administer electrical stimulation and massage prior to attempting chiropractic adjustment.

Individual chiropractors use a range of techniques based on their education and personal preference. Some of the more commonly used treatments involve the Thompson technique (which relies on a drop table and detailed procedure protocols), activator technique (which uses a spring-loaded tool to deliver adjustments to the spine), Gonstead technique (which emphasizes evaluation of the spine along with specific adjustments that avoid rotational vectors), and diversified technique (full spine manipulation). Medicine-assisted manipulation is a form of chiropractic manipulation in which manipulation is done under anesthesia, provided by an anesthesiologist.

During treatment, measurable improvement in the patient's pain and function should occur. On average, treatment consists of 6 to 12 sessions. Treatment should stop if there is no lasting improvement.

Vertebral subluxation – the core concept in the chiropractic philosophy that the spine is the origin of disease – remains unsubstantiated. Chiropractic treatment may be helpful as an integrative option for musculoskeletal pain.

In general, chiropractic manipulation is safe when performed by a professional in an appropriate manner. Absolute contraindications to spinal manipulation therapy include rheumatoid arthritis and conditions known to result in unstable joints. Although unlikely, spinal manipulation – particularly of the cervical spine – can cause complications that can result in disability. Manual manipulation of the cervical spine in some reports is associated with vertebrobasilar dissection, leading to a neurologic deficit.

CASE STUDY

Case

A 53-year-old man with back pain once came to see you, and you diagnosed lumbar facet joint pain. You initially prescribed an anti-inflammatory for pain and reviewed lifestyle modification techniques such as weight reduction, proper posture, and proper back support at work. The man returns and says that although the changes he has made since the first visit have been helpful, he continues to have back pain and does not want to be on medication.

You begin to present interventional options but the patient stops you, saying that he does not want to undergo any injections. Your patient wants to know what alternative options he has. You explain the basics of chiropractic treatment.

REFERENCES

1. Keating JC Jr. A brief history of the chiropractic profession. In: Haldeman S, Dagenais S, Budgell B, Grunnet-Nilsson N, Hooper PD, Meeker WC, Triano J, eds. *Principles and Practice of Chiropractic.* 3rd ed. New York, NY: McGraw-Hill; 2005: 23–64.

2. McDonald WP, Durkin KF, Pfefer M. How chiropractors think and practice: The survey of North American chiropractors. *Seminars in Integrative Medicine.* 2004;2(3):92–98.

3. Lawrence DJ, Meeker WC. Chiropractic and CAM utilization: A descriptive review. *Chiropr Osteopat.* 2007;15:2.

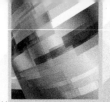

CHAPTER **35**

Avoiding Opioid Abuse

CURTAILING ABUSE AND DIVERSION
▶ Determine if the Patient Needs an Opioid
▶ Realistic Expectations, Prescribing Opioids, and the
  Narcotic Agreement
▶ Monitoring Patients Taking Opioids

HANDLING ABUSE AND DIVERSION ONCE DISCOVERED
▶ Addressing Violations of the Narcotic Agreement
▶ Discharging Patients from the Practice

A fundamental principle in medicine is to do no harm. Practitioners need to know how to prescribe opioids without doing harm – how to treat pain without the fear of contributing to addiction and abuse, how to provide medical pain management in a proper setting that protects the patient, and how to establish an environment and treatment plan that protects the doctor and his or her practice.

There is great demand in the medical community for guidelines on how to properly prescribe opioids and prevent abuse. A majority of this interest has come from the recognition that there is widespread opioid abuse. Substance abuse is a leading cause of preventable illness and death in the United States.[1] The prevailing perception is that substance abuse involves illegal drugs only; however, more Americans abuse medical prescriptions than use cocaine, heroin, hallucinogens, and inhalants combined.[2] Between 1997 and 2001, in the state of North Carolina, deaths from illegal drugs decreased whereas deaths involving prescription opioids increased 300%.[3] In 2002, in the entire United States, controlled prescription drugs played a role in 29.9% of drug-related emergency department deaths (opioids accounted for 18.9% of those deaths).[2] In 2007, overdose because of opioids caused 11,499 deaths more than heroin and cocaine combined.[4] Currently, Americans face an opioid abuse epidemic. Americans constitute 4.6% of the world's population but consume 80% of the world's opioids. They use 99% of the world's supply of hydrocodone.[5]

Failing to treat pain is not the answer to preventing opioid prescription abuse. Opioids can be extremely beneficial and positively life altering for patients with intractable pain but are extremely dangerous in the hands of abusers. The goal is to curb abuse and diversion of opioids while maintaining their availability for patients who properly benefit from their use to treat pain. Patients are far more likely to seek treatment for their pain from a general practitioner or other health care provider than from a pain management specialist.

CURTAILING ABUSE AND DIVERSION

Safe medical pain management using opioids can be accomplished by following this algorithm:

1. Determine if an opioid is necessary.
2. If so, prescribe an opioid in a well-informed manner (see chapter on opioids), establish realistic expectations, and have the patient sign a narcotic agreement.
3. Monitor the patient using regular follow-ups, checking pain management levels and functionality, conducting urine drug screens, and checking the narcotic database regularly.

Determine if the Patient Needs an Opioid

For acute pain in hospitalized patients, the use of an opioid as a first-line agent is reasonable. For outpatients in acute and chronic pain, other first-line agents are available. A patient who presents with pain does not automatically need an opioid. Practitioners can use nonopioids and/or procedures to combat pain before resorting to opioids. It is also appropriate to refer patients to a pain management specialist and not prescribe opioids. Several examples may be illustrative. For arthritis of the knees, a nonsteroidal anti-inflammatory drug (NSAID) or possibly a knee injection may be effective. For lumbar radiculopathy (sciatica), a neuro-pathic pain medication and possibly a lumbar epidural steroid injection may be beneficial. For axial cervical or lumbar spine pain, a facet injection may be warranted. For muscle strains, an NSAID or muscle relaxants may work. For fibromyalgia, opioids have never been shown to be helpful. Instead, try a medication approved by the Food and Drug Administration (FDA) for fibromyalgia: Pregabalin (Lyrica), duloxetine (Cymbalta), or mil-nacipran (Savella). For diabetic peripheral neuropathy, a trial of a neuropathic pain medication on a titration schedule may prove beneficial. For a multimodal approach to multiple pain alignments, physical therapy may be necessary.

If you encounter a patient who wants narcotics only and refuses other treatment modalities, you are under no obligation to prescribe them. If you encounter a patient who was prescribed opioids by another pro-vider and you do not feel that opioids are appropriate for the treatment plan, again, you are under no obliga-tion to prescribe them.

Realistic Expectations, Prescribing Opioids, and the Narcotic Agreement

If the decision to prescribe an opioid is made, realistic expectations should be established. Opioid-based treat-ment plans are doomed from the start if patients expect to be completely pain free. The goal is to develop a meaningful degree of pain relief and thus improve qual-ity of life. Rarely do patients become pain free – if this is the expectation then the development of a success-ful, nonabusive therapeutic treatment plan is unlikely. Unreasonable expectations lead practitioners to titrate up to 12 Percocet a day: The opioid is incrementally increased in the attempt to obtain a pain-free state. When the therapeutic relationship inevitably breaks down, the patient is referred to the pain management specialist. This is the classic "pump and dump."

Before beginning opioid treatment, the physician should completely review the chapter on opioids. Then he or she should discuss the narcotic agreement with the patient, and both patient and provider should sign it. The narcotic agreement is required for patients to be treated for chronic pain or for those needing their second refill on an opioid prescription for acute pain.

The narcotic agreement is critical because it estab-lishes a paper trail that protects both patients and practitioners. It lays out the rules so that patients are clear about what is expected of them. Pain practitio-ners consider the agreement advantageous because it outlines standards of care, initiating opioid therapy in an atmosphere of mutual trust and full disclosure. The document is an "agreement" rather than a "contract"; the latter implies a stronger legal relationship and suggests a greater obligation. It is important to per-sonalize the narcotic agreement based on the practi-tioner's practice and the laws of the state in which it is located. In addition, it should include the following points:

● The patient may receive prescriptions for opioids from this practice only and can use one pharmacy only, which must be documented. [*This is a criti-cal component of the opioid treatment agreement, mandating that a sole provider control all access to opioids and all opioids come from one phar-macy.*]
● It is the patient's responsibility to safeguard medica-tions. Medications may not be replaced if they are lost, damaged, destroyed, left on an airplane, and so on.
● Available alternatives to treat pain have been reviewed with the patient and the patient would like to proceed with opioid therapy.
● Opioid therapy can result in dependence, tolerance, and/or addiction.
● At each medical visit the patient must make a com-plete and honest self-report of pain relief, adverse effects of treatment, and function.
● Aberrant behaviors constituting noncompliance with the agreement include selling or lending of medica-tion, obtaining unauthorized prescriptions, altering prescriptions, using illegal street drugs, and escalat-ing dosages.
● Regular appointments must be kept to review the treatment plan.
● The patient must consent to random urine drug test-ing and pill counts.
● The patient agrees to waive privacy so that his or her provider may contact other providers to discuss patient care.
● The patient must disclose visits to a hospital emer-gency department and receipt of controlled sub-stances. The patient may receive opioids from the emergency department doctor if that doctor deter-mines that opioids are needed for acute care. How-ever, it is essential that the patient reports this.
● A breach of any of these conditions will result in ces-sation of opioid prescribing and possible discharge from the practice.

It helps to include a statement to the effect that opi-oids will be prescribed only during normal office hours.

Monitoring Patients Taking Opioids

It is imperative that patients have regular follow-ups. Most practices require that patients taking opioids be seen every 2 months, but the time span can range between 1 and 3 months. At each visit, the provider must check and document three items: Analgesia activ-ity, side effects, and aberrant behavior.

Analgesia Activity: Documentation of the patient's pain level should occur at every visit. A questionnaire is useful; the patient may complete it upon arrival, before the consultation; it includes a numeric analog scale, with 0 being no pain and 10 representing the worst pain imaginable. The number does not have to be 0 for the treatment to be considered effective – what is important is that the patient has meaningful pain reduction. To determine if pain reduction has been significant, it is essential to ask the following questions:

- Is current pain relief sufficient to make a real difference in the patient's quality of life?
- Are activities of daily living improved?
- How does current pain level and functional status compare with start of treatment and subsequent visits?

If the patient's pain level remains a 10/10 on a numeric analog scale with no meaningful pain relief and no increased function despite medication changes, opioid efficacy is highly questionable. In this circumstance, it is important to seriously consider weaning the patient completely off opioids.

In addition, it is essential that the potential for addiction be monitored at all follow-ups. Nonaddicted patients gain function and quality of life if their pain medication is properly adjusted. These patients will reduce the opioid dosage if adverse effects develop. Addicted patients lose function and quality of life with narcotics. Even adverse effects do not cause addicted patients to stop taking their medication.

Side Effects: Opioids can cause a number of side effects, including sedation, constipation, pruritus, and nausea. The previously mentioned questionnaire should contain an item asking patients if they experience any side effects; if so, what they are; and if they limit the use of the medication.

Aberrant Behavior: Aberrant behavior are actions that break the narcotic agreement. Evidence of the behavior will come from both patients themselves and third parties: For example, the patient will reveal aberrant behavior by calling to say that the medication ran out 10 days early. The patient may miss follow-ups. A third party will call you, such as a pharmacist, to inform you that your patient is trying to fill a narcotic script from another provider. Beyond these events, there are a number of other ways to monitor your patients by implementing the following steps.

Urine Drug Screens: One way of checking for aberrant behavior is by performing random urine drug screens. The drug screen tests for the presence of the prescribed opioid(s) as well as absence of unauthorized drugs. The urine drug screen reinforces the stability of

the treatment plan agreed upon by a patient and provider. It also protects your medical practice by documenting objective measures you are making to curb opioid abuse and diversion.

A number of companies would gladly make a no-cost site visit to set up a urine drug screening service. You will be able to personalize the test to your particular practice, but all urine drug screens contain some basic components. Federal workplace drug testing monitors the "federal five": Amphetamines, cocaine, opiates, marijuana, and phencyclidine (PCP). Most office-based urine drug screens do not commonly test for PCP, which is responsible for only 0.2% of substance abuse treatment admissions but they do test for the other four. There are minimum cut-offs for illegal drugs; nondirect exposure will not show up in the urine. For example, if a patient is socializing with people smoking marijuana but not partaking with them, marijuana will not be detectable in the patient's urine screen. It is important that the drug screen test for all the major opiates individually: Hydromorphone, hydrocodone, oxycodone, morphine, fentanyl, methadone, and tapentadol.

Urine drug screens address three basic issues. The first is the presence of illegal drugs, the second is the presence of the prescribed opioid, and the third is the presence of a nonprescribed opioid (e.g., one that you did not prescribe).

One, illegal drugs vary in terms of how long they stay in the system. Table 35-1 lists the clinical averages.

Two, if a patient has been compliant with the medication you are prescribing, the drug should be in the urine. Each opioid stays in the urine for an approximate amount of time (Table 35-2).

The product tested for in the urine is the metabolite of the parent drug the patient takes. Some opioids have different metabolites than the parent drug ingested (Table 35-3).

It is important to remember that if the patient is on codeine it metabolizes to morphine and that hydrocodone metabolizes to hydromorphone. Thus if the patient is on Vicodin (hydrocodone/acetaminophen) and hydromorphone shows up in the urine, it is most likely a metabolite of hydrocodone.

TABLE 35-1 Illegal Substance Detection Window in Urine Drug Screen Tests

Illegal Substance	Detection Window
Amphetamine	1–4 d
Cocaine	2–3 d (7 d for heavy or long-term use)
Marijuana	5 d (30 d for long-term use)
Phencyclidine	2–7 d (14 d for long-term use)

TABLE 35-2 Opioid Detection Window in Urine Drug Screen Tests

Opioid	Detection Window (d)
Methadone	2–4
Morphine	2–3 (possibly longer if chronic use)
Oxycodone	1–3
Hydrocodone	1–2
Hydromorphone	2–3
Codeine	2–3
Fentanyl	2–3
Tapentadol	2–3

At the time of urine collection the patient should report the last time the prescription medication was taken. If the patient reports taking the medication within the last 2 days, it should test positive in the urine drug screen. One important point to confirm is that your drug-screen parameters include specific immunoassay screens for each of the medications you are prescribing. If the patient is on the long-acting opioid OxyContin for chronic pain twice a day, the metabolite oxycodone should be in the urine.

If the patient is on Percocet (oxycodone with acetaminophen) one tablet every 6 hours as needed (120 tablets a month) and fills the prescription every month, this medication is being taken around the clock. The medication is needed everyday and that is why the patient refills the prescription for 120 tablets every month. Oxycodone should be present in urine.

On occasion a patient is not on a standing medication but uses the medication more sporadically on an as-needed basis. The urine drug screen comes back

TABLE 35-3 Parent Drugs and Their Metabolites Monitored in Urine Drug Screens

Parent Drug	Parent Drugs and Metabolites Found in the Urine
Methadone	Methadone and EDDP (2-ethylidene-1,5-dimethyl-3,3-diphenylpyrrolidine)
Morphine	Morphine and hydromorphone
Oxycodone	Oxycodone, oxymorphone, noroxycodone
Hydrocodone	Hydrocodone and hydromorphone, norhydrocodone
Hydromorphone	Hydromorphone
Codeine	Codeine, morphine, hydrocodone
Fentanyl	Fentanyl, norfentanyl
Tapentadol	Tapentadol

showing no opioid in the urine. The patient may state that either the medication was not needed recently or that the supply ran out days before the drug screen because they were overtaking it (a violation of the narcotic agreement). In these circumstances, a pill count at the next urine drug screen is necessary. I recommend retesting the patient within 2 weeks of detecting the abnormal drug screen to address the situation promptly. Based on the number of pills remaining, you can assess whether the patient truly has been using the medication appropriately. Here are two scenarios:

Scenario A: Based on when the prescription was issued more tablets left over than would be expected if the patient took the medication around the clock. This pill count would explain why no opioids were seen in the urine.

Scenario B: The patient has the appropriate number or less tablets then expected if the medication was taken to the daily maximum limit prescribed. No opioids in the urine indicates the patient is diverting the medication.

The third basic issue, it is necessary to determine whether a nonprescribed opioid (e.g., one that you did not prescribe) is present in the urine. If a patient is taking long-acting morphine for pain and both morphine and oxycodone test positive in the urine, the patient is obtaining opioids from more than one source. It is also important to keep in mind that pharmaceutical impurities can confound results. For example, morphine contains up to 0.5% codeine. Detection thresholds are typically established to account for this.

Prescription Monitoring Programs: Most states now participate in prescription monitoring programs, which consist of a database that tracks opioid prescriptions to individuals (each state has a different database design). As a health care professional you are able to register and then go to your state's prescription monitoring web page and look up patients by name and date of birth to see when they have had narcotic prescriptions filled, how much was filled, and who prescribed the medication. This should be routinely checked. The mid levels or doctors in our practice occasionally may find patients in their care for opioid treatment with a signed narcotic agreement who have filled five different opioid prescriptions in 1 month from five different providers.

HANDLING ABUSE AND DIVERSION ONCE DISCOVERED

One of the most difficult situations to handle is a patient who is breaking the narcotic agreement. Careful management is critical for the safety of the patient, the community, and the practice. Some cases call for a clear, direct course of action, but most situations mandate a judgment call. This section is designed to make the judgment call easier.

A small percentage of patients display aberrant behavior that points directly to the need to stop medication and refer to detoxification. Examples include the patient who has changed information on the prescription, one who has received six different prescriptions from six different providers while under narcotic agreement with your practice, and one who has survived an overdose. However, most situations are more ambiguous. The patient who finishes medication 3 days early and wants a refill or the patient who misses two appointments in a row. There are no hard-and-fast rules on how strictly to enforce the narcotic agreement. A physician must make his or her own professional decision. I will outline my decision-making process as a guide to formulating a system that may work well for you and your practice.

Initially, it is necessary to risk-stratify patients into one of two categories when prescribing opioids: High risk or low risk. The best available data indicate that all patients are not equally likely to abuse prescription opioids and break the narcotic agreement. Patients with addictive tendencies most often engage in multiple aberrant behaviors. Based on this critical piece of information, it is possible to risk-stratify patients and tailor their care to achieve the best results. The goal of classifying patients into these two groups is not to isolate and deny high-risk patients pain treatment with opioids but rather to increase the likelihood of a good clinical outcome. There is no consensus regarding risk factors that are most predictive of drug abuse. However, there is consensus about which factors put patients at higher risk for drug abuse. These factors include the following:

- History of substance abuse[6]
- Social patterns of drug use[7]
- Psychological stress[7]
- Poor social support[8]
- A focus on opioids[9]
- Exaggeration of pain[9]

If patients exhibits a risk factor from the list, they are in the high-risk group.

Addressing Violations of the Narcotic Agreement

Several examples are a good way to show how to handle patients who violate the narcotic agreement.

Example 1: A patient runs out of medication 5 days early. It is important to remember that any opioid that is altered and/or consumed in defiance of medical direction has the potential to be deadly.

- Low-risk patient: Refill the prescription early. Inform the patient that you will not be filling the prescription early again.

- High-risk patient: Do not refill the prescription early. Inform the patient that medications will not be filled early and that if this occurs again, opioid treatment will cease.

Example 2: A patient is taking Percocet. The laboratory reports that both hydrocodone and Percocet are in the patient's urine.

Low-risk patient: This "first offense" may warrant a warning, based on the situation and circumstances. The practitioner discusses the issue with the patient. If the situation recurs, discharge from the practice is appropriate. Even if it does not recur, the patient should have more frequent urine drug screens.

High-risk patient: Immediate discharge from the practice is warranted.

Example 3: A patient's urine test is positive for cocaine.

Low-risk patient: Immediate discharge from the practice is appropriate.

High-risk patient: Immediate discharge from the practice is appropriate.

Example 4: How often should a urine drug screen be performed?

Low-risk patient: The patient should have a urine drug screen once or twice a year.

High-risk patient: The patient should have a urine drug screen at least three times a year, especially if he or she exhibits strong potential for aberrant behavior, in which case it may be necessary to perform a drug test and do a pill count at every visit which I do with some of my patients.

Example 5: A patient is taking Percocet 7.5/325 one tablet tid p.r.n (90 tablets a month) and picks up the prescription every month. The urine drug screen shows no opioids.

Low-risk patient: The office calls and asks the patient to come in for a pill count and urine drug screen in the next 72 hours. If the patient is a no-show, discharge from the practice is warranted. If the result of the pill count or drug screen is not appropriate, continuation of opioids depends on the situation. A patient still in possession of all pills with a negative drug screen may be hoarding medication – it is essential that the dangers of this situation be addressed with the patient. A patient with no pills and a negative urine drug screen warrants discharge from the practice. A patient who is a few pills short with a positive drug screen receives a narcotic violation for overtaking the medication and notice that recurrence of the situation will result in discharge.

High-risk patient: The office calls and asks the patient to come in for a pill count and urine drug screen in the next 48 hours. If the patient is a no-show discharge from the practice is appropriate. If the patients pill count is short discharge from the practice is appropriate. If the patient has all their pills this situation requires further conversation.

Example 6: A pharmacy calls and states that a patient is trying to fill a prescription from another provider for an opioid (e.g., one that you did not prescribe). The patient never informed you that another provider has issued a prescription.

Low-risk patient: Check the database to see whether the patient has been receiving prescriptions from other providers while under narcotic agreement with the original prescribing physician. If the patient has obtained opioids using multiple prescriptions, immediate discharge from the practice is warranted. If this is the first and only time, do not allow the pharmacy to fill the prescription, and tell the patient that this is a narcotic violation. Gather information regarding the situation.

High-risk patient: Immediate discharge from the practice.

Discharging Patients from the Practice

I want to reassure the health care provider that clinicians are not obligated to put their medical license and practice at risk by providing opioids to patients who do not follow directions, which includes breaking the narcotic agreement in any way. One question that often arises: Is it the clinician's responsibility to taper opioid therapy if the treatment must be discontinued? Legal direction on this is purposely vague – saying generally that when possible, offer to assist patients in safely discontinuing medications. In my practice, we offer a 1-month tapering dose for patients when it is safe for them and those with whom they interact. Patients who sell their medication, take cocaine, alter prescriptions, or obtain pills from other providers are not safe to themselves or others.

If you are going to discharge a patient from the practice, it is essential to promptly notify the patient of the termination of the provider–patient relationship. To cover all bases, it is good to both call patients and send them a letter to have paper documentation. When patients receive the call letting them know they are being discharged, most are very accepting and know why. However, a practitioner's involvement with the patient is not over; it is necessary try to find adequate care elsewhere for the discharged patient. Sending the patient a list of practices in the area as well as rehabilitation–detoxification programs suffices.

REFERENCES

1. Stewart WF, Ricci JA, Chee E, et al. Lost productive time and cost due to common pain conditions in the US workforce. *JAMA.* 2003;290(18):2443–2454.
2. Under the counter: The diversion and abuse of controlled prescription drugs in the U.S. National Center on Addiction and Substance Abuse at Columbia University (CASA), New York, NY; 2005.
3. North Carolina Department of Health and Human Services. Findings and recommendations of the task force to prevent deaths from unintentional drug overdoses in North Carolina, 2003. Division of Public Health, Injury and Violence Prevention Branch, Raleigh, NC.
4. Okie S. A flood of opioids, a rising tide of death. *N Engl J Med.* 2010;363(21):1981–1985.
5. Wang J, Christo PJ. The influence of prescription monitoring programs on chronic pain management. *Pain Physician.* 2009;12(3):507–515.
6. Webster LR, Webster RM. Predicting aberrant behaviors in opioid-treated patients: preliminary validation of the Opioid Risk Tool. *Pain Med.* 2005;6(6):432–442.
7. Savage SR. Assessment for addiction in pain-treatment settings. *Clin J Pain.* 2002;18(4 Suppl):S28–S38.
8. Dunbar SA, Katz NP. Chronic opioid therapy for nonmalignant pain in patients with a history of substance abuse: report of 20 cases. *J Pain Symptom Manage.* 1996;11(3):163–171.
9. Atluri S, Sudarshan G. A screening tool to determine the risk of prescription opioid abuse among patients with chronic non-malignant pain [abstract]. *Pain Physician.* 2002;5(4):447–448.

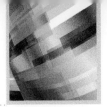

Index

Note: Page number followed by f and t indicates figure and table respectively.

A

Abdominal adhesions, and pain, 45–46
Abdominal pain, 44–45
  abdominal wall neuroma and, 45
  Carnett test in, 44, 45f
  case studies on, 47–48
  chronic, 44–45
    abdominal surgery and, 45–46
  history examination in, 44
  referred, 46, 46f
  somatic, 45, 45f
  stress and, 44
  treatment of, 46
    abdominal wall pain generator, 47
    lifestyle modification, 46
    neuropathic pain, 46
    nonspecific pain, 46
    referred pain, 46–47
    severe pain, 47
    spasm, 46
  visceral, 45
Abdominal strengthening exercises, 253
  abdominal crunch, 253, 253f
  half V sit-ups, 253, 253f
Acetaminophen, 80
  action mechanism, 80
  adverse effects of, 80
  case study on, 81
  ceiling effect, 80
  contraindications to, 80
  indications for, 80
  use of, 80
Acromioclavicular arthritis, 4, 4f
Acupuncture, 256–257, 256f
Acyclovir, in postherpetic neuralgia, 22
Addiction, methadone in, 102
Adhesions, 45
  abdominal, 45–46
  intestinal, 46
Adhesive capsulitis, 5–6, 6f
Advil. See Ibuprofen
Alcohol abuse, and nerve damage, 90. See
    also Neuropathic pain
Amitriptyline, 89
  side effects of, 92t
  starting doses and titration schedule, 91t
Androderm, 104
Antidepressants. See also specific drug
  case study on, 92
  contraindications to, 92
  and cross-tapering, 92
  dosage and titration schedule, 91, 91t
  drugs interactions, 92

for fibromyalgia, 90–91, 91t
indications for, 90–91
for neuropathic pain, 88–92
side effects of, 92, 92t
tricyclic, 89, 90f
uses of, 90–91, 91t
Antiepileptic (antiseizure) drugs.
    See also Carbamazepine;
    Gabapentin; Pregabalin
  action mechanism, 94–95, 94f, 95f
  case study on, 97
  contraindications to, 96
  for fibromyalgia, 95
  indications for, 95
  for neuropathic pain, 93–97
  side effects of, 96, 96t
  starting doses and titration schedule for,
    95–96, 96t
Appendicitis, 45, 45f
Arthritis
  in elbow, 7
  hip, 12–13, 12f
  knee, 16–17
  in shoulder, 3–4, 4f
Artificial disc replacement (ADR), 218,
    218f
Avascular necrosis (AVN), 67

B

Back pain, low. See Low back pain
Baclofen, 87t
  action mechanism, 85, 85f, 85t
  dosing for, 86, 86t
  side effects for, 87, 87t
  uses of, 86
Balance exercises, 251
Biofeedback, 257
Bisphosphonates, 68
Botox. See Botulinum toxin injections
Botulinum toxin injections, 194. See also
    Headache, injections for
  areas of injection and recommended
    doses, 196t
  indication for, 195
  procedure for, 196–198, 196t, 197t, 198t
  sites for, 197
    cervical paraspinal muscles, 198, 198f
    corrugator, 197, 197f
    frontalis, 197, 197f
    occipitalis, 197, 197f
    procerus, 197, 197f
    temporalis, 197, 197f
    trapezius, 198, 198f

Breakthrough pain, 37, 103. See also Cancer
    patients, pain in
  management of, 103, 103t
Bunion. See Hallux valgus
Bupivacaine, 242
  for epidural use, 116, 117
  for joint and bursa injections, 163, 163t
  for nerve blocks, 201–202, 201f, 202t
    (see also Nerve blocks)
Bursa, 3
  ischiogluteal, 15–16, 15f
  olecranon, 7, 7f
  subacromial, 3, 3f
  trochanteric, 14–15, 15f
Bursitis, 162. See also Joint and bursa
    injections
Buttocks, pain in, 14
  greater trochanteric bursitis and, 14–15,
    15f
  ischiogluteal bursitis and, 15–16, 16f
  sacroiliac joint and, 14, 14f

C

Cancer patients, pain in, 37
  brain tumors, and headache, 38–39, 39f
  case study on, 43
  metastatic bone pain, 37–38, 37f
  neurolytic celiac plexus block for,
    179–180
  neurolytic ganglion impar block for, 184
  neurolytic superior hypogastric block
    for, 183
  neuropathic pain, 38
    chemotherapy and, 38, 39f
    radiation and, 38, 39f
  preexisting painful condition, 41
  programmable intrathecal pump for, 237
    (see also Intrathecal pain pumps)
  spinal cord compression and, 39–40, 40f
  surgery and
    mastectomy, 40–41, 41f
    thoracotomy, 40, 40f
  treatment of, 41
    cancer blocks, 43
    radiation therapy, 43
    spinal cord compression, 42, 42t
    WHO analgesic guidelines, 41, 42t
  visceral pain, 38, 38f
Capsaicin, 82, 83t
  action mechanism, 82
  forms, strengths, and application of, 83, 83t
  side effects of, 83
  use of, 82–83